Courageous Well-Being for Nurses

Courageous Well-Being for Nurses

• STRATEGIES *for* RENEWAL •

Donna A. Gaffney

•

Nicole C. Foster

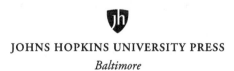

JOHNS HOPKINS UNIVERSITY PRESS

Baltimore

© 2023 Johns Hopkins University Press
All rights reserved. Published 2023
Printed in the United States of America on acid-free paper
2 4 6 8 9 7 5 3 1

Johns Hopkins University Press
2715 North Charles Street
Baltimore, Maryland 21218
www.press.jhu.edu

Library of Congress Cataloging-in-Publication Data

Names: Gaffney, Donna A., author. | Foster, Nicole, 1996– author.
Title: Courageous well-being for nurses : strategies for renewal /
Donna A. Gaffney, Nicole C. Foster.
Description: Baltimore : Johns Hopkins University Press, 2023. |
Includes bibliographical references and index.
Identifiers: LCCN 2022038713 | ISBN 9781421446684 (paperback) |
ISBN 9781421446691 (ebook)
Subjects: LCSH: Nurses—Mental health. | Nurses—Health and hygiene. |
Self-care, Health. | Resilience (Personality trait) | Stress management.
Classification: LCC RC451.4.N85 G34 2023 | DDC 610.73—dc23/eng/20221223
LC record available at https://lccn.loc.gov/2022038713

A catalog record for this book is available from the British Library.

Special discounts are available for bulk purchases of this book.
For more information, please contact Special Sales at specialsales@jh.edu.

Perhaps it is unusual to begin a dedication by
describing a tree. We'd like to tell you about the
Rowan tree—a fitting metaphor for nursing.

◆

Rowans are found in the far reaches of the Northern Hemisphere, most commonly in Ireland and Scotland. The ancient Celts considered the Rowan to be a symbol of protection and transformation and believed that it could turn adversity into creative opportunity. It thrives in the most hostile environments, such as mountainous hillsides and rock-laden riverbeds.

Parched for water and nutrient resources, the Rowan's extensive network of roots reaches deep into the ground for nourishment. Its strength is matched only by its graceful form and its potential for healing and hardiness. It is known as the Tree of Life.

The Rowan is thought to protect and give courage and strength to those walking the path of spiritual growth and enlightenment. It calls us to be inspired, to be encouraged, to grow.

Perhaps these pages will come to be an amulet for nurses and the nursing profession—to protect and ground you ... with *tenacity*. Like the Rowan, we hang on, dig in, and spread our roots in whatever circumstances come our way.

◆

We dedicate this book to you, dear reader.

Contents

Forewords

Two colleagues offered to each write a foreword for our book: Dr. Anne Hofmeyer and Dr. Susan Salmond. They are extraordinary nurses who played instrumental roles in shaping the pages you are about to read, beginning with a webinar series titled "Healing Ourselves while Healing Others" during the earliest days of the pandemic, to the launch of the virtual Schwartz Rounds series, an online forum for connecting health care colleagues who face challenging situations while caring for themselves and others.

Dr. Anne Hofmeyer, Adelaide, South Australia

I am delighted to write a foreword to this timely book for nurses written by Donna Gaffney and Nicole Foster. *Care for the carer* was a common catchphrase when I was working as a nurse in hospice/palliative care more than five decades ago. Role strain, dealing with heavy workloads, exhaustion, personal distress watching patients suffer and die, and inadequate resources and training were but a few of the daily stressors. We were expected to care for ourselves so we could care for others. In other words, it was a solo endeavor. This expectation sparked my life-long interest in "self-care" practice, what it meant to colleagues, and research into empathy, self-care, well-being, resilience, connectedness, and self-compassion. I am convinced that *care for the carer* is definitely not a solo endeavor and is now more important than ever before.

The global SARS-CoV-2 pandemic has deeply affected the personal, professional, and political lives of nurses and health care providers. Some have called the pandemic the greatest challenge to the world since World War II. Nurses understand that their well-being influences their ability to serve others. But the fatigue, grief, moral distress, helplessness, burnout, and guilt (about not doing enough) experienced by nurses during the pandemic run deep. Rushton (2021)* said nurses must confront their limitations with the same compassionate words they would say to others and honor what they *did do* for their patients.

---

*Rushton, C. H. (2021). Preserving integrity and staying power as a nurse in a pandemic. *American Journal of Nursing* 121(3): 68–69. https://doi.10.1097/01.NAJ.0000737332.30793.91

They continued to turn up. Nurses need to acknowledge they can neither "carry" nor fix unsolvable system problems. Going forward, nurses
must find ways to care for themselves and connect with others so they
can continue to care for their patients.

Ashcraft and Gatto (2018) describe self-care as "deliberate decisions
made and actions taken by individuals to address their own health and
well-being" (140).* This is a timely reminder that if we rely on motivation alone to care for ourselves, we are less likely to persevere when
we feel exhausted and distressed. It reminds us that we need deliberate decision-making (planning), discipline, and routine to sustain
our resilience and well-being. There are countless research articles,
evidence-based resources, self-care books, and podcasts designed for
nurses during the pandemic because self-care practices ease fatigue.
The question is how to devise a flexible plan to nurture your resilience
(i.e., flexibility, self-regulation, optimism, and curiosity) so you can keep
going through the best and worst of workdays, and sustain the belief
that you will get through.

What sets this book apart is the theoretical interpretation of clinical
nurses' powerful stories about their caregiving experiences in the pandemic front lines, the impact on their well-being, and what practices
sustain them. We can learn these lessons and integrate these proven
practices into our self-care plan going forward. In this landmark book,
Gaffney and Foster use storytelling as a way to present the meaning
nurses assign to their experiences, grief, and journeys of personal healing. Storytelling has the capacity to unite nurses worldwide because
they may recognize themselves in these stories. Nurses can develop a
plan that incorporates self-care practices that have sustained others'
well-being. The commonality of the compelling stories provides an
entry point for nurses who feel alone (and maybe guilt). It encourages
nurses to recognize their common humanity and feel less alienated
in these troubled times. Drawing on scientific literature, the wisdom
from some of the world's leading researchers, nurses' stories, and professional expertise, Gaffney and Foster present a series of chapters to
foster personal understanding, self-compassion, and self-care practices

*Ashcraft, P. F., & Gatto, S. L. (2018). Curricular interventions to promote self-
care in prelicensure nursing students. *Nurse Educator* 43(3):140–44.

to sustain well-being. They use Carol Ryff's model of psychological well-being as the conceptual framework for the book.

In this book, Gaffney and Foster provide critical information to help you explore:

- Who you are (self-awareness and insight), to understand and acknowledge what you carry (baggage, struggle, bias) into your relationships and work.
- What is self-compassionate self-talk and why it is essential to your well-being.
- Proven resources to manage stress, sleep, nutrition, and movement.
- How to deliberately fit restorative practices into busy work schedules. Intentional practices help maintain emotional and physical balance in difficult circumstances.
- How to manage moral adversity and heal moral pain and emotional distress.
- When counseling services could be helpful and steps to take.

The authors explain insights, well-being practices, and supportive routines that have worked for nurses in difficult and disruptive times. You may find ideas in this book to help you devise a flexible plan to sustain you through the best and worst of days, and nurture hope for your future. This journey of discovery and learning takes you through the basics such as nutrition, sleep, exercise, social connections, and mental health. The first step is self-awareness. You are in the best position to customize your well-being plan by choosing practices that could support you in a crisis and on better days. Caring for yourself is more than mindfulness, nutrition, sleep, exercise, debriefing, and solitude. Acting in creative and curious ways can boost your sense of well-being, gratitude, and peace. But it becomes more difficult to follow your well-being plan when feeling depleted. Thus it is important to plan how you will keep going during tough times, which is vital to your well-being and career success.

Professor Kristin Neff reminds us that self-compassion (treating yourself as you would treat a friend who is having a hard time) means having sensitivity toward your own suffering along with a deep wish to alleviate that suffering. Self-compassion requires us to acknowledge we are suffering (mindfulness), that we are all in this together (common humanity), and that we need to be kind to ourselves (self-kindness) before we have the strength to do the same for others. Importantly, self-compassion helps us to maintain boundaries in our caring of others so we do not become overwhelmed. These insights can foster hope and strengthen our capacity to care for ourselves, our colleagues, families, and the communities we serve.

No discussion would be complete without highlighting the shared responsibility to foster well-being at the individual and organizational levels. The world needs resilient health care leaders who are empathic and engaged, who possess the skills and capabilities to support staff through volatile times related to "living with COVID" now and in the future. With the unrelenting challenges to do more with less, and calls for ongoing renewal through personal and professional development, I expect this book will be essential reading for current and future generations of nurses in clinical practice, education, and leadership. It offers practical knowledge that can be used by individuals, managers, and leaders to build a stronger, resilient workforce. Caring for yourself is self-preservation and relevant for everyone. We are stronger together.

I am delighted to recommend this book. It is a powerful suite of clinicians' stories about their caregiving experiences during the pandemic and beyond that is also skillfully embedded in current theory and evidence by the authors. Keep this book to reread, because enhancing your well-being is a lifelong practice and investment in yourself and your professional career. Further, I encourage you to buy another copy for a colleague. Your kind gift could be pivotal in enhancing their well-being and sense of hope.

Anne Hofmeyer, RN, PhD
Adjunct Senior Research Fellow
Rosemary Bryant AO Research Centre
University of South Australia
Adelaide, South Australia

Dr. Susan Salmond, Newark, New Jersey, United States

Nurses were exhausted. I saw it in so many of my colleagues. I saw it in my daughter Erin, who had followed my career path into nursing. At the time—spring of 2020, the height of the pandemic in this part of the United States—she was a nurse responsible for running a COVID ward.

Our hospitals were at capacity with patients who were dying; there was no vaccine in sight, and wouldn't be for almost another year. The virus was barely a few months from discovery, we did not know how to care for those who were infected, and we certainly did not have experience on how to advise women who were pregnant and at risk of COVID infection. And Erin was pregnant—a long-awaited pregnancy.

Most evenings I went with my other daughter and her four children to stand outside Erin's house. We banged pots to cheer her and other health care workers, left signs, and talked with her while we stood on the street and she stood on her front patio. She was afraid. I was afraid.

For me and so many other nurses, the pandemic was personal; it affected my family and my nursing colleagues personally. As an educator, I made the switch from in-person learning to online learning and continued to prepare the next generation of nurses, but I felt like I was not doing enough for frontline nurses. In so many ways, Erin symbolized for me the risks that nurses were taking and the stress that it put on them, their families, and maybe even their futures. I wanted to give back and help nurses "get through."

Taking my motivation to help frontline nurses, I gathered with some of my colleagues and developed a proposal to repurpose a grant that I had received from the Robert Wood Johnson Foundation to advance nurses' knowledge of population health. We argued that nursing was now an at-risk population and needed support. Proposing to advance initiatives to support the emotional well-being of nurses, the foundation approved the change in purpose, and we were able to launch virtual Schwartz Rounds for New Jersey nurses, giving them an outlet to share their stories, connect with colleagues, and learn approaches to help cope with the many challenges. As a complement to the virtual Schwartz Rounds, we provided trainer sessions in Stress First Aid to facilitate individual and organizational approaches to more effectively cope with the emotional stressors of care during the pandemic and beyond. Our third initiative, to complete the triad of interventions, was to obtain a seed grant to support the development of a nurse-to-nurse hotline for individuals in crisis seeking support and possible referral for mental health services.

In the rollout of both Schwartz Rounds and Stress First Aid, I was witness to the amazing strength and commitment of nurses. The stories that nurses told of rapid patient deterioration, frequent death, and lack of personal protective equipment, along with the uncertainty of not knowing how to treat COVID-19, appeared to be the perfect storm for burnout and secondary traumatic stress. Within all of this, however, nurses showed their strength, resilience, and creativity. Gathering in circles after a patient died to hold hands and pray together allowed them to connect with one another as well as to something greater than themselves. With strict visitor restrictions, nurses were the conduit between the patient and the family, sharing their own cell phones and iPads (before hospitals bought their own devices) so patients could connect with loved ones, often saying goodbye. Nurses told of staying with dying patients in the last moments of life. The alternative—dying alone—wasn't an option. The frontline workers were scared for their loved ones, some choosing to live in a hotel to protect their families from possible infection that they could unintentionally bring home. Many who did go home stripped their clothes in the garage and went straight to the shower before greeting loved ones, ever fearful of spreading the illness at home.

The creativity of nurses was so evident in the shared stories. Plagued with uncertainty and making up protocol along the way, nurses, working in multidisciplinary teams, were part of the development of innovations such as the use of long intravenous tubing, keeping IVs out in the hall. Innovations to share scarce respirators, perform proning rounds, develop virtual rounding tools, create color-coded signs to improve communication, and deliver rapid skills training to prepare nurses from other specialties to care for COVID-19 patients all gave testimony to the ingenuity and commitment of nursing. Yet despite this innovation and ingenuity, nurses also verbalized distress that they were not able to care for patients as they wanted to, as they were trained to do, leaving many with the trauma of moral distress alongside the trauma of loss and the trauma of wear-and-tear injury. Our nurses were being challenged, and their emotional well-being was a concern to all.

Nurses were the true heroes of the early COVID pandemic; they were hailed for both saving lives and putting their own lives on the line. Deservedly, there was amazing support from the community, who were truly in awe of the efforts of nurses and other health professionals. As we moved into the second wave, the context was different. In the first wave, all non-COVID services were shut down to maximize the number of health care providers caring for patients with COVID. During the second wave, things were somewhat back to normal in terms of operations. Without the extra staffing, nurses caring for COVID patients were doing about the same job with fewer resources, both physically and emotionally. The community was tired of COVID, and the outpouring of support for frontline workers was drying up. Still, nurses were facing the same challenges, with a demanding workload and continued risks to their personal health and their family's health. The phrase "from heroes to zeros" was used to capture this phenomenon. Many nurses felt unsupported by their organizations and their communities. They pleaded with their friends and family to wear masks and to get vaccinated while still caring compassionately for critically ill unvaccinated patients.

During our Schwartz Rounds, we continued to hear stories from nurses of being exhausted and questioning whether their organizations were truly aware of the stresses they were under. Some panelists and participants shared stories of exceptional administrative support and focus on nurse well-being, and they offered ideas for others who were not receiving this support: new staffing patterns, break rooms repurposed as relaxation rooms to decrease stress, resiliency teams, and implementation of Stress First Aid programs on units. Not all nurses received this support, however, and they reported feeling abandoned.

Today, more than three years into the pandemic (or shall we call it an endemic), nurses still face issues around COVID care, and new challenges are testing their strength and resolve, such as rising incivility, workplace violence, and resistance by the community to adhere to masking and visitor restriction policies. Just as nurses had to be the ones during the first surge to tell family members at the doors of the emergency department that they had to leave, we now have school nurses trying to intervene with angry parents over stay-at-home policies, and staff nurses trying to enforce masking requirements. Instead of being thanked, as happened during the first COVID wave, they are the recipients of our community's frustration and growing lack of patience.

Nurses are tired, worn down, and pessimistic, yet they continue to do what nurses do—care with compassion. If we are going to have a healthy nursing workforce, there must be a true commitment at the organizational level to promote healthy work environments that enhance emotional well-being, and that assist nurses and teams of nurses to work together to manage stress. During the pandemic, a recurring theme was the supportive strength that nurses received from their colleagues. This is a positive outcome and needs to be nurtured, as strong team support is critical to ongoing emotional well-being. Stress was certainly not unique to the pandemic—stress is inherent in what we do as nurses, as well as in the environments in which we practice. It is time for nursing as a profession, and the organizations in which we work, to invest in a culture that supports emotional well-being. This will require an investment of resources into structures and programs that promote physical and emotional health: resilience teams, chief wellness officers, and programs such as Stress First Aid and Psychological First Aid. Organizations have a responsibility to promote self-care and team care within the workplace.

Our professional values of stoicism, selflessness, and loyalty assist us in enduring hardship while leading us toward not taking care of ourselves and sacrificing our own self-care needs for the needs of others. As we moved into the second wave of the pandemic, nurses talked about the emotional toll that the first wave had brought, and they had a new realization of the importance of constructively dealing with stress in their lives through purposeful self-care. This book of personal and professional stories and strategies highlights the value of self-care, and provides tangible examples that can be adopted and adapted for your own personal well-being.

Despite the stresses of being a nurse, I wouldn't trade it for the world. But I do believe that we, as nurses, owe it to ourselves to master the skills we need to deal with stress, and to take care of ourselves as we advise others to do the same. We owe it to ourselves, to the next generation of nurses, to our families, to our children. And yes, Erin did, in the fall of 2020, give birth to a full-term, healthy baby boy. We are blessed, and at our house we have one more reason to take care of ourselves.

Susan Salmond, RN, EdD, ANEF, FAAN
Professor and Executive Vice Dean
School of Nursing
Rutgers, The State University of New Jersey
New Brunswick, New Jersey, United States

Preface

• *An Invitation* •

The photograph still haunts me. I remember it as if it was yesterday—the layers of PPE, her direct and honest gaze. Facebook became a young nurse's confessional, as she pleaded with her followers to understand why she could no longer cope with the ravages of the pandemic, all the uncertainty, and the fear that her family would contract the deadly virus. She apologized because she felt she couldn't do her job. But I felt I should have been the one apologizing. I was flooded with remorse that I could not be there for her. I immediately posted on her feed: I support you. I am praying for you. I know exactly how you feel. I am afraid, too. There were hundreds of others saying the exact same words. Facing my own moral distress, and recognizing I couldn't work beside these nurses and somehow lighten their burden, I was overwhelmed by the magnitude of my colleagues' suffering.

As a nurse and psychotherapist, I am accustomed to listening to people's stories—to *nurses'* stories. That initial Facebook post would be the first of hundreds of social media entries I read in the early months of the pandemic. This chorus of nurses' voices rang out loudly, and in a way I hadn't heard before. I collected and curated their stories from social media, phone interviews, and email correspondence. Their challenges and needs were overwhelming.

I felt a sense of urgency unlike at any other time in my professional life—as a nurse or psychotherapist. I have always provided support, psychotherapy, and education for students, registered nurses, and mental health professionals—during the Gulf War, Hurricane Katrina, and the earthquake in Haiti. But not even during the 10-plus years I worked with 9/11 families had I ever witnessed anything like this.

Barely three weeks after the first COVID diagnosis in the New York–New Jersey epicenter, my good friend and colleague Ann Marie Mauro called early on a Saturday morning with an invitation. She was on the faculty at Rutgers University School of Nursing and asked if I would be willing to create a webinar for them on coping with the pandemic. Sue Salmond, the executive vice dean, knew that she had to provide something for her undergraduates, graduate students, alumni, and faculty. I knew a single webinar would not be enough.

Three nurse colleagues joined me in developing an eight-session webinar series. Anne Hofmeyer from Australia had researched compassion and empathic distress. Peg Pipchick, a marriage and family therapist, addressed the stress on relationships. Milagros Elia provided mindfulness and stress-reducing practices at the end of every session. Rereading those emails to my colleagues in March of 2020 is almost too painful. I was frantic. I wrote to Anne:

> The narratives and conversations I've heard from nurses are horrifying, sad and filled with hopelessness. I am on the phone every night/ day with a nurse who is on the edge. I would love it if you could be a part of this project. I fear there will be long-term consequences in our profession from this ever-changing and rapidly evolving situation. I am so worried about the nurses on the front lines.
>
> We have to move fast. And Now.

And so it began. The series was posted free of charge on the Rutgers website three weeks later. We learned from nurses attending the webinars how much they needed the well-being and stress management strategies we presented. They wanted to know more. I realized that the best way to ensure they were equipped for the future, no matter what health crisis struck our communities or our profession, was to pull together a book of information, perspectives, and strategies nurses could rely on to serve them as a resource to guide and protect them from the challenges of their work.

Coming Together

Two months after the webinar series concluded, I met my coauthor, Nicole Foster, a newly minted masters-prepared health and wellness coach from Columbia University. We are separated by years (many of them), different disciplines, and 3,000 miles. Yet when I read Nicole's *Well-Being in the Waiting: Finding Presence during Unprecedented Times,** I discovered her deep commitment to human health and wellness, and I

---

*Foster, N. (2020). *Well-Being in the Waiting: Finding Presence during Unprecedented Times.* https://nicolecfoster.com/product-page/well-being-in-the-waiting-ebook-download

knew she would add so much to this project. Ours was a fortuitous meeting: I was familiar with nurses and nursing and the effects of stress and trauma on their mental health, and Nicole was committed to explore the intersection of psychology, spirituality, and mind-body practices.

It seemed necessary that information on well-being could and should be organized in one place for nurses. There are hundreds of books on mindfulness, stress reduction, healthful eating, and personal growth, and we cite and suggest many of them to our readers. While it's impossible to provide such an enormous body of work on well-being in one book, we thought, "Why not introduce readers to well-being with an overview of topics and a sampling of different strategies—the traditional and the unique, the well-established and the newer cutting-edge research?" We decided to try out our ideas, and in late summer of 2020, we piloted an early e-book version of this text. Not only did the nurses tell us they liked the content and format, they gave us more ideas for what they wanted us to include.

By mining the most current research on well-being, as well as what I've learned from my clinical practice over the past three decades, I added to the foundation. Nicole and I collaborated on the organization of the book and the flow of the chapters. We each took the lead on content that fell within our areas of expertise. Nicole helmed the chapters on sleep, exercise, and nourishment, and contributed to the chapter on mindfulness and meditation. We read each other's words, exploring, contemplating, and ultimately deciding how to best organize the great body of well-being research and practices.

Sharing Stories

It wasn't until we met an extraordinary group of nurses, however, that the real purpose of this book took shape. More than 30 nurses in different settings, from different countries, inspired us as they told of the most challenging situations they've encountered in health care: disasters, short staffing, demanding work conditions, epidemics, and, yes, the coronavirus pandemic. Without their stories and their wisdom, this book could not have come into existence. We are indebted to them in more ways than we ever imagined. "Thank you" doesn't seem like enough. But giving these incredible professionals a platform to tell their stories is the best place to start—for all of us—to connect, to learn, and to heal, so we all can continue to grow as we care for others.

We knew this book would not be your garden variety "self-care" book. Consider it a trail guide of sorts—our gift to nurses and nursing. Yet somehow, through their words and actions, we are the ones who have received the gift. These nurses are among the smartest and most courageous people we know.

The chapters in this book do not necessarily follow a linear path. That was purposeful. We want you to choose your own path and start at the best place for *you*.

Outline of the Book

Introduction

The chapters of this book unfold with stories from nurses who tell us, in their own words, not only about their professional and personal challenges, but also about how they found workable practices that enhanced their well-being. In addition to current international evidence-based science, Carol Ryff's model establishes the framework for the chapters that follow. Her six core elements of well-being include self-acceptance, the establishment of quality ties to others, a sense of autonomy in thought and action, the ability to manage complex environments to suit personal needs and values, the pursuit of meaningful goals and a sense of purpose in life, and continued growth and development as a person.

Chapter threads weave together various concepts, including collective well-being of family, relationships, and colleagues, work and life balance, and the impact of work stress on family and family stressors on work. The influence of the structure and environment of the health care system does not go unnoticed. The burden of health and well-being is not the sole responsibility of individual nurses, but a shared responsibility with health care organizations.

Chapter 1. Becoming Self-Compassionate

This chapter provides a basis for turning toward oneself for compassion and turning down the noise on the critical voices inside of our heads. Utilizing evidence-based strategies from top researchers in the field of self-compassion and mindfulness, including Kristin Neff and Tara Brach, you are guided through exercises to let emotions flow, drop self-judgment, and employ self-compassion. The strategies introduced can be practiced in a variety of settings. We specifically detail how to use them at work, home, and almost any place in between.

Chapter 2. Managing Stress

The second chapter offers ways for professional nurses to navigate the realities of stress at work and home. While stress can be unavoidable in many situations, the manner in which one responds to it can either enhance or inhibit well-being. Through a unique reflective practice, the reader makes an inventory of what they are "carrying" in their work and relationships. The strategies focus on families, colleagues, and friends, allowing readers to navigate their fears and uncertainties of going home and communicating with their children, family members, and other important people in their lives. Many of the practices and exercises are trauma informed.

Chapter 3. Exploring Mindfulness and Meditation

Complementing the intentionality of well-being, this chapter provides a brief introduction to mindfulness and meditation and why it is useful in reducing stress and promoting well-being. Resources in this section feature activities and meditations led by experts in the fields of mindfulness, psychology, and alternative or complementary health care practices, including Jon Kabat-Zinn, Andrew Weil, and Sharon Salzberg.

Chapter 4. Sleeping Well

In this chapter, you discover the benefits of sleeping well. We provide solutions and strategies to enhance sleep, which in turn affects all functioning and well-being. Following World Health Organization (WHO) recommendations for sleep and longevity, we provide evidence-based strategies that promote better sleep, including aromatherapy, herbal tea, supplements, environmental accommodations, and mindfulness.

Chapter 5. Nourishing Well

In this chapter, Nicole uses her passion for and depth of knowledge in plant-based eating to provide simple, vibrant recipes and meal solutions that are nourishing and completely accessible. Along with recipes, we include new research in the field of nutritional psychiatry, illustrating how your brain responds to different foods, both positively and negatively.

Chapter 6. Implementing Daily Movement and Exercise
Following the foundation of the importance of sleep, this chapter promotes regular exercise for improving overall physical and mental well-being. Guidelines from the WHO are provided as a baseline suggestion, followed by an extensive list with modes of movement and exercise, presenting a variety of options alongside discussion of their effectiveness.

Chapter 7. Embracing Nature and the Outdoors
While movement, meditation, and sleep are commonly prescribed to mediate the effects of stress, the content of this chapter provides evidence-based solutions to improving well-being by connecting with nature. Cited research studies emphasize the physiological and psychological benefits of being immersed in nature, in green and blue spaces. Resources include organizations that are leading the "nature as medicine" movement: Park Rx in the United States, Reconnect in Nature in Wales, as well as a network of Shinrin-yoku (forest bathing) practitioners through the International Nature and Forest Therapy Alliance in Australia.

Chapter 8. Finding Sanctuary in Words, Images, and Sounds
In addition to practicing nursing, many of our storytellers shared their creative sides—how they began, and how and why they continued to explore and enrich their creative pursuits. We introduce you to these writers, artists, singers, and photographers who show us how their creativity became the wellspring that not only gave them respite and joy, but also enhanced their well-being. The works of James Pennebaker, Louise DeSalvo, and Hilde Lindemann Nelson provide tools for readers as they write their own stories—healing trauma and stress or creating tales from far-off lands. Bibliotherapy, or reading books as a means to treat stress, is another powerful tool. When reading, we can walk in another's shoes, experience other events, and even feed our own need

to escape to other times and places. The arts and music are standouts in this chapter as we take you on a journey with nurses who capture their world on film, in song, and on paper.

Chapter 9. Seeking Empowerment through Advocacy and Activism

The previous chapters of this book lead readers to a greater sense of well-being, which can ultimately enhance their empowerment at work and at home. We have seen how nurses who are advocates and activists contribute to their profession and to the world around them. Yet there is an even greater benefit—one that is personal. Taking action in one's profession or community is a potential antidote to vicarious trauma. We share nurse colleagues' stories of resilience and strategies for empowerment.

Chapter 10. Navigating the Challenges of the Health Care Landscape

How do we confront the tumultuous health care environment? So often, burnout, vicarious trauma, empathic distress, grief, and moral distress are left in its wake. How do we restabilize when our boundaries become blurred with those of patients and families, when empathy goes off course, resulting in loss of focus and distress? Weariness, disengagement from work, and other signs of burnout are explored, as well as tools and strategies for renewal and rekindling. Finally, this chapter outlines how moral distress and actual or perceived powerlessness in clinical settings has, more than ever, complicated the practice of professional nurses.

Chapter 11. Continuing the Journey of Transformation and Healing

We've all heard the words, "Maybe you should talk to someone." The benefits of professional support make sense—it's another approach to improving your well-being, with purpose and focus. This final chapter offers guidance, valuable strategies, and resources that are easily accessible and often without cost. Suggestions will contribute to your well-being and help you heal when facing crisis, trauma, loss, or overwhelming stress. In the aftermath of crisis, there are often lessons learned. Instinctively, we apply this new knowledge again when we need it most. But sometimes previous lessons don't work in new, more intense situations. I specifically focus on the questions I've heard many times during and even before the pandemic: How do I know when I need professional help? What does it entail, how much does it cost, and where do I find it? Readers can explore this new terrain, step-by-step, with helpful self-assessment tools and the latest work on collective resilience approaches to healing. We are all relational beings; our interdependence on each other is indispensable. Healing is forged over time, within each of us, and in community.

Resources and Glossary

We hope that this book will be useful to you. Included is a list of resources, gathered from nurses and experts in related fields. These books, websites, podcasts, videos, and webinars illustrate ways to promote compassionate coping and enhance your well-being. The book also includes a glossary.

◆

We would like to share one final thought. Manifestations of courage appear and reappear on the pages you are about to read. You will sense it in the stories shared by our collaborators—incredible nurses all. We are not talking about heroes. We are talking about the very essence of courage: the ability to pursue goals or a purpose despite risk or fear. The courage to be yourself, or a better version of yourself, may lead you on the ultimate journey to well-being.

Courageous Well-Being for Nurses

Prologue

"We have a possible COVID-19 patient, and she will be assigned to you. You will only have this one patient for the day ... and we are assigning her to you because you are the youngest."

IN THEIR OWN WORDS

My COVID-19 journey began with being the first nurse in my hospital to care for a "suspected COVID-19 patient." I had started working in October of 2019, my first job as a nurse. It was now the beginning of March 2020, before the shutdown, before COVID-19 started ramping up in the United States. We were hearing rumors of a case or two in New York, but nothing that people were concerned about. I will never forget walking into work that day. When I came to the nurses station to get my assignment, the entire night shift stopped talking and stared at me. I knew at that moment that we had a COVID-19 patient on the floor. What I did not know was that they would look at me and say, "Good morning, we have a possible COVID-19 patient, and she will be assigned to you. You will only have this one patient for the day ... and we are assigning her to you because you are the youngest."

In that second, I had three choices. First, I could be offended. I was the youngest—what did that mean? Healthier? Less likely to get it? Less likely to be affected by a virus we literally knew NOTHING about? Or ... I had the choice to say "no" because I was too scared. I had been a working nurse for only five months, I had just finished orientation with my preceptor six weeks prior ... I had no clue how to handle a critical patient on this level, let alone a possible COVID-19 diagnosis! Or ... I could take a deep breath, do my normal routine of chart reviews, and work my hardest to make sure my patient was the first priority. And that's just what I did.

That day was a rush of emotion—it felt like every single director, educator, vice president, supervisor, etc., had come to the unit to have a say in the care of the patient. It made me angry to see so many people talking around and around. I understood that everyone was concerned, nervous, and scared. I have no doubt that everyone just wanted to be safe. But that day I was the only person for hours to enter that patient's room. I was the only one who held her hand and tried to comfort her. She was on a BiPap for her breathing. She was also deaf; I made sure I located the iPad with the sign language interpreter app, so that we could communicate. Our ICU intensivist came later that morning. He was the only person who came into the room with me that day. I remember sitting in the room with him, both of us holding her hands as he spoke to her about how she could have possibly contracted the coronavirus. I remember how he made sure the iPad interpreter got every word he said. He also made sure our patient understood the next steps—going to the ICU. She signed to us, "Am I going to die?" We all looked at each other silently for a moment. I'm sure there was fear in our eyes.

After we left the room and took off our PPE, the crowd of administrators outside the room began to talk around me once again, but I felt *relieved* and was finally able to take a deep breath now that my patient was going to the ICU. I was exhausted from the buildup of emotion and fear that I had tucked away throughout the morning in order to do my job properly and with a level head. Little did I know that day was going to become my and countless other nurses' new normal.

> "I had been a nurse for only 6 months, dealing with multiple
> deaths of patients every week. In the past year, I had seen
> more deaths than my aunt, who has been a nurse for over
> 30 years. How was I supposed to deal with all of this?"

I will never forget one patient, John. He was suffering for days: grasping, breathing, dripping sweat, in and out of consciousness, suffering from this wicked virus. His family was amazingly kind to us, and we tried our best to FaceTime with them as much as possible. Unlike my first day with a COVID patient, today there were no iPads to be found. We used our own cell phones, securely taping them in plastic bags. My friend Susan was caring for John that day. We had just finished our med passes and finally sat down at the nurses station when our telemetry monitor started going off. His heart rate was decreasing. We stood up at the same time, and Susan said, "I can't let him die alone." She stopped and looked at me as I followed her toward his room, "It's okay. You don't have to come." We all feared going into these rooms more than we had to. I grabbed her hand and said, "And you don't have to do this alone." We squeezed hands, gowned up, and both held our patient's hands, one on each side, as we talked with him, repeating his family members' names to him (whose faces and voices we knew so well), letting him know it was okay to let go, that they didn't want him suffering anymore. After what seemed like hours watching him struggle for breath, he took his last one. Our masks were soaked with tears, our face shields fogged; sweat collected head to toe under our gowns and scrubs. Though nothing can compare to our patients' suffering, those days were our darkest.

I cried extra hard that day on the way home; really, I should have pulled over. I had been a nurse for only six months, dealing with multiple deaths of patients every week. In the past year, I had seen more deaths than my aunt, who has been a nurse for over 30 years. How was I supposed to deal with all of this?

No way was I going to risk being around my own family without knowing what I could bring home. Before I left work, I would change my clothes and shoes, and then change my shoes again before getting in my car. Once I got home, I would wipe down my car and strip down my clothes in the garage. My fiancé waited at the back door with a laundry basket for my scrubs and driving clothes. He went directly to the laundry room to wash my clothes. Yes, we were neurotic, and it was overkill, but how could we not be? It was exhausting. My eyes were raw right at the corner of my tear ducts for weeks because of the tears; my cheekbones were indented and slightly bruised from wearing a mask for 13 hours. Before bed, I put Vaseline on those areas to get rid of the pain and heal the rawness. Those marks were daily reminders of what we had to face on the next shift.

My family was my saving grace, even though we couldn't be together under one roof. There were countless times that I'd come from work and dinner was in our outdoor fridge. Or there was a basket on my front porch with sweets, so I knew they were thinking of me. On the day Susan and I lost our patient John, I came out of the shower, and my fiancé said to come to the garage to eat dinner. It was 40 degrees outside, and I thought, "What?" I bundled up, and there in my garage, in the freezing cold, was my family. It was 9 o'clock at night and my dad, sister, brother-in-law, and stepmom were sitting in chairs six feet apart, each with dinner in their lap. They had all come over just to have dinner with me. That was my life as a nurse—only being able to see my family from a distance. So, I cried when I saw them because it meant so much that they were there; all of us doing the best we could during that time. We had many dinners like this, in the driveway, on the back patio . . . being together but only from a distance.

I remember hugging my dad for the first time on Father's Day in 2020. We had decided to go on the boat for the day, with the wind and outdoors keeping us distanced. My dad got out of his car, both of us with our masks on; he walked straight up to me and just hugged me. I can't tell you how emotional that hug was—it was a very long three months of not giving my dad a hug. We probably stayed in that hug for five minutes, my sister crying in the background. But it meant everything to me. And then we went right back to our safe ways. Our hugs were limited for a long time, not nearly what they used to be.

It's hard to see the world "getting back to normal." I want so much to welcome it with open arms, but I catch myself all the time questioning what I am doing. When I am asked to go to lunch, to finally have a nice time enjoying my friends' company, I look up to see the waitress' mask not over her nose. I sit up straighter, immediately annoyed. When I am at the food store and see people halfway through the entrance door before they finally decide to put on a mask, or when I overhear someone say, "I hate these masks, they are pointless," I get so angry so quickly. It is a deep down anger that lingers no matter how hard I fight it in my mind. Because what I want to say is, "If you only knew! If you only knew how that mask could have saved hundreds of my patients. Why don't you walk a day in my shoes, or better yet a day in my patient's shoes, or don and doff hundreds of gowns a week, sitting on the phone with countless family members trying to explain how their loved one isn't going to recover." But instead, I close my eyes, take a deep breath, and walk away. I get asked a lot how I deal with it all. But what people don't realize is that I am still dealing with it. Because while the world is moving forward (and trust me, I want it to),

I don't think I will ever recover from what I have seen. I will always remember the lives that were lost, every hand that was held. I will always try to be the safest I can be, for myself, my loved ones, and for all the strangers around me. We all owe that for the COVID-19 lives that were lost.

March–June 2020: Elyse Bennett Burch, BSN, RN, Critical Care Unit and Progressive Care Unit, Freehold, New Jersey, United States

Note: This powerful story sets the tone for our book and for our world, because this *specific* story has so many elements of *every nurse's* story. Hopeful. Young. Fresh. And in the end, there is still hope.

Introduction

*"There were a lot more just like me doing the same thing.
I did not feel brave. I did not feel like a hero. I felt like a nurse."*

IN THEIR OWN WORDS

My test results said positive for COVID in early March 2020. Scared to death, I was already experiencing the symptoms: coughing felt like fire roaring up my chest, headaches were a pickaxe pounding my frontal lobe, and insane fatigue and malaise were defeating. The scariest was the chest pressure and shortness of breath. It was like I had a belt tied around my chest and a spider living in my bronchioles and my lungs. I was a slave to its every move with every breath I tried to take. How many times have I helped a patient in respiratory distress? Too many to count, but now that patient was myself. Weeks two and three I became hypoxic and started to hallucinate my mother's voice. All I could think was, "Am I going to die?"

I got better. I knew I needed to go back, even though I felt far from healed. Why go back into the thick of it? I could not take seeing my colleagues fight this and not helping in some way. It seemed egregious for me to sit at home and do nothing. Nursing is my calling. Paired with my care and concern for my colleagues, it demanded I return to the floor. I put IVs in patients, got blood work, brought food trays in and out, and spent time with patients. I spoke with them, tried to alleviate their fears, and allowed human contact that COVID had stolen from everyone. It was mind-blowing.

What COVID demanded from nurses took not only clinical prowess, but also comfort measures and care we rarely have the opportunity to give to patients. I thought I must have some immunity after my illness, but I was not stupid, and I rigorously protected myself. This

6

made me feel like I could stay in the room, comfort patients, and relate to their fear and worry.

What was different was that I could touch them physically. COVID is a thief, and it steals everyone away from you. You cannot get close, touch, or feel. But I could stay in the room longer and do things for the nurses and patient care technicians who had not contracted the virus. I felt like I had some kind of immunity because of how sick I had been. Honestly, if I was scared, I do not remember it. I went into a nurse mode that was unlike anything I have ever felt.

The moments with patients were powerful. One patient, a nurse, was fit as a fiddle only three weeks before—and training for a marathon. She used what little breath she could catch to gasp, "I...I...I'm having...I want to catch...my...breath." I sat with her and had her close her eyes. Together we visualized her running her marathon next year, thinking about the sun in her face and her breath powerfully moving her through the space. The common theme over and over was to be grateful for your breath. A deep, slow, confident breath.

Someone asked me if anything surprised me about my experience and practice during this time. I felt it grounded everything I know about life, nursing, and leadership. When you lead with kindness, thoughtfulness, and love, it will always steer you right. This is who I am as a nurse. There were a lot more just like me doing the same thing.

I did not feel brave. I did not feel like a hero. I felt like a nurse.

March 20, 2020: Kevin T. Moore, BSN, RN, COVID Unit,
New York City, United States

THE JOURNEY BEGINS
•

Before you begin any journey, it's essential to know where you're going. Your destination is not a singular point. It's an evolving state of life-long well-being that keeps you afloat and supports you in all aspects of your life. Well-being is not the absence or prevention of illness, or even health. It is comprehensive, multidimensional, and considers the whole person—body and mind. There must be the presence of some-thing positive: self-acceptance, growth, positive relationships, auton-omy, purpose, and environmental mastery. Dr. Carol Ryff's model of psychological well-being identifies these six essential elements (1989). This model is considered to be one of the most valuable and scientifically verified explorations of well-being. We'll talk more about Ryff's concept, as we think it is the right fit for understanding well-being and all of its intricacies.

So, what is well-being? Well-being is about discovering the roots of what is fundamental and fulfilling to you. To prioritize your well-being is to compassionately care for yourself through kindness, stress reduction, and behaviors that promote both your physical health and emotional growth. Well-being can also be revolutionary; the practices described in this book extend far beyond traditional approaches of what it means to be healthy and well. We want you to embrace this definition of well-being unapologetically, and then apply it to every aspect of your life.

THE UNSPOKEN CONSEQUENCES OF NURSING

◆

Stress is an inevitable and undeniable part of the human experience. It means we are aging, growing, and experiencing new things. And while moving through life without experiencing stressors isn't possible, the way we cope with the tough stuff life throws our way is within our control. If you are a nurse or health care provider, it is important to understand how stress works, because you *know* that stress comes with the job. After a long day, it can be tempting to wind down with several hours of television, your go-to comfort food, and a boozy beverage. But these ways of coping—or, really, numbing the emotions your stress churns up—are not only unsustainable but also unhealthy.

Coping with stress in your life means taking the time to learn effective strategies that enhance your well-being and allow you to perform better, even as more stress comes flying your way. This is what some call self-care. Whether this term inspires you to roll your eyes in annoyance or jump for joy, self-care can be highly effective, and this is especially true for professional nurses. It's about enhancing your well-being. That is the goal.

You might be asking why we are focusing on well-being and not self-care. The answer was apparent to us: Nurses all around the world have told us that the idea of self-care doesn't accurately address the real issues in health care affecting those in the nursing profession. During workshops, professional support groups, and across every social media platform, nurses have voiced concerns and skepticism about the idea and the practice of self-care. The pandemic amplified these unsettling realities. We commend you for speaking up, and we agree. The way most people talk about self-care doesn't even begin to cover what is required to both do your jobs and take care of yourselves.

One exchange on Twitter was especially powerful: "I've been reading and writing a lot about nursing and self-care, and I've come to the realization that it might be a wonderful idea and needed practice, but I don't think it's truly supported or even attainable for most nurses without significant changes." Another nurse responded, "Totally agree, and it feels like we are pitted against the people we serve. Workplaces can be inhumane. We shouldn't have to adapt to tolerate them."

One nurse recognized the value of self-care but acknowledged that "nurses don't necessarily have control of their work situations," and in some cases, the very environment that is supposed to promote health and healing for patients is toxic for those who are providing life-saving care. Another nurse explained that self-care as a solution imagines a problem that the individual alone can fix. So many problems are systemic, and as a result require multifaceted, systemic approaches.

Nurses have shared with us how the lack of personal protective equipment (PPE) and supplies that made headlines everywhere during the global pandemic isn't the only risk they face on a daily basis. In a crisis like the one COVID-19 presented, there is no time—for food, water, or even bathroom breaks. Most nurses told us they resorted to grabbing a handful of crackers to keep their blood sugar up. It is impossible for anyone working under such conditions to sustain their physical or mental well-being. As the first, second, and third waves of the pandemic surged in countries across the world, the assault on nurses grew. PPE was still in high demand and often unavailable, leaving nurses with less-than-optimal protection. The volume of patients exploded in emergency departments and hospitals. Staffing levels were depleted. The issues became even more complicated. Once again, nurses posted on social media outlets and wrote opinion pieces. In a controversial decision made by a governor of a US midwestern state at the behest of hospital administrators, nurses who tested positive for COVID-19 and were asymptomatic would still be allowed to work. That action symbolized what so many nurses told us, which is that they felt expendable—and that their needs would immediately be ignored for the good of the system. Thankfully, the nurses' association from that state rejected the new policy and appealed to the state to try every other strategy first. Four days later, a statewide mask mandate was issued.

Perhaps the most disappointing truth acknowledged by so many of you is the realization that during the height of the pandemic, some hospital administrations offered token self-care gifts or sent out mass emails to employees reminding them to take care of themselves while doing little (or nothing at all) to improve the conditions that depleted staff. Like the small treats given to nursing staff during Nurses Week, these were seen as nothing more than a "bone" that employers threw at nurses to appease or calm them. One nurse even pointed out that there is a tendency to victim-blame: "When we do self-care incorrectly, or don't do it enough, it's our fault. Not the employer who doesn't manage staffing shortages or doesn't train managers for leadership." It was clear from our interviews and discussions with nurses that the problem does not solely lie with the individuals; we must address the system while simultaneously encouraging nurses to enhance and maintain their well-being.

We want you to know that we hear you. We have pushed aside the limited model of self-care and have built an approach to well-being that is far more comprehensive, and maybe even unique. The material and practices in this book, which have been thoroughly researched and go beyond the "typical" self-care tools, contribute to and enhance well-being. Consider this approach a consciousness-raising of sorts. We want you to see the path to your well-being in ways that you never imagined.

THE SCIENCE OF WELL-BEING

◆

All human beings want to live meaningful and fulfilling lives, and cultivate what is best within themselves. They also want to experience happiness, satisfaction, and contentment, known as subjective well-being (Diener et al., 2009). Leading authorities in the field of positive psychology and resilience have studied the strengths that enable individuals and communities to thrive. If we trace the concept of well-being back to the ancient Greeks, Aristotle in particular, we'll come across the word *eudaimonia*, which is a state of living well and actualizing one's human potential. Essentially, eudaimonia is more than happiness. It's not about outcomes or end results, but a process of fulfilling or realizing our nature—our potential—and the life we were intended to live (Deci and Ryan, 2008).

Ryff's (2018) psychological well-being model was founded on the concept of eudaimonia. Her groundbreaking work was done at University of Wisconsin–Madison, where she is also founder of the Midlife in the United States (MIDUS) project. Based on an extensive and diverse theoretical foundation, the multidimensional model of positive psychological functioning was thoroughly researched by Ryff and Keyes (1995), who observed that many theorists across the globe were writing about similar human characteristics. In this work, they compared, contrasted, and evaluated Abraham Maslow's concept of self-actualization, Carl Rogers's theory of the fully functioning person, Gordon Allport's conception of maturity, and Carl Jung's construction of individuation. They also considered theories of human development: Erik Erikson's stages of psychosocial development, Charlotte Bühler's concept of life fulfillment, and Bernice Neugarten's description of healthy aging. Using Marie Jahoda's criteria of positive mental health, they shifted away from defining well-being as the absence of illness. Instead, they answered the question of what it means to possess positive psychological health. The points of convergence in the abovementioned theories comprise the six core dimensions of the model of well-being.

Ryff's model is a dynamic, multifaceted concept that includes subjective, social, and psychological dimensions of well-being as well as health-related behaviors. The Ryff Scales of Psychological Well-Being are theoretically sound, measuring the multiple facets of psychological well-being. The instrument has been validated in hundreds of studies and has survived across cultures and translations. It consists of either 84 questions (the long form) or 54 questions (medium form), and takes just three to five minutes to complete.

The six core elements include self-acceptance; the establishment of quality ties to others; a sense of autonomy in thought and action; the ability to manage complex environments to suit personal needs and values; the pursuit of meaningful goals and a sense of purpose in life; and continued personal growth and development.

Ryff's model offers us opportunities to understand how core experiences in our adult lives are related to people's perceptions of themselves as living by their own convictions (autonomy); being capable (environmental mastery); being meaningfully engaged (purpose in life); having connections with others (positive relationships); realizing one's potential (personal growth); and experiencing positive self-regard (self-acceptance).

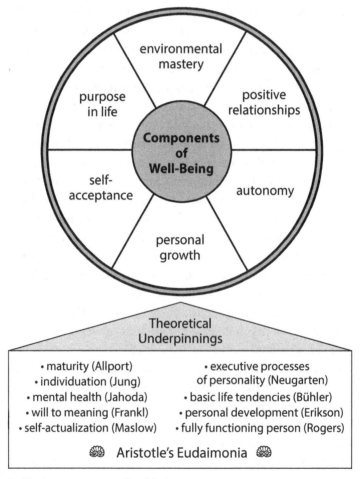

Ryff's six components of well-being.
Used with permission from the Andrew W. Mellon Foundation

Epidemiological studies have found that well-being, especially a greater sense of purpose in life, can be a protective factor against illness and disabilities, reducing later-life risk for cognitive impairment, Alzheimer disease, cardiovascular disease, stroke, and osteoporosis (Boyle et al., 2010; Kim et al., 2013a, b).

Numerous studies have shown that eudaimonia is linked with better physiological regulation of stress hormones, inflammatory markers, glucose, cardiovascular risk factors, and allostatic load (Zilioli et al., 2015; Ryff, 2018). Research within the field of neuroscience has found that there is better emotional recovery from negative events when we possess a greater sense of purpose in life. Eudaimonic well-being is involved in activation of brain regions involving emotion and executive function. Multiple scientific communities have used Ryff's model of psychological well-being to come together and embrace integrative science, giving all researchers a better understanding of what factors affect health and well-being.

As nursing professionals know, inequalities in health care are profound. Nothing has proven this more than the dual pandemics of COVID-19 and racism. In the United States, where medicine and health care are not socialized, health disparities exist partly because of the systemic inequalities faced by marginalized populations. Health care is a profitable industry, and those in positions of power are often considering the bottom line more than the well-being of the average citizen. Sadly, as we have seen throughout this pandemic and the racial injustices coinciding with it, the well-being of the few who can afford and have access to care is prioritized over the well-being of the many who cannot. Ryff advocates for future research to explore this reality and how decisions in leadership affect the well-being of those below them in status hierarchies. "The key task is to explicate what the manifestations of greed at the top means for others—specifically, how do the behaviors and values of self-serving versus beneficent leaders matter for the eudaimonic well-being of those over whom they wield great influence?" (Ryff, 2018). This quote illustrates that there are real barriers that get in the way of eudaimonic well-being and stunt growth that might otherwise be possible, if the systems in place were improved. This is not meant to discourage or make you feel like any steps taken toward improving individual well-being are for naught. Rather, the opposite is true. Being aware that there are components of well-being that are currently out of your control can be empowering. This knowledge can motivate you to gather the tools, skills, and strategies that help in the moment, and propel you to be an advocate and activist for yourself and others who deserve more from their leadership.

What are some forces for eudaimonia? What elements of life enrich and nourish the realization of human potential? One promising direction points to the pivotal role of the arts and humanities in promoting and achieving better health care, health education, and subsequent well-being (Wyn Owen et al., 2013). Key ideals of eudaimonia are to be virtuous and grow. Applied to the science of well-being, these ideals require caring about the things that make human lives, and the world in which we live, better. The arts and humanities, with their infinite capabilities of creativity and understanding of the complexity of the human soul, are just those things.

Ryff (2018) summarizes the urgency of this moment with her thought-provoking words, "Socially relevant research must consider the pernicious forces that work against eudaimonia and fuel unjust societies, while also attending to the beautiful and sublime aspects of life that nurture experiences of purposeful engagement, meaningful living, and self-realization" (246).

THE SIGNIFICANCE OF EVIDENCE

♦

It feels important to say from the outset that our book is evidence-based. The information and effectiveness of the content and practices have been thoroughly investigated by numerous researchers from a wide range of disciplines. In other words, these strategies and practices are *proven* to work.

The process of identifying relevant research to support the topics and practices in this book began with reading and rereading the work of pioneers and authors of classic research. We dug deep into the literature for the most current and groundbreaking work of scholars and researchers across the globe. We asked them to read our chapters, add new references and research, ask questions, and offer new ideas and suggestions. In an effort to be as inclusive as possible, we asked our international colleagues to focus on global inclusivity and to help us identify any blind spots or oversights. Each chapter contains an overview of the relevant research along with full references to books, research articles, and other resources.

We wrote this book for nurses, inspired by the wisdom and spirit you embody in your profession, the evidence-based practices that inform your work, and with your stories in our hearts and minds.

THE STORYTELLERS

◆

It became clear to us that nurses' voices from across the globe should shape the framework of this book. Their stories are told in their own words, powerful and detailed, and serve as anchors for every chapter. Beginning with a nurse storyteller's narrative, the stage will be set for the rest of the chapter. Their voices will be heard above all else.

Read the words below, and listen with your heart.

IN THEIR OWN WORDS

Well, I guess I am just going to let it all out, Facebook. Right here. Right now.

Who knows how I will feel in 10 minutes, because I feel so fragile and unstable. I am having a hard time coping with this pandemic. I'm being hit in every direction. So, my anxiety rises, the fear rises, and at times I feel almost paralyzed by these emotions.

It is the uncertainty that overwhelms me. And everyone that I've spoken to.

I just try to put myself at ease, but we don't know when this will end or how. Will it affect me personally—not only seeing such sick patients but also possibly getting the virus myself, or someone I love getting it? What will it look like six months from now, one year from now? When do we go back to "normal"? No one has these answers yet, but the thought of not knowing is a lot.

A former coworker and friend, younger than me, was intubated in the ICU today. It all hit me at once, and I cried for the first time since all this started. Now there is fear in addition to the uncertainty.

Tonight, my shift ended with a brutal code. We fought hard for this one. The virus was too much, and they were far too young. We're never going to be the same after this pandemic, are we?

There may not be a word for what we're experiencing right now.

My administration sends out emails reminding us to take care of ourselves. "Self-care" always felt a bit strange to me, and I wasn't sure why. Then I realized it's a nice thing for hospitals to say, easier than actually doing something to improve our conditions—like giving us more supplies, additional staff, extra breaks, and days off. The issue is that a lot of people think that self-care can fix these overwhelming problems. An individual alone can't fix them because many, many problems are systemic and require multifaceted organizational approaches.

But we don't need to push through—we need to stop, regroup, communicate, and ask for support and solutions. We need to evaluate and then take appropriate action. Speak up, collaborate with colleagues. Speak up again.

In the meantime, how do I protect my well-being?

There's got to be a way.

April 7, 2020: Anonymous Facebook Post,
Women's Health, Mid-Atlantic United States

Health care providers, and nurses in particular, became the acclaimed storytellers of 2020 and continue to be to this day. We've heard them describe the painful realities and rigors of nursing not only during the pandemic but also before. Although they struggled, they lifted their voices, and in many cases they effectively solved problems and found ways to heal themselves and each other.

To illustrate how nurses not only struggle but also survive the challenges of this profession and begin to make change, we invited nurses from around the world to share their stories. Each chapter in this book is anchored by one or more of those stories—about nursing, about the pandemic, or other circumstances that test the mettle of professional nurses. Although their struggle is part of the story's message, the real focus is on the solution, and how strategies and practices changed their lives and professional experience. This book can be described as part anthology, part guide to well-being. We'll walk you through a wide range of strategies and experiences that are based on the strength of the research behind optimizing well-being and improving health. You'll explore how to integrate these practices into your own life.

You can start anywhere you like in the book. If writing is your thing, go to the chapter on finding sanctuary first. If eating healthier is your goal, dive right into the chapter on nourishment. Most importantly, we'll encourage you to find what works best for you. Know that by investing in yourself through these practices, you are improving how you show up in the world as a person, a professional nurse, a partner, a parent, a mentor, and a friend. You'll have the foundation and skills to move forward, find your path, and be the change. Even better, we'll help you do all of that all while tending to your mind, body, emotions, and spirit.

WHY NOW IS THE BEST TIME TO START

◆

Professional nurses possess a depth of knowledge and empathic understanding that allows them to provide extraordinary individualized care to their patients—often at times of great distress, such as during the novel coronavirus pandemic. Even if you are not working in the most acute and intense settings of health care or directly caring for patients with COVID-19, you are just as likely to experience collateral damage from this global pandemic. Maybe you're a psychiatric nurse who counsels those who were reeling from the anxiety of isolation, or you're an oncology nurse whose patient has had his chemotherapy delayed. Perhaps you're a pediatric nurse who works with families who are unable to get their children immunized on schedule, or you work on the labor and delivery floor, caring for women who are terrified of giving birth during such a tumultuous time. You might be a public health nurse or school nurse trying to adjust to changing policies, new vaccinations, and the demands of the public. Or maybe you're a hospice nurse who sees her dying patients alone in their final hours on earth.

No matter your area of practice, you'll experience stress at some point in your career. And when you bear witness to the trauma and pain of your patients—not to mention navigate the overwhelming changes happening in clinical settings around the world—it can take a long-lasting toll, no matter how well prepared you are.

A major literature review in 2022 confirmed that empathy is the cornerstone of health care, linked to better clinical outcomes and positive patient care experiences (Nembhard et al., 2022). But for nurses, empathy can also put one at risk for empathic distress, which comes at a high price. How can you face such urgency and uncertainty in a multitude of health care settings while also building resilience? How can you become empowered to live your best life, both professionally and personally? How can you make the changes that are so desperately needed in both health care as a whole and in the nursing profession in particular? Self-compassion is the starting point and the foundation of this work. It enhances your resilience, and resilience fuels empowerment. These actions serve a dual purpose: They inoculate against stress and serve as an antidote to the ravages of trauma. They are the foundation of how we can succeed individually and make contributions to health care collectively.

Recognizing how to best protect yourself from the emotional demands of the nursing profession, and then acting on it, does not come easily. In fact, it takes courage. We are just as disheartened as you are that these elements of professional development are not often viewed as essential in many organizational, academic or practice settings. This may be the reality of nursing now, but it doesn't have to be in the future.

We're not just talking about the self-care activities suggested when you're almost past the point of no return. Case in point: One emergency department nurse described a particularly tense change of shift, one she couldn't wait to leave after 12 grueling hours. She was looking forward to meeting her boyfriend for a rare but well-intentioned walk in the park, but the relief nurse was late. Five minutes went by, then ten. When the relief nurse finally showed up nearly half an hour late, the nurse shouted a tirade of words and accusations. When she left the room, she wasn't thinking about that well-intentioned walk. Instead, she carried regret and shame for how she reacted. She knew she wasn't wrong in what she said, but she did know that how she said it could've been more professional. That day, the walk served as a time to vent to her boyfriend and feel his support. The next day, walking allowed her to reflect. In the weeks after, this nurse's post-work walks became a non-negotiable routine to transition back to her life outside of work. While walking, yoga, meditation, and stress management can be helpful in times of chaos, well-being is rooted in consistent, sustainable solutions that build internal strength over time.

You may have tried any number of "self-care" strategies and still feel it's not enough, it's not working, or that these actions don't address the real problems in the health care system. You might feel bombarded by messaging from employers, the media, and best-selling books, leading you to a cycle of judgment and self-blame—a far cry from the contentment you're after. This is not your fault. But you don't have to resign to feeling disempowered. Instead, you can be part of the solution. As you read this book, you will gain a much broader, more comprehensive way of thinking about enhancing and building on your well-being.

First things first. There is no one-size-fits-all approach. There is no singular tool that holds the answer for your well-being. At its core, we are talking about a tough-minded practice of being aware of your needs and priorities, and respecting your own unique situation. Our hope is that this book helps you create space for your well-being—physically, emotionally, socially, professionally, and spiritually—especially during times of stress. In the following pages, you will find practices, tools, and strategies to help you along your journey. Bring them with you as you navigate your way to optimal well-being.

WAYFINDING: THE SECRET TO THRIVING AND SUCCEEDING AS A NURSE

•

In 2016, the animated film *Moana* was released by Walt Disney Pictures. The protagonist of the story is a young Polynesian girl trying to find her courage and direction in the world. Highlighted in the film is the song "We Know the Way," written by Lin-Manuel Miranda. This song, about wayfinding, is a combination of Samoan, Tokelauan, and English languages and includes the following lyrics:

> At night, we name every star
> We know where we are
> We know who we are, who we are

It serves as a celebration of voyaging and the pride that comes with South Pacific natives being the world's first great navigators.

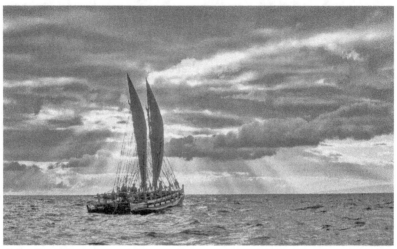

© Monte Costa / Photo Resource Hawaii

Wayfinding is much more than the hopeful message conveyed by this song. According to Maori scholar Chellie Spiller, coauthor of *Wayfinding Leadership* (2015), this ancient tradition began with Polynesian navigators who didn't have the benefit of equipment to navigate across the oceans. Instead, they used a number of non-instrument tools such as mental mapping, which allowed them to estimate latitude to within half a degree of error from the angle of stars in the sky.

Traditional Polynesian ocean voyaging is also known to have health benefits. In 2021, a Hawaiian research team (Mau et al., 2021) interviewed medical officers who participated in a three-year worldwide voyage aboard a traditional wa'a kaulua, a dual-hulled canoe. They found that immersion in ocean voyaging improved multiple dimensions of holistic health—relationships, mental focus, greater awareness of natural surroundings, and overall well-being.

Wayfinding is every bit as important in today's world. After all, wayfinding is built on the practices of mindfulness and presence. Spiller emphasizes that a wayfinder has the ability to respond rather than react, especially when confronted with enormous challenges. In Spiller's work with nurses, she talks about how the concept of wayfinding speaks to our experiences at a deep level, saying, "We can tap our inner navigator in times of uncertainty and change in our personal lives, as well as becoming more intuitive and adaptive leaders professionally."

It's proof of our remarkable ability to show vulnerability and courage, and to lean on our communities.

Wayfinding has everything to do with nursing. Consider the health care crisis endured by so many clinicians around the world during the COVID-19 pandemic. One's educational background, technical prowess, and nursing skills were not enough to sustain professionals through the storm. The health care paradigm was constraining. A dramatic shift was needed. It was clear that the tools necessary to survive were lacking.

The contents of this book will help you find your way to well-being, while acknowledging the shortcomings of the world around you. Set your sights on your needs and desires. Establish where you are looking to land. Know where you are. Know who you are. As a wayfinder, your inner wisdom allows you to set sail and intuitively navigate your journey to enhanced well-being.

READY TO LAUNCH: YOUR JOURNEY
TO WELL-BEING STARTS HERE
◆

We hope this book will not only help you learn more about yourself, but also help you find the strategies, tools, and practices that will make the most difference in your life. Remember, there is no singular way to enhance your well-being. But there may be a *best* way that meets your needs. We want you to explore, experiment with, and ultimately incorporate the most helpful practices into your daily life so you can strengthen and enhance your mental health, and start to experience truly glorious well-being.

We dedicate this book to you, the reader,
and this moment of meeting we share.
Half the work is yours.

REFERENCES
Boyle, P. A., Buchman, A. S., Barnes, L. L., & Bennett, D. A. (2010). Effect of a purpose in life on risk of incident Alzheimer disease and mild cognitive impairment in community-dwelling older persons. *Archives of General Psychiatry* 67(3): 304–10. https://doi.org/10.1001/archgenpsychiatry.2009.208

Deci, E. L., & Ryan, R. M. (2008). Hedonia, eudaimonia, and well-being: an introduction. *Journal of Happiness Studies* 9(1): 1–11.

Diener, E., Scollon C. N., & Lucas R. E. (2009). The evolving concept of subjective well-being: the multifaceted nature of happiness. In: Diener, E., ed. *Assessing Well-Being: The Collected Works of Ed Diener*. New York: Springer, 67–100.

Kim, E., Sun, J., Park, N., Kubzansky, L., & Peterson, C. (2013a). Purpose in life and reduced risk of myocardial infarction among older US adults with coronary heart disease: a two-year follow-up. *Journal of Behavioral Medicine* 13: 124–33.

Kim, E. S., Sun, J. K., Park, N., & Peterson, C. (2013b). Purpose in life and reduced incidence of stroke in older adults: "The Health and Retirement Study." *Journal of Psychosomatic Research* 74(5): 427–32. https://doi.org/10.1016/j.jpsychores.2013.01.013

Mau, M. K. L. M., Minami, C. M., Stotz, S. A., Albright, C. L., Kana'iaupuni, S. M., & Guth, H. K. (2021). Qualitative study on voyaging and health: perspectives and insights from the medical officers during the Worldwide Voyage. *BMJ Open* 11(7). https://doi.org/10.1136/bmjopen-2021-048767

Miranda, L. M. & Foa'I, O. (2016). We Know the Way. On *Moana*. Digital recording. Los Angeles, CA: Walt Disney Records.

Nembhard, I. M., David, G., Ezzeddine, I., Betts, D., & Radin, J. (2022). A systematic review of research on empathy in health care. *Health Services Research*. https://doi.org/10.1111/1475-6773.14016

Ryff, C. D. (1989). Happiness is everything, or is it? Explorations on the meaning of psychological well-being. *Journal of Personality and Social Psychology* 57(6): 1069–81.

Ryff, C. D. (2018). Well-being with soul: science in pursuit of human potential. *Perspectives on Psychological Science* 13(2): 242–48. https://doi.org/10.1177/1745691617699836

Ryff, C. D., & Keyes, C. L. M. (1995). The structure of psychological well-being revisited. *Journal of Personality and Social Psychology* 69(4): 719–27.

Spiller, C., Barclay-Kerr, H., & Panoho, J. (2015). *Wayfinding Leadership: Ground-Breaking Wisdom for Developing Leaders*. Wellington, New Zealand: Huia.

Wyn Owen, J., Phillips, R., Thorne, P., Camic, P., Clift, S., Crane, N., & Donaldson, D. (2013). Arts, health and wellbeing: beyond the millennium. London: *Royal Society for Public Health* 201(3).

Zilioli, S., Slatcher, R. B., Ong, A. D., & Gruenewald, T. L. (2015). Purpose in life predicts allostatic load ten years later. *Journal of Psychosomatic Research* 79(5): 451–57. https://doi.org/10.1016/j.jpsychores.2015.09.013

CHAPTER 1

•

Becoming Self-Compassionate

"I decided I didn't want to feel like this anymore."

IN THEIR OWN WORDS

It was April 8th 2020. I came into work at 7 pm and found out that one of my patients became a Do Not Resuscitate during the day. At 9 pm, his family wanted to FaceTime—to say goodbye. When I reached them on the phone, they asked about his status. I had to tell them that he wasn't doing well. Then I showed them their dad on camera. He was completely unconscious, still breathing, but really just gasping for air. The family cried while they told him they loved him, appreciated his sacrifices, and that he was the best dad.

My goggles were fogging up because I started crying with them. I told them I was holding his hand for them and that my heart was with them. I was squeezing his hand hoping that would arouse him enough to open his eyes for them, but he didn't. The family thanked me, but I knew it wasn't what they deserved. They would never see their dad any other way again. After I ended the call and left the room, I ripped off my masks and goggles so I could breathe. I wasn't able to get myself together; I just kept sobbing and headed back to the nurses station. My nurse manager and another nurse asked what happened, and through my sobs I said, "I had to FaceTime a family." All my manager said was, "We have the Employee Assistance Program." I didn't know what to say in response, so I sat down and drank the water that one of the nurses got for me. I tried to collect myself so that I could take care of my other five patients.

April 8th was one of my hardest days during the COVID pandemic, and while many terrible things happened that day, it was the FaceTime that made me sob during that shift. My anger was growing toward everyone, some of it more irrational than the rest … my patients for not keeping their oxygen on, my friends and family for trying to understand, and the higher-ups in the hospital recommending EAP. Throughout the year, my coworkers and I became more exhausted. We kept saying to each other that we felt so burnt out, but we weren't doing anything about it. I opened up the EAP link on my hospital's website a couple of times, and every time I saw that 1-800 number, I just closed the window.

On January 9th 2021, my mom sent me the Emotional PPE Project website. I looked into it and kept the tab open to a therapist on my iPad for three months. On April 7th, about one year after my hardest day, I decided I didn't want to feel like this anymore and emailed that therapist. I cried nonstop throughout that first phone call, and then she told me about self-compassion. I might get a poster of Kristin Neff to put on my wall; I am a huge fan. Just the thought of being kind to myself helps. There were times I felt my coworkers would judge me for going to therapy. Then I took a chance and started telling everyone I was in therapy and that it's freeing. I've even shown the Emotional PPE Project website to a couple of my coworkers. I can't shut up about therapy and self-compassion. They are so important.

April 8, 2020: Maryrose Huryk, MSN, RN, CNL, Medical-Surgical Telemetry / COVID Unit, Livingston, New Jersey, United States

SELF-COMPASSION AND WELL-BEING

◆

As noted in the introduction, well-being is not simply the absence of illness, nor is it only defined by happiness and life satisfaction. Noted well-being researcher and pioneer Carol Ryff (1989) constructed and defined the six theory-guided dimensions of well-being: meaning and purpose in one's life; autonomy; a sense of personal growth; managing one's environment; quality relationships; and self-acceptance. Self-compassion, both tender and fierce, contributes to these essential elements.

TENDER SELF-COMPASSION

•

One of the greatest gifts we can give to ourselves is self-compassion. This goes well beyond popular or trendy self-care tools like at-home facials and soaking tubs (although these can be most enjoyable). When we talk about self-compassion, we're talking about the foundation of how we treat ourselves, moment by moment. Kristin Neff, psychologist and self-compassion researcher, describes self-compassion as extending compassion to one's self, especially during times of perceived inadequacy, failure, or general suffering. She clarifies that self-compassion is not self-pity or self-indulgence or self-esteem. As the age-old sentiment goes, it is treating ourselves with the same kindness and care we would give to a friend.

There's a frequently cited analogy about the importance of self-compassion that has to do with an airplane's oxygen mask. You've heard it before: The luggage is stowed, the tray table is in its upright and locked position, and the seat belts are fastened. We are asked to give our full attention to the flight attendant, at which point we are reminded to put on our own oxygen masks before placing a mask on another person, even our children. It seems counterintuitive, but if you can't breathe, you won't be able to help others.

Neff points out, however, that the oxygen mask analogy doesn't go far enough. Not only do we need oxygen before and during the emergency, but we also need it afterward. Self-compassion is the essential "oxygen," and the need for it doesn't stop when the event is over. Since the start of the pandemic in late 2019, we've heard a number of nurses and essential personnel tell us, "I'll wait until this is over and then I'll deal with all of the stress." Practicing self-compassion effectively means that we deal with stress and trauma before, during, and after the situations that challenge us.

Neff describes the three elements or pillars that comprise self-compassion: self-kindness, common humanity, and mindfulness. Unless all three exist, self-compassion is incomplete, leaving us vulnerable to negative thinking, which in turn leads to stress, anxiety, and burnout. While these pillars may seem straightforward and easy to apply, implementing these elements often goes against our natural inclinations of self-judgment, isolation, and identification. Practicing self-compassion is truly turning down the volume on those negative thoughts and voices in our minds, stepping back, and offering a softer, gentler, and more realistic approach to life.

Through extensive research, Kristin Neff identified three essential elements that comprise self-compassion. On her website, Self-Compassion.org, Neff defines these three elements as follows:

1. Self-Kindness

"Self-compassionate people recognize that being imperfect, failing, and experiencing life difficulties is inevitable, so they tend to be gentle with themselves when confronted with painful experiences rather than getting angry when life falls short of set ideals."

2. Common Humanity

"The very definition of being 'human' means that one is mortal, vulnerable, and imperfect. Therefore, self-compassion involves recognizing that suffering and personal inadequacy is part of the shared human experience—something that we all go through rather than being something that happens to 'me' alone."

3. Mindfulness

"Mindfulness is a non-judgmental, receptive mind state in which one observes thoughts and feelings as they are, without trying to suppress or deny them. We cannot ignore our pain and feel compassion for it at the same time. At the same time, mindfulness requires that we not be 'over-identified' with thoughts and feelings, so that we are caught up and swept away by negative reactivity."

An illustration may be helpful to better visualize how the three pillars relate to each other. Look carefully at the graphic below. Can you see your own experience in each of the three pillars of self-kindness, common humanity, and mindfulness?

Take a few moments to write down examples from your own life. Answer the following questions: Am I kind to myself? When was the last time I treated myself with kindness? And then ask yourself: If I am suffering, who is suffering with me? Look around you. You are

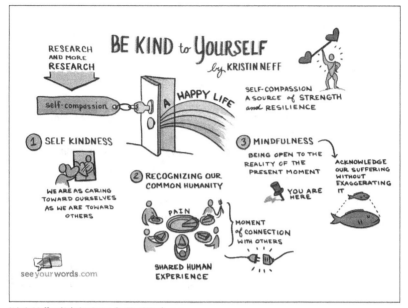

Kristin Neff and Johnine Byrne, SeeYourWords.com

not alone. Finally, ask yourself how aware you are of your emotions in the present moment. Do you acknowledge your emotions without judgment? Or as Jon Kabat-Zinn (2009) reminds us, "Just watch this moment, without trying to change it at all. What is happening? What do you feel? What do you see? What do you hear?" See below for more on the newest research on the effectiveness of mindfulness.

THE SCIENCE OF SELF-COMPASSION

Researchers have found that treating yourself with self-kindness and mindfulness is a significant predictor of other health-promoting behaviors. Kristin Neff, the pioneer in the field of self-compassion, found that self-compassion is positively correlated with happiness, optimism, and wisdom. It also enhances your resilience and ability to cope.

Self-compassionate health care professionals report less stress and sleep disturbances, as well as greater resilience and mental health. Kotera et al.'s (2021) study on sleep, shame, mental health problems, and self-compassion among UK nursing students found

(continued)

that those with increased self-compassion, as measured by Neff's Self-Compassion Scale, were less likely to experience mental health problems, even if they had sleep problems. Other researchers have also found that self-compassion is negatively correlated with mental health distress among nursing students in China (Luo et al., 2019) and positively associated with emotional intelligence in Turkish nursing students (Şenyuva et al., 2014). Canadian researchers (Vaillancourt and Wasylkiw, 2020) also found that high self-compassion in nurses was associated with greater job satisfaction, better sleep, and lower rates of burnout.

A systematic review of more than 200 studies by Conversano et al. (2020) confirmed that mindfulness strategies, among the most frequently used interventions, improve self-compassion. A 2020 study of 1,700 health care providers in New Zealand (Dev et al., 2020) found that increased work stress consistently predicted burnout and lower quality of life, while greater self-compassion predicted lower burnout and better quality of life. Delaney (2018) enrolled nurses into an eight-week mindfulness self-compassion program. Upon completion of the program, the nurses reported increased self-compassion, greater resilience and compassion satisfaction, and less burnout and secondary trauma.

Neff adapted and shortened the mindful self-compassion program to meet the needs of health care professionals. The Self-Compassion for Healthcare Communities (SCHC) program is considerate of health care professionals' schedules and continues to emphasize that self-compassion strategies can be practiced anywhere and any time, in the moment that pain or suffering arises. Neff's research team evaluated the effectiveness of this program in two studies. In the first study, those who participated in the full program of six one-hour sessions had a significant increase in self-compassion and well-being, which was maintained for three months. The second study found that in addition to enhanced self-compassion, the program attendees experienced less secondary traumatic stress and burnout (Neff et al., 2020).

References

Conversano, C., Ciacchini, R., Orrù, G., Di Giuseppe, M., Gemignani, A., & Poli, A. (2020). Mindfulness, compassion, and self-compassion among health care professionals: what's new? A systematic review. *Frontiers in Psychology* 11(1683): https://doi.org/10.3389/fpsyg.2020.01683

Delaney, M. C. (2018). Caring for the caregivers: evaluation of the effect of an eight-week pilot mindful self-compassion (MSC) training program on nurses' compassion fatigue and resilience. PLoS One 13(11): 0207261.

Dev, V., Fernando, A. T., & Consedine, N. S. (2020). Self-compassion as a stress moderator: a cross-sectional study of 1700 doctors, nurses, and medical students. Mindfulness 1–12.

Kotera, Y., Cockerill, V., Chircop, J. G. E., & Forman, D. (2021). Mental health shame, self-compassion and sleep in UK nursing students: complete mediation of self-compassion in sleep and mental health. Nursing Open 8: 1325–35. https://doi.org/10.1002/nop2.749

Luo, Y., Meng, R., Li, J., Liu, B., Cao, X., & Ge, W. (2019). Self-compassion may reduce anxiety and depression in nursing students: a pathway through perceived stress. Public Health 174: 1–10. https://doi. org/10.1016/j .puhe.2019.05.015

Neff, K., Knox, M., Long, P. & Gregory, K. (2020). Caring for others without losing yourself: an adaptation of the Mindful Self-Compassion Program for Healthcare Communities. Journal of Clinical Psychology 76: 1543–62.

Şenyuva, E., Kaya, H., Işik, B., & Bodur, G. (2014). Relationship between self-compassion and emotional intelligence in nursing students. International Journal of Nursing Practice 20(6): 588–96. https://doi. org/10.1111/ijn.12204

Vaillancourt, E. S., & Wasylkiw, L. (2020). The intermediary role of burnout in the relationship between self-compassion and job satisfaction among nurses. Canadian Journal of Nursing Research 52(4): 246–54.

The golden rule of treating others how you would like to be treated is a reminder to treat ourselves with compassion through the lens of the other. Nurses, however, need to be reminded of the reverse—to treat yourself with as much compassion and care as you would treat your patients. As with most tools, this is a practice that improves and builds over time. The ultimate goal is for this to become second nature, actually rewiring the way our brains work.

Unfortunately, for many of us, it is easy to be self-critical and engage in negative thinking and self-talk. Thoughts that are judgmental or labeling can be followed by a downward spiral of more negative thinking and behaviors. When we succumb to negative thinking, we become our own worst enemy—blaming ourselves and maybe even feeling shame when things don't go right. You might have gone down this path yourself or heard others say, "I should never have done that! Why didn't I catch that?" or "Really? I could have been more organized." You deserve better than the rage of the bully in your brain. Unfortunately, the health care climate fosters this kind of negative thinking. We think we should be able to do it all. During pandemic surges, hospital administrators needed staff to take extra shifts to cover patient care. Nurses have asked us, "Can I say no?" To that, we say, "Yes!" Yes. Yes. Yes. You *can* say no. You are always worthy of self-compassion and the opportunity to make a decision that meets your needs.

Neff emphatically points out that self-compassion is not self-pity, self-indulgence, weakness, selfishness, narcissism, or complacency. Self-compassion does not excuse horrific work situations or allow you to "roll with it" or make you "immune" or "hardened." Self-compassion is the foundation for a more honest appraisal of who you are and, ultimately, what you can do to respond to difficult situations.

FIERCE SELF-COMPASSION
◆

In 2021, Neff introduced a more comprehensive interpretation and application of self-compassion; namely, that there are two aspects of this well-researched concept—tender and fierce. Borrowing from ancient Chinese philosophers, Neff describes the yin and yang of self-compassion: the quieter, more nurturing force of yin, or tender self-compassion, and the goal-oriented, dynamic yang of fierce self-compassion. The two forces are not only interconnected but also move in concert, striving for balance, complementing each other at different points in our lives, surfacing when needed the most. The yin and yang of self-compassion have been revealed more fully as the pressures of the world, especially for women, emerged. Neff speaks about gender and gender stereotypes, sexism, and even the #MeToo movement. Women have been socialized to be more yin-like; just take a look at Neff and Byrne's illustration of fierce self-compassion below. In the lower right corner, there we are, "steeping" in the rules that society has imparted to women and men. Yin, or tender self-compassion, is the softer, nurturing, mother bear. Fierce self-compassion seems to come more readily to men.

The nurses we've talked to throughout the pandemic era bring into focus the fierce self-compassion nurses are now practicing. Outraged by the health care system's inadequacies and missteps in the face of

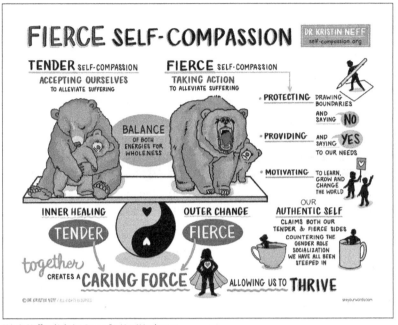

Kristin Neff and Johnine Byrne, SeeYourWords.com

an alien virus, both health care providers, particularly nurses, and their patients had been left to suffer in the wake of the coronavirus. Perhaps during earlier times, nurses quietly made change and changed the system too, but 2020, the Year of the Nurse and Midwife, as christened by the World Health Organization (2019), brought a megaphone to the plight of nurses and those they cared for. Enough was enough. Nurses were vulnerable, frustrated, anxious, angry, sick, and ready to leave the profession. They were and still are suffering, as are their patients.

How is fierce self-compassion different from its tender counterpart? What does it look like? Can one practice both tender and fierce self-compassion? The answer is yes; in fact, it is necessary for balance in our lives. We need to call on a full range of actions when we are in need or suffering. The circumstances of our suffering affect how we choose to respond.

Fierce self-compassion also possesses the three pillars, but they are framed in a somewhat different manner. If tender self-compassion nurtures and blankets us with kindness, then fierce self-compassion calls up a completely different response: seeking protection, taking action to meet our own needs, and becoming motivated to relieve not only our own suffering but that of others. Fierce self-compassion is driven by action. The difference relates to the purpose of self-compassion—at a specific moment. Neff makes the comparison clear. When we need to be more accepting of ourselves, we are still, quiet. The purpose of tender self-compassion is "being with" our emotions, thoughts, or suffering. Not changing anything.

Fierce self-compassion has at least three action pathways. Each of those is expressed through the pillars of self-kindness, common humanity, and mindfulness. Let's look at all of these elements together. When we are called to the action pathway of protection, we seek clarity and truth to know what we must do (mindfulness); we muster the courage to take action (self-kindness), such as enforcing boundaries; and finally, we can find strength in numbers, aligning ourselves with others who share our concerns (common humanity). This one pathway clearly illustrates how nurses not only survived but also had the potential to thrive during the pandemic.

A second action pathway of fierce self-compassion focuses on meeting our own needs. We mindfully come to understand these needs with honesty and authenticity. With kindness, we recognize what we must do to fulfill those needs, and finally we acknowledge our common humanity, our colleagues, and patients. Yet we must balance what we give to our patients or colleagues and to ourselves.

Finally, we ask ourselves, What am I supposed to learn from this situation, and how can I see what needs to change? In essence, we create a vision for our future, and maybe for the future of the nursing profession. We are motivated to make change in our own lives or in the greater community. With kindness, we encourage ourselves to grow and learn. Assessing our common humanity, we come to understand that we learn from our mistakes, revealing a newfound wisdom.

One can't help but wonder if Dr. Neff's latest development, fierce self-compassion, was specifically created for professional nurses. Look at the illustration by Neff and Byrne above. Where do you see yourself in those images? What have you learned? How must your life change? What are your goals? How will you project yourself? What are your acts of kindness? Acts of courage?

THE PRACTICES

◆

The following tools and strategies will help you more fully understand and assess your own measures of tender and fierce self-compassion. Consider these short practices a starting point. They are adapted from Self-Compassion.org; additional links are in the Resources section at the end of this book.

Small steps. Big payoff.

To perform a self-assessment, visit Kristin's 12-Point Self-Compassion Scale.

For a meditation practice, listen to Kristin lead you through a nine-minute practice, titled Self-Compassion for Caregivers.

To learn more about fierce (motivating) self-compassion, read the overview at Self-Compassion.org.

In order to get a sense of how we can practice self-compassion, we must identify how we are compassionate toward others and how it benefits us. In the exercise below, bring to mind a friend from your personal life or, better yet, your work life. Reflect on your relationship and how you've been there for that person during times of struggle, frustration, or pain.

THE SCIENCE OF COMPASSION

Studies over the past decade have found that positive feelings of caring, fulfillment, and connectedness are generated by compassion. New research on empathic distress by Klimecki and Singer (2012) reports that others' suffering can be tiring, but compassion doesn't make you feel fatigued. In fact, it serves as a buffer against empathic fatigue.

Reference
Klimecki, O., & Singer, T. (2012). Empathic distress fatigue rather than compassion fatigue? Integrating findings from empathy research in psychology and social neuroscience. In: *Pathological Altruism*. New York: Oxford University Press, 368–83.

Treat Yourself as You Would a Friend

Goal: To cultivate self-compassion

Time and place: Approximately 5–10 minutes, a quiet space

On a separate piece of paper or in a journal, reflect on the following.

- First, think about times when a close friend feels bad about themselves or is struggling in some way.
  - How would *you* respond to your friend in this situation? (Imagine that you are at your best.)
  - What would you typically do and say in this situation? Write down your response. Think about *how* you would say those words, your tone and nonverbal expressions.
- Now, think about times when you are feeling bad about yourself or are struggling.
  - How do you typically respond to yourself in these situations?
  - Write down how you typically respond. What you do, say, and what tone it is in?
- Did you notice a difference?
  - If so, with kindness, ask yourself why. What factors or fears come into play that lead you to treat yourself so differently from others?
- Write down how you think things might change if you responded to yourself in the same way you typically respond to a close friend or colleague when you're suffering. Why not try treating yourself like a good friend and see what happens?

This exercise is adapted from Neff (2022), with permission.

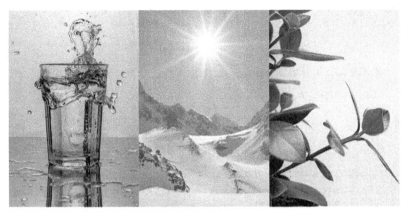

By Nicolas Ruiz, Hendrik Morkel, and Annie Spratt on Unsplash

"Drink Water. Get Sunlight. You are just like a houseplant
with more complicated emotions."—Unknown

Bringing awareness to your inner world—your thoughts and emo-tions—is a significant step in improving well-being, reinforcing self-compassion, and tapping into mindfulness. If there is one thing to know before beginning this exercise, it is this: thoughts are simply thoughts. They do not define our lives with critical or catastrophic undertones. At the underbelly of every thought there is a feeling—an emotional response that can reinforce a negative mindset. The following exercise encourages you to tap into those underlying feelings, reroute thoughts and emotions that are not beneficial to you, and welcome compassion and comfort instead. Some of these exercises may sound familiar, as they share elements of cognitive behavioral theory.

Four Steps to Rerouting Negative Thoughts

Goal: To bring awareness to your emotions, both positive and negative

Time and place: Approximately 3–5 minutes, a quiet space

STEP 1: NOTICE AND NAME THE EMOTION
I am feeling sad.
Is it sadness, fear, frustration, anxiety, anger, shame, disgust, or guilt?
    You will know the feeling.
Don't try to fight it . . . just start by observing and labeling it.

STEP 2: STOP WHATEVER YOU ARE DOING
Literally just stop. Take three deep breaths and say, *I want to be kind
    to myself.*
Don't try to fight it, or argue with it, or ignore it.
Now say to yourself, *I want to be kind to myself . . . to do what I can to feel
    better.*

STEP 3: OBSERVE WHAT YOU ARE THINKING
Identify the unkind thought (for example, *I can't do this work; I shouldn't
    have done that; Nothing goes right for me;* or *I'll never feel right again*).
Simply observe the thoughts; don't blame yourself for having them.
    They may be mantras you repeat a lot, or maybe they're new
    unkind thoughts.
Say to yourself, *These are thoughts that are keeping me feeling bad.*

STEP 4: FIND A KINDER THOUGHT THAT YOU CAN BELIEVE OR ACCEPT
You might simply say, *I want to be kind to myself* or *Let me be kind to myself.*
Or choose something more concrete like, *Although I've made some
    mistakes, because I am human, I've also done a lot of things right in the past,
    and I can do them again in the future.*

Having trouble coming up with kind thoughts to tell yourself?
Ask yourself, *What would I say to a friend?*
Now, say those words to yourself instead of the unkind thoughts.

MINDFUL SELF-COMPASSION PRACTICES
◆

Mindfulness is an important part of self-compassion. Below are several practices that will make it easier to enhance your appreciation of a wide range of emotions.

RAIN Technique

Bringing awareness to our emotions depends on mindfulness, which is precisely what inspired Tara Brach (2017) to develop this technique. Based on the practices of Buddhist teachers, this mindfulness tool can be used when you're in the trenches to help you sort through any difficult emotions in a simple, nonjudgmental way.

Oftentimes, we resist experiencing our moment-to-moment realities and get stuck on autopilot. By enlisting this technique, we let go of feeling like we need to control everything, and instead we let our hearts and minds connect to the present moment. In four simple steps (using the RAIN acronym), you'll be on your way to acknowledging emotions and embracing the life you are living.

R: Recognize what is happening

A: Allow life to be just as it is

I: Investigate inner experience with kindness

N: Nurture with self-compassion

PUTTING IT INTO PRACTICE

RAIN Technique

Goal: To bring awareness to your emotions and reroute negative thoughts

Time and place: Approximately 3–5 minutes, in a quiet space

RECOGNIZE WHAT IS HAPPENING
Ask yourself, *What is happening in this moment? What am I feeling? What sensations do I notice in my body?*

ALLOW LIFE TO BE JUST AS IT IS
Tell yourself, *I can allow these thoughts and feelings to just be, even if they are uncomfortable.*

(continued)

INVESTIGATE INNER EXPERIENCE WITH KINDNESS

Ask yourself, *What causes me to feel this way? Is it really true? Where is the evidence?*

NURTURE WITH SELF-COMPASSION

Intentionally nurture your inner life with self-care. Intentionally offer yourself a gesture of kindness that comforts, softens, or opens your heart.

This exercise is adapted from Tara Brach's website, with permission.

Here is another way you can increase your consciousness of emotions. Try the following writing practice, especially if you are fond of poetry.

"The Guest House": A Writing and Creative Exercise
Consider what the thirteenth-century Persian poet Rumi was saying when he wrote the poem "The Guest House." There is an overarching theme of gratitude and acceptance throughout the poem. It also reminds us that we do not have to fight against the thoughts and emotions passing through us. Rather, we can meet them with respect and courage. We encourage you to try the practice below.

PUTTING IT INTO PRACTICE

Your Guesthouse

Goal: Recognizing and allowing your emotions to be present

Time and Place: Approximately 15–20 minutes in a quiet space

Jackie Hawken (2015) at Mindfulness Bristol in the United Kingdom combines Rumi's poem "The Guest House" and Tara Brach's RAIN exercise. We are indebted to Kabir Edmund Helminski, the translator of Rumi's work, for allowing us to use four of the seven verses in the poem.* Hawken has given us permission to adapt and share her practice with you. See Mindfulness Bristol (2022) for Hawken's original exercise.

The Guest House

Darling, the body is a guest house;
every morning someone new arrives.
Don't say, "O, another weight around my neck!"
or your guest will fly back to nothingness.
Whatever enters your heart is a guest
from the invisible world: entertain it well.

Every day, and every moment, a thought comes
like an honored guest into your heart.
My soul, regard each thought as a person,
for every person's value is in the thought they hold.

If a sorrowful thought stands in the way,
it is also preparing the way for joy.
It furiously sweeps your house clean,
in order that some new joy may appear from the Source.

It scatters the withered leaves from the bough of the heart,
in order that fresh green leaves might grow.
It uproots the old joy so that
a new joy may enter from Beyond.

With Rumi's poem in mind, meet any emotion that arises within you by seeing it as a visitor knocking at your guesthouse door, and use RAIN to help yourself mindfully deal with it:

Recognize that the emotion is knocking at the door of your guesthouse.
Allow the emotion to be present. Do not suppress it, but accept it is there, right in front of you.
Inquire and investigate where in your body you feel this emotion, along with any specific characteristics that accompany the feelings that are there.
Nurture with self-compassion by offering yourself a gesture of kindness that comforts, softens, or opens your heart.

(continued)

By accepting that "this too shall pass"—the guest will eventually leave the guesthouse— you will be able to face your emotions and feelings with more courage and optimism. In Jackie Hawken's original exercise, she uses the first three verses from "The Guest House," and the final verse is from a different Rumi poem, "The Mouse and the Camel." It is not unusual for people to take different Rumi translations or verses and put them together.

This exercise is adapted from Bristol Mindfulness, with permission from Jackie Hawken.

Let's take a look at how a school nurse found self-compassion in the midst of a tumultuous year and a career crisis.

IN THEIR OWN WORDS

"Thank you for saving my life."

Not words you hear very often as a middle school nurse.

In March 2020, schools shut down, and I wasn't sure of my role. Parents, students, and staff were supported via emails, notes, and phone calls. I wanted to do more than that. I was hired to work a few evenings/week in a local emergency department, and contact tracing became my second job.

As a contact tracer, assisting during the pandemic while school was remote and then hybrid, it was rewarding having the opportunity to be a lifeline for many people who developed COVID and weren't sure what to do or how to manage their illness. One of my contacts, the wife of the speaker of the words above, called me for advice because her husband's oxygenation had slipped below 90. Remaining calm, I asked her to hang up the phone and call 911. Several weeks later, after being extubated, leaving the ICU, and eventually returning home, he called— to thank me.

Throughout that summer, talk was underway for what a return to school would look like. The satisfaction I experienced working with patients and families over the spring and early summer months was replaced with stress, anxiety, and uncertainty. Facts shared fell on deaf ears, as many staff members and parents were fueled by fear. A decision was made in my district to return to school in a hybrid model. Right before the year was to get underway, an email from the teacher's union president fanned the flames of fear. I had to speak up.

There were those who accused me of not taking COVID seriously enough. There were nasty emails and angry phone calls—something I was unaccustomed to. My therapist reminded me time and time again that we only have control over our intent, not someone else's interpretation. She encouraged me to watch Dr. Kristin Neff's TEDxTalk, "The Difference between Self-Compassion and Self-Esteem."

The pandemic has brought about the best in people, and the worst. The past 18 months have been a time of reflection, disillusionment, and discovery about myself and others. Entering the field of nursing over 35 years ago with a mission to help others, there was no encouragement to first take care of myself. I have since learned the importance of self-compassion: "Treating myself with kindness, care, and concern, as I would treat others."

Practicing self-compassion this year has taught me that it is time to make changes in my professional life. I am not sure what the next steps will be, but for my own mental health, I cannot stay. My family and I have been spared the trauma of losing someone we love to the disease. But my family and I are starting to lose me: I am not the same person I was 18 months ago. When asked years ago what I love about being a school nurse, my answer was, "Every day I have a chance to make a difference in the lives of children." That belief has not changed, but I have started to question if I am still making a difference. And if I am, at what cost to me?

Contact tracing stoked my long-held aspiration of becoming a nurse educator. A master's degree achieved at the age of 54 has gotten me that much closer to making that dream a reality. I'm scared to death about next steps, but I am grateful to work in a profession where there are myriad opportunities.

My faith assures me that God has a plan: It is time to see where He wants me to go.

August 29, 2021: Susan Hanly, MSN, RN, former Stony Brook Middle School Nurse, Westford, Massachusetts; Now Adjunct Clinical Instructor at Quinsigamond Community College, Massachusetts, United States

Confronted with the stressful and sometimes painful experiences of our patients and even our colleagues, empathy is our greatest asset. It is the ability to share the emotions of another or anticipate how someone else is likely to feel in a particular situation. But finding and embracing self-compassion comes first.

PUTTING IT INTO PRACTICE

Bringing Emotional Awareness into Focus

Goal: To visualize your emotions in words and images

Time and place: Approximately 10–15 minutes, in a quiet space

If you are an artist at heart, open your sketchbook and draw your own guesthouse.

- What emotions are arising right now or appear frequently in your life?
- Where do they reside within the home?
- Are they out in the open, or hidden away?
- What does your final drawing represent?

If writing is your thing, take a few moments to journal about this experience, implementing the RAIN technique.

- Reflect on this experience, and describe what emotions appeared.

    In your mental guesthouse image, what emotions are visible, and which ones are you hiding? How do you feel after noticing how your emotions manifest in your guesthouse?

A DAILY DOSE OF COMPASSIONATE CARE FOR YOU

•

Nurses, health care providers, and other professionals who help others for a living are more prone to experiencing burnout and distress, as they often take on the feelings of people in their care. In recent years, COVID-19 has brought that undercurrent of burnout to the surface in ways we never imagined. It is not sympathy when we feel *for* another person. Carl Rogers (1975) believes empathy is the "cornerstone of the human relationship" and can be a driving source of connection.

According to Tania Singer (2015), feeling too much empathy can cause distress, especially when the boundaries between ourselves and others become blurred. When we take on more of an emotional burden, we think, *What if this were me?* Soon, we develop an aversion to our work and pull back, causing us to experience what is called empathic distress fatigue. The toll of our work can stay with us unless we recognize what we are experiencing, especially if we do not have an opportunity to debrief. Yes, it is our job to care—but when we are on the heavier end of the empathy spectrum, where we are caring too much for others and too little for ourselves, caring can be harmful.

Compassion is the feeling that surfaces when we witness another person's distress *and* have a strong desire to help relieve that person's suffering. We feel warm toward this person, and naturally we want to help. It is this desire to help, and to take action to relieve others' suffering, that separates caregivers from those who express empathy but stand on the sidelines. We actually do not become fatigued from being compassionate; quite the opposite. Researchers have found that compassion increases activity in the areas of the brain that contribute to feelings of reward and connectedness, enhancing positive emotions. In other words, we feel better when we are taking action in the face of another's pain. This is the primary reason why self-compassion is so critical to health and well-being.

SELF-COMPASSIONATE CARE IN YOUR POCKET

♦

Fierce self-compassion thrives when you are able to identify and prioritize your own needs *consistently*. Beth Hudnall Stamm (1995, 2010) has studied compassion and offers several suggestions. In March 2020, she along with her colleagues revised a tool for clinicians to carry with them. You can print out and carry with you the ProQOL Pocket Card (see below and in the Resources section). This small but concrete reminder can help you stay on track with activities that promote compassion for yourself and others.

Professional Quality of Life (ProQOL) Pocket Card for the COVID-19 Crisis

1. Thank your body with restful sleep
2. Nourish your body with enough food
3. Vary the work that you do
4. Move your body with some light exercise
5. Find something that sparks joy
6. Acknowledge what you did well today
7. Accept mistakes with nonjudgment
8. Find humor in the mundane of daily life
9. Take time to pray, meditate, or relax
10. Support a friend, colleague, or loved one

Reprinted by permission.

Professional nursing is more than caregiving for others. It requires caring for yourself as well. It is the foundation for all you do, personally and professionally. It doesn't replace your professional goals or self-advocacy to make change in your career or the profession. Self-advocacy is the cornerstone that allows you to do what's best for yourself in any arena. The ProQOL Pocket Card reminds and encourages you to keep these suggestions in mind at all times. You might even consider creating a personalized pocket card with some of the exercises on these pages that resonate with you the most. The choice is yours. Creating consistency with these skills and activities helps to strengthen and maintain resilience so that you are able to do your work with care, energy, and self-compassion.

REFERENCES

Brach, T. (2017). The RAIN of self-compassion: a simple practice for clients and clinicians. In: Loizzo, J., Neale, M., & Wolf, E. J., eds. *Advances in Contemplative Psychotherapy*. New York: Routledge, 146–54.

Hawken, J. (2015). *Mindfulness for a Broken Heart, Self-Compassion for Negative Mind-States*. Seattle: Create Space.

Kabat-Zinn, J. (2009). *Wherever You Go, There You Are: Mindfulness Meditation in Everyday Life*. New York: Hachette.

Mindfulness Bristol. (2022). The Guest House Mindfulness Exercise. Accessed September 4, 2022, https://www.mindfulnessbristol.co.uk/about-mindfulness/the-guest-house-mindfulness-exercise/

Neff, K. (2021). *Fierce Self-Compassion: How Women Can Harness Kindness to Speak Up, Claim Their Power, and Thrive*. New York: Harper Wave.

Neff, K. (2022). Definition of self-compassion. Self-Compassion.org. Accessed July 21, 2022. https://self-compassion.org/the-three-elements-of-self -compassion-2/

Rogers, C. (1975). Empathic: an unappreciated way of being. *Counseling Psychologist* 5(2): 5.

Rumi, J. (1993). "The Guest House." In *Love Is a Stranger*, trans. Kabir Edmund Helminski. Putney, VT: Threshold Books.

Ryff, C. D. (1989). Happiness is everything, or is it? Explorations on the meaning of psychological well-being. *Journal of Personality and Social Psychology* 57(6): 1069–81.

Singer, T. (2015). Empathy is not compassion: showing evidence for differences in their neuronal and experiential signatures as well as their plasticity. Presented at the International Convention for Psychological Science (ICPS), Amsterdam, March 12–14, 2015.

Stamm, B. H. (1995). *Secondary Traumatic Stress: Self-Care Issues for Clinicians, Researchers and Educators*. Lutherville, MD: Sidran Press, xvii–xviii.

Stamm, B. H. (2010). *The Concise ProQOL Manual*, 2nd ed. Pocatello, ID: ProQOL .org.

Stamm, B. H., Higson-Smith, C., Hudnall, A. C., & Stamm, H. E. (2020). The Professional Quality of Life Pocket Card, General Helper and for the COVID-19 Crisis. https://proqol.org/helper-pocket-card

World Health Organization. (2019). Executive Board designates 2020 as the "Year of the Nurse and Midwife." Accessed August 19, 2021. https://www .who.int/news/item/30-01-2019-executive-board-designates-2020-as-the -year-of-the-nurse-and-midwife-

CHAPTER 2

•

Managing Stress

"What's done is done, leave work at work,
and it is time to go home."

IN THEIR OWN WORDS

As news started to break that COVID-19 had entered my hospital, everyone was on edge. It was March 2020, and we had known about the virus for a few months now, but as cases were making their way from overseas into the United States, I knew it was only a matter of time before the virus was going to come to the East Coast. Around this same time, I entered my management job as an assistant nurse manager in the Coronary Care Unit and in the Surgical and Trauma Intensive Care Units. As I gained my footing during orientation in my new leadership role, COVID was still on my mind.

Then it came.

We finally had our first few cases enter the health care system. To add to my stress, my orientation was cut short by a few weeks because my manager had to be quarantined for three weeks after being exposed to someone who recently tested positive for COVID. It was unnerving, and now, there I was, on my own as patient after patient tested positive for the virus. I had to enforce the constantly changing guidelines with the staff to comply with the latest hospital and government policies.

Nurses are often hardworking, but for me, I always took things personally and worked extra hard. For the past five years, I brought work home with me to see how else I could improve. As weeks continued to pass, it started to weigh on me more and more.

The real tipping point came when I became a code responder and helped with rapid-sequence intubations. I was leaving work at 3 am, with my next shift beginning at 7 am.

It was mentally and physically draining; it was the same routine each day.

Check the numbers. Monitor staffing. Determine if we had enough supplies, and try to deal with constant changes and fear.

Early during the pandemic, I thought all of those extra hours were helping me get better at my practice, but my management responsibilities were affecting my sleep. For a few weeks, I was constantly waking up during the night because I was worried about what was happening at work. I took so much work home with me, I never really had a clean separation between work and home. As the stress levels continued to rise, I knew I had to make a change. I needed my rest. I yearned for that restart. I had to find a solution. Through self-help applications and trial and error, I found what worked for me.

It was important for me to create a new norm and establish a flow that would allow me to establish that separation. I learned to take a five-minute pause after work and use the mantra, "What's done is done, leave work at work, and it is time to go home." During this time, I focused on de-stressing. I listened to peaceful sounds or music to establish a flow as I left work, and reset before I arrived home. After a few days of getting used to this flow and tailoring it to my situation, I've found it to be really beneficial—creating that separation, to just leave work and know that nursing is not 24 hours—for me.

October 13, 2020: Fredrick P. Apostadero, MSN, RN,
Resource Nurse, Coronary Care, Surgical,
and Trauma Intensive Care Units,
Hackensack, New Jersey, United States

WELL-BEING AND STRESS

•

Carol Ryff (2014) found that mastery of our environment and personal growth are two of the six key elements of well-being. There is no denying that being a health care professional takes a toll on mental, physical, and emotional well-being, and at the very least it is a "stressful" profession. How can one master their environment, and feel competent and able to control a range of activities that may be new or frightening? Mastery includes effective use of surrounding opportunities. Personal growth depends on continued development through openness to new experiences. We realize our potential and witness improvement and greater self-knowledge.

At the height of the pandemic, there were few opportunities other than working more hours and caring for patients who were catastrophically ill. There was barely time to grow and learn. Many new nurses pointed out that they knew being a nurse during the pandemic would be hard, but they had no idea it would be "pandemic hard." More seasoned nurses wept as they listened to the stories of their younger colleagues. While the stress may be a sacrifice well worth the benefits of this challenging yet rewarding role, it does not give us permission to exempt ourselves from reducing stress. In fact, the more stress you experience, the more stress management you will need.

THE SCIENCE OF STRESS AND THE HUMAN RESPONSE TO STRESSORS

Early in the twentieth century, scientists began to develop a strong interest in stress and how it affects human beings. Initially studying rats in 1936, pioneer researcher Hans Selye discovered the general adaptation syndrome—the human body's response to actual or threatened stressors (Selye, 1950). Selye classified steroids, now known as glucocorticoids, and emphasized the role of the hypothalamic-pituitary-adrenocortical (HPA) axis (Szabo et al., 2017). After two world wars besieged the globe with death, trauma, and anxiety, the public finally understood how stress was manifested in their bodies. Selye was quoted in a *New York Times* article: "When England was bombed and everybody in a threatened city fled to a shelter, more cases of stomach ulcers were detected than usual. In fact, people talked of air raid ulcers" (Kaempffert, 1946, E11).

Since then, the study of stress has expanded and taken a circuitous and sometimes controversial route through the sciences (Selye, 1973). Many researchers see stress as either a response, as Selye believed, or a process, as Lazarus and Folkman (1984) do. They contend that it is the individual's role to determine whether a situation is threatening, a cognitive appraisal approach. They emphasize that there is "a particular relationship between the person and the environment that is appraised by the person as taxing or exceeding his or her resources and endangering his or her well-being" (19).

Lazarus and Folkman (1984) describe their transactional theory of stress as consisting of two stages of cognitive appraisal. How individuals respond during each of those stages determines whether they experience distress. First, an individual performs a primary appraisal: Is this situation relevant to me, and does it affect my well-being? Secondary appraisal takes place as the situation continues. The question now becomes: Do I need to take action and deploy coping strategies? At this time, there's also an assessment of available resources and behaviors that may be called into service that can be new or learned (Lazarus and Folkman, 1984). There are three types of stressful appraisals. The first two, *harm/loss* and *threat*, are often accompanied by negative emotions. A third appraisal category is *challenge*, which can have elements of positivity. In this case, one might ask: What can I learn from this situation? (Lazarus, 2006).

A significant body of research links stress to health consequences (Glaser and Kiecolt-Glaser, 2005; O'Connor et al., 2021). Autonomic and neuroendocrine responses to stressors can directly affect health, as Selye saw in rats and human beings. As noted in the 1946 *New York Times* article, cardiovascular disease is a known correlate to stress. Diabetes, allergies, chronic pain, and musculoskeletal issues are among the many other consequences. Mental well-being is also compromised, leading to depression and anxiety. As illustrated by anecdotal reports from nurses during the pandemic, changes in behaviors associated with stress—inadequate sleep, poor diets, and minimal exercise, to name a few—can indirectly and negatively influence health.

Developments in stress research acknowledge that there are both positive and negative aspects of stress (Crum et al., 2020). Selye (1978) called positive stress "eustress" some 75 years ago to differentiate from the negative of "distress." Folkman (2011) suggests that positive emotions can serve to downregulate, reduce, or suppress responses to a stressor and support coping strategies.

(continued)

Epel, Crosswell, and colleagues at the Stress Measurement Network at the University of California, San Francisco, developed a classification of terms to more clearly define stress, stressors, and stress response. They suggest that stress is not a unitary concept but rather "a set of interactive and emerging processes" (Epel et al., 2018, 147).

Stress can be classified by type of exposure and psychological/behavioral responses to stressors. Exposure is described as the time span in which the stressor occurs (short-lived, a daily occurrence, or chronic, lasting months or years); the life period (in utero, childhood, adulthood); the window in which stress is measured (once, daily, or retrospective); characteristics of the stressor (duration, controllability, severity, and life domain, e.g., work, relationships, money); the focal point of the stressor; and the capacity of the stressor to cause destructive emotional responses (Epel et al, 2018).

Psychological and behavioral responses to stressors fall into three categories. The first is a global subjective feeling of stress. The second is related to a specific life domain, such as work, family, or caregiving. The third is subjective and/or behavioral responses to specific stimuli. These responses can include emotions, cognitive assessment, worries, and coping behaviors (Epel et al, 2018). The authors also consider the impact of cultural contexts and individual vulnerability/resilience. To learn more about the work of the Stress Measurement Network, go to https://www.stressmeasurement.org/.

References

Crum, A. J., Jamieson, J. P., & Akinola, M. (2020). Optimizing stress: an integrated intervention for regulating stress responses. *Emotion* 20(1): 120.

Epel, E. S., Crosswell, A. D., Mayer, S. E., Prather, A. A., Slavich, G. M., Puterman, E., & Mendes, W. B. (2018). More than a feeling: a unified view of stress measurement for population science. *Frontiers in Neuroendocrinology* 49: 146–69.

Folkman, S. (2011). Stress, health, and coping: synthesis, commentary, and future directions. In: S. Folkman, ed. *The Oxford Handbook of Stress, Health, and Coping*. Oxford: Oxford University Press, 453–62.

Glaser, R., & Kiecolt-Glaser, J.K. (2005). Stress-induced immune dysfunction: implications for health. *Nature Reviews Immunology* 5(3): 243–51.

Kaempffert, W. (1946). Victories in the battle to prevent diseases caused by the stress and strain of life. *New York Times*, October 27, 1946, E11.

Lazarus, R. S. (2006). *Stress and Emotion: A New Synthesis*. New York: Springer.

Lazarus, R. S., & Folkman, S. (1984). *Stress, Appraisal, and Coping*. New York: Springer.

O'Connor, D. B., Thayer, J. F., & Vedhara, K. (2021). Stress and health: a review of psychobiological processes. *Annual Review of Psychology* 72: 663–88.

Selye, H. (1936). A syndrome produced by diverse nocuous agents. *Nature* 138: 32.

Selye H. (1950). *The Physiology and Pathology of Exposure to Stress: A Treatise Based on the Concepts of the General-Adaptation-Syndrome and the Diseases of Adaptation.* Montreal: Acta.

Selye, H. (1973). The evolution of the stress concept: the originator of the concept traces its development from the discovery in 1936 of the alarm reaction to modern therapeutic applications of syntoxic and catatoxic hormones. *American Scientist* 61(6): 692–99.

Selye, H. (1978). On the real benefits of eustress. *Psychology Today* 11(10): 60–70.

Szabo, S., Yoshida, M., Filakovszky, J., & Juhasz, G. (2017). "Stress" is 80 years old: from Hans Selye original paper in 1936 to recent advances in GI ulceration. *Current Pharmaceutical Design* 23(27): 4029–41.

STRESS MANAGEMENT

◆

We wish we could "stress-proof" the nursing profession and the impact it has on our personal and professional lives, but that is impossible. So, we will work toward the next best thing: managing and hopefully reducing work-related stress. We cannot forget, however, that our personal lives can affect our work lives as well—family issues, relationships, and other commitments can take their toll. We'll talk more about this later.

As you may have seen in the work you do, stress can be a contributing factor to illness and hinder the healing and recovery process. As the classic quote from Robert Frost says, "the only way out is through," and this is especially true for reducing stress. First, we must acknowledge it with stress-managing exercises like the ones on these pages.

The weight of stress goes far beyond the aching tension that you may hold in your shoulders and jaw; its impacts on your health are limitless. A self-assessment of the stresses in your life can help you identify how they are affecting your well-being.

WHAT WE CARRY

◆

The Things They Carried, by Tim O'Brien (1991), is an anthology about soldiers and their experiences in Vietnam. The title essay in particular holds significance for nurses. Before we talk about how to use an excerpt from O'Brien's essay to understand our own stress-laden burdens, we'd like to pause for a caveat. It is not lost on us that the work of nurses, especially during the pandemic, has been described using militaristic terms. Hospitals are described as war zones, the virus is the enemy, we fight the unseen enemy on battlegrounds, and nurses are on the front lines. And they're called heroes. Some authors believe that using military language and imagery is not appropriate or justified and could increase anxiety, adding to our stress (Freshwater, 2020). We agree. In fact, many nurses tell us emphatically that they are *not* heroes. But there are other potent similarities that have more to do with who we are and not what we are doing.

O'Brien's (1991) words allow us to focus on how we visualize and think about the "things we carry" at work and in our lives—physical, spiritual, or psychological; heavy or light; joyful or stressful. The following excerpt from "The Things They Carried" may best describe how nurses feel when they are working in the most critical care areas.

> They carried the sky. The whole atmosphere, they carried it, the humidity, the monsoons, the stink of fungus and decay, all of it, they carried gravity. (14)

Gravity and the enormity of the moment. The overwhelming sights and sounds—ventilator noise that drowns out human voices, beds, carts, gurneys, equipment, and no place to move. Every person is covered from head to toe in layers of paper, plastic, and fabric; they are unable to see each other. It is the camouflage of critical care.

O'Brien's soldiers and today's nurses share much in common. The above excerpt prompts us to see that both nurses and soldiers carry things that have physical space and weight. Soldiers have their helmets, nurses wear face shields and N95 masks. And they both carry necessities. Military dog tags and watches for the soldiers and hospital IDs, hand sanitizer, pens, and watches for nurses. Photos, Bibles, and religious medals seem to be in everyone's pockets. These objects hold special meaning. And present for all is the weight of a complex breadth of emotions, worries, fears, anxieties, and memories.

The following exercise can help you reflect on what you are carrying. In your backpack and in your pockets. On your shoulders and in your hearts.

For this exercise, you will think about what you carry on your shoulders or in your heart, and you'll take several minutes to write. Please remember to take care of yourself during this exercise. Although this excerpt is a compelling and evocative prompt appropriate for adults and high school or college students, if you are a veteran or active duty service member or have one in your life, this could be a triggering experience. Please see the resources at the end of the book for similar exercises for young people, who may enjoy the children's poetry book *What a Day It Was at School!*, with the poem "My Backpack Weighs a Thousand Pounds." You can also visit Jim Lommasson's online photography exhibit, "What We Carried, Fragments and Memories from Iraq and Syria," presented by the Arab American National Museum for the Ellis Island National Museum of Immigration.

What Do You Carry?

Goal: To reflect on what you carry in your pockets, on your shoulders, and in your heart

Time and Place: Approximately 20 minutes, or longer when sharing with another person, in a quiet space

First read the excerpt above from Tim O'Brien's book, *The Things They Carried*. If possible, read a longer passage from O'Brien's title essay, on pages 2 and 3. Some universities offer this essay online as well.

O'Brien lists what several of the men in the story carry in their packs, everything from foot powder to love letters to fear.

Think, talk, and write about what you carry in your backpacks or pockets. Use these prompts to stimulate your thoughts.

What do I carry with me?
What do I carry...in my backpack?
What do I carry...in my pockets?
What do I carry...on my shoulders?
What do I carry...in my heart?

(continued)

Pause and reread your words, or share with a colleague or family member.

Understanding *what we carry* helps us identify our stressors, allowing us to take action and manage them. Here are some of the powerful words we've heard from nurses when asked to think about the things they carry.

> "I carry my prayers and thoughts for those on the front lines. I have empathy that I feel for their struggle and am grateful to be able to hold them in my heart. I recall the memory of the hard work I did during the AIDS pandemic."

> "Stress. My patients dying alone at the bedside. My family. My coursework. My mark on society."

> "I think I carry my emotions and constant thoughts about my friends and family. For example, in this dark time I am constantly paranoid of the health and wellness of not only myself but also my loved ones. I can't even imagine losing any one of them."

> "On my shoulders, I carry my family, my future as a nurse, and all my dreams and goals. In my heart, I carry God, compassion, and understanding."

Think about what you carry. Once you identify your stressors, you can plan a course of action to manage that stress. Stress reduction is more than just another item on your to-do list that you're eager to check off and complete. It will take time, practice, and dedication.

You've likely heard meditation and exercise are great ways to reduce stress, which they are (see chapters 3 and 6). Detailed on these pages are stress-reduction activities that are tailored specifically to your unique needs as a nurse. They will help you clear your mind and shed some of the unnecessary stress that may follow you home.

Before we describe the practices, let's consider some of the important research on mindfulness-based interventions (see box opposite).

If you struggle to detach from your work life as many people do, a visualization technique might be the missing piece in determining how to let go of work-related stress while at home. Rather than meditation, which typically encourages you to "empty your mind," visualization is a more active process. During this time, the breath and mind are guided toward the desired outcome, which can be a mindset, a bodily sensation, or a feeling.

THE SCIENCE OF MINDFULNESS-BASED STRESS REDUCTION

The impact of chronic stress in our lives has been well documented—from the physical effects on blood pressure, weight, and even skin conditions to the psychological consequences of anxiety, depression, and chronic stress. Health care professionals, nurses in particular, are especially prone to the ravages of occupational stress, and the COVID-19 pandemic increased those consequences dramatically (Chersich et al., 2020). Skoda et al. (2020) studied the effects of the pandemic on health care professionals in the international community. Mindfulness, a technique of emotional regulation, can help to manage stress and transform negative emotions (Vitale, 2021). The effectiveness of mindfulness-based stress reduction (MBSR) programs has been well established since 1979, when it was originally conceived by Jon Kabat-Zinn (1982). Traditionally, an MBSR program is based on an eight-week-long training program, with individual weekly 2.5-hour face-to-face sessions followed by a one-day retreat (Kabat-Zinn et al., 1992). Each session offers different forms of meditation, such as yoga, breathing exercises, social support, or exposure and resistance to stressors. MBSR interventions not only reduce stress but also contribute to improved physical health in a variety of ways (Kabat-Zinn, 1993). MBSR programs are structured to provide content and practices that teach participants attitudes of nonjudgment, trust, nonstriving, acceptance, letting go, and patience (Kabat-Zinn, 1990). Over the course of the pandemic, many of these programs and others like them have been offered virtually.

Research on mindfulness training (Evans et al., 2018) confirms that these programs even pave the way to added self-compassion and empathy (Birnie et al., 2010), while also finding that those who participated in the program had significant reductions in stress-related symptoms and disturbances in mood. Mindfulness programs have been adapted to shorten the original eight-session program and include

(continued)

other mindfulness practices, yoga, and self-guided materials. A clinical trial of Malaysian nurses with mild to moderate levels of stress, anxiety, and depression (SAD) found that the hybrid face-to-face and web-based mindfulness workshop they attended significantly reduced their anxiety and stress (Ghawdara et al., 2020). A recent analysis by Suleiman-Martos (2020) of MBSR studies confirmed that MBSR interventions reduce stress and ultimately burnout levels among nurses. A study of Italian nurses directly involved in the care of COVID-19 patients found that mindfulness practices significantly improved their mental state (Vitale, 2021). The researchers' findings also confirmed what has already been reported by the World Health Organization (2020) and by the Centers for Disease Control and Prevention (2020) that encouraged mindfulness practices during the pandemic. In a study of 270 Iranian nurses who reported job stress, half of the nurses received eight sessions of MBSR; the other group received no intervention. The results showed that while job stress before the intervention was not significantly different between the nurses, those who participated in the MBSR program were less anxious and stressed.

References
Birnie, K., Speca, M., & Carlson, L. E. (2010). Exploring self-compassion and empathy in the context of mindfulness-based stress reduction (MBSR). *Stress and Health* 26: 359–71.

Centers for Disease Control and Prevention. (2020). Coping and stress. Last reviewed March 25, 2022. https://www.cdc.gov/mentalhealth/stress-coping/cope-with-stress/

Chersich, M. F., Gray, G., Fairlie, L., Eichbaum, Q., Mayhew, S., et al. (2020). COVID-19 in Africa: care and protection for frontline healthcare workers. *Globalization and Health* 16(1): 46. https://doi.org/10.1186/s12992-020-00574-3

Evans, S., Wyka, K., Blaha, K. T., & Allen, E. S. (2018). Self-compassion mediates improvement in well-being in a mindfulness-based stress reduction program in a community-based sample. *Mindfulness* 9(4): 1280–87.

Ghawadra, S. F., Lim Abdullah, K., Choo, W. Y., Danaee, M., & Phang, C. K. (2020). The effect of mindfulness-based training on stress, anxiety, depression, and job satisfaction among ward nurses: a randomized control trial. *Journal of Nursing Management* 28(5): 1088–97. https://doi.org/10.1111/jonm.13049

Kabat-Zinn, J. (1982). An out-patient program in behavioral medicine for chronic pain patients based on the practice of mindfulness meditation: theoretical considerations and pre-liminary results. *General Hospital Psychiatry* 4: 33–47.

Kabat-Zinn, J. (1990). *Full Catastrophe Living: Using the Wisdom of Your Body and Mind to Face Stress, Pain and Illness.* New York: Delacorte.

Kabat-Zinn, J. (1993). Mindfulness meditation: health benefits of an ancient Buddhist practice. In: Goleman, D., & J. Gurin, eds. *Mind/Body Medicine.* Yonkers, NY:
Consumer Reports Books, 259–75.

Kabat-Zinn, J., Massion, A. O., Kristeller, J., Peterson, L. G., Fletcher, K.,
Pbert, L., Lenderking, W. R., & Santorelli, S. F. (1992). Effectiveness of a
meditation-based stress reduction program in the treatment of anxiety disorders. *American Journal of Psychiatry* 149: 936–43.

Skoda, E. M., Teufel, M., Stang, A., Jöckel, K. H., Junne, F., et al. (2020). Psychological burden of healthcare professionals in Germany during the acute phase of the
COVID-19 pandemic: differences and similarities in the international context.
Journal of Public Health 42(4): 688–95. https://doi.org/10
.1093/pubmed/fdaa124

Suleiman-Martos, N., et al. (2020). The effect of mindfulness training on burnout
syndrome in nursing: a systematic review and meta-analysis. *Journal of Advanced
Nursing* 76(5): 1124–40.

Vitale, E. (2021). The mindfulness and the emotional regulation skills in Italian
nurses during the COVID-19 pandemic: a descriptive survey-correlational study.
Journal of Holistic Nursing 39(4): 345–55. https://doi.org/10.1177
/08980101211015804

World Health Organization. (2020). Coronavirus disease (COVID-19) advice for
the public. Last updated May 10, 2022, https://www.who.int
/emergencies/diseases/novel-coronavirus-2019/advice-for-public

Visualizations are an act of mental imagery, allowing you to "walk" through a scene while your eyes are closed and your body is in a calm, safe state. Engaging in these visualization techniques can be incredibly helpful in combating stress, as you allow yourself to create a new perspective in your mind. Further, Varvogli and Darviri (2011) have shown that mental imagery is related to many cognitive processes in the brain, including motor control, attention, perception, planning, and memory, which is why its stress-reducing effects are so powerful.

The practices below can reduce stress, inviting you to leave your worries behind once you depart work. You will learn how to:

- Establish a Coming-Home Ritual
- Create a Sanctuary at Home to have a space just for you
- Find Sanctuary at Work through visualization and writing

Discover the strategies that best serve you, and use them whenever you may need them. You can choose to go through these practices in whatever order you like, customizing them to meet your needs. Before you begin, first read through the script. Then proceed step-by-step to engage in the following visualizations.

It's easy to say you'll leave your workday behind you, but it is far more challenging to accomplish that feat. Rituals are important for grounding us and establishing stress-reducing behaviors. A Coming-Home Ritual is an opportunity to use these important practices every time you leave work.

PUTTING IT INTO PRACTICE

Reducing Stress

ESTABLISH A COMING-HOME RITUAL

Goal: To shed work-related stress

Time and place: As long as you need, at work and at home

Sending-off. Before you leave work for the day, check in with a colleague. Connecting at the end of the workday is a way to support each other and can help you prepare for unwinding at home.

Visualizing. Next, bring a visualization to mind—imagine you are shedding layers of stress of work-related activities. With every step, think of removing a heavy coat or sweater. You'll begin to feel lighter.

Listening. Whether you drive, take public transportation, or walk home, listen to music for the journey. Choose songs or instrumental pieces that bring a smile to your face or relax you.

Arriving. When you walk in the door, shed your work clothes in a convenient place, such as a basket or bag near the entrance or directly into the laundry. Leave your shoes at the door.

Cleansing. Shower if you can. As the water streams over you, visualize it taking away the angst of the day—down the drain.

Renewing. Change into your most comfortable "home" clothes.

Nourishing. Have a meal or something to eat or drink, perhaps a soothing or refreshing nonalcoholic beverage.

As with any stress reduction practice, this exercise is not a cut-and-dry prescription for well-being. It is important to listen to the voice within to decide what works for you and create a realistic, sustainable ritual. At first, the Coming-Home Ritual might be uncomfortable or feel silly, but there is value in leaning into this discomfort and creating a ritual that allows you to let go of your work life when at home.

If this practice does not resonate with you, reflect on what might work. What can you do to switch roles from on-the-job nurse to the person you are at home? What adjustments can be made to this exercise that will be best for you and your life?

CREATE A SANCTUARY AT HOME

Goal: To create a physical space at home, away from work, that serves to shelter, calm, and relax you

Time and Place: 20–30 minutes to begin but will require additional time as you continue to refine your sanctuary

Our bodies are our ultimate home, a fact that may have contributed to your decision to choose a profession helping others care for theirs. Yet we have to consider how the physical spaces that surround us are a close second and can also affect our well-being. Creating a home environment, or at least one space in your home, that is calming, relaxing, and free from your work life is an opportunity to unplug from the stress that tends to follow us home after we leave the office or hospital.

Consider creating a physical space in your home that is just for you. It can be a corner of a room, the top of a nightstand, or perhaps an entire bedroom. No matter your space limitations, there's always room to establish a sanctuary. This place of refuge or worship holds a sacred presence within it.

Why is it important for you to create a sanctuary? Creating a sanctuary at home will allow you to have a physical place just for you, and it can be filled with reminders of what brings you peace, joy, and comfort. Your sanctuary serves as a place to anchor for prayer, meditation, and reflection; or perhaps it simply allows you to enjoy a quiet resting place after a long day.

(continued)

DISCOVERING MEANING IN YOUR SANCTUARY

Goal: To contemplate the intentions for your sanctuary

Time and Place: However long you need, in your sanctuary

Set an intention for what this sanctuary means to you: Is it a place to rest or find energy?

What items will be present to help you find comfort and grounding?

Add one element that relates to each sense—perhaps something comforting and soft, fragrant, and calming to see and hear.

Consider including elements that have meaning to you, whether it be photographs of loved ones and friends, religious or spiritual items, or even a favorite souvenir from a trip.

What items and energy will be forbidden from entering your space?

Is this space solely for you and not anyone else who lives with you?

Will you allow digital devices into your space? Decide what works for you.

What will you do in this space?

Will you pray, meditate, or write in a journal?

Will you allow yourself to simply rest and reset?

FIND SANCTUARY AT WORK: A WRITING EXERCISE

Goal: To take comfort in stressful times or to find a special healing space within

Time and place: 5–10 minutes in a quiet space

As you'll read later in this book, writing about deep and traumatic matters is not only psychologically healing but also good for our physical health. Sexton and Pennebaker (2009) have found that vivid writing stimulates specific areas in the brain. Our pulse and blood pressure become lower, our T-cells increase, and our immune system is boosted.

By writing, we air what is on our minds and share it with the page. As soon as the words are written down, they no longer have the same power over us. Author Lee Smith (2006) makes this point clear: "Simply to line up words one after another upon a page is to create some order where it did not exist, to give recognizable shape to the sadness and chaos of our lives" (374).

A sanctuary is a place that brings relief and a sense of calm. To find your own sanctuary, imagine an inner landscape where you can go at any time.

Get ready: Sit comfortably, feel your bottom as you sit on the chair. Place your feet on the floor in front of you. Your head lifting up towards the sky.

When you think of a sanctuary that you know or would like to know, begin with a sensory experience:

What do you see?
What can you touch and/or feel?
What do you hear?
What do you smell?
Can you taste anything and what is it?
Let an image of a special place, your own healing place, come to you.
When you see it and feel it, walk around in it. Take a good look from every perspective.
Now pick up your journal or writing tablet and begin to write. Allow as many senses as you can to be involved.
Write for five minutes.

DISCOVERING YOUR OWN CARING STRATEGIES

◆

The *Oxford English Dictionary* defines "self-care" as "the practice of taking action to preserve or improve one's own health." It is the act of selflessly caring for your well-being—be it physical, mental, emotional, or spiritual.

As self-care has become a popularized term, its meaning has often been confused with luxuries rather than necessities. For most of us, these practices are much simpler to access and implement. It might be as simple as brewing a cup of chamomile tea and enjoying it before bed, or taking a daily walk around your block. Whatever it is, self-care is meant to benefit you and enhance your overall well-being.

In the exercise below, we will uncover what self-comforting practices resonate with you. Once you determine these strategies, consider them to be part of your complete self-compassionate care toolbox. Use them daily or as needed depending on what works for you.

FINDING YOUR COMFORT STRATEGIES

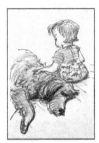

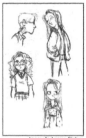

Images by Lauren Airriess

Fold the paper in half, length-wise. First fill in the "childhood" side.

THEN: Think back to your childhood—what made you feel better when you were sick or sad or lonely (a place, story, person, food, etc.). Write them on the lines below . . . at least 3 to 5 things that gave you comfort.
Then fill out the "Now" side of the page.
CHILDHOOD:

1._____

_____

2._____

_____

3._____

_____

4._____

_____

5._____

NOW: Think about the *last time* you were upset, stressed out, sad, or just plain out of sorts. List the things that give you comfort NOW (a book, person, music, poem, movie, song, etc.). Write them on the lines below. Include as many ideas as you can.
TODAY:

1._____

_____

2._____

_____

3._____

_____

4._____

_____

5._____

Compare the comfort strategies you used as a child to the strategies you use today. Revisit the practices of your younger self to heal and comfort you from today's stresses!

Several years ago, Donna used the exercise above with a multidisciplinary group of forensic nurses, social workers, and law enforcement officers. One of the most common responses to this exercise focuses on water—swimming, showers, baths, and fish tanks. One gentleman sitting in the back of the classroom raised his hand and chuckled as he offered his own strategy, "I like water too, especially with my scotch!"

This brings us to an important conversation on how certain strategies may not be helpful or healthful. Food can offer us comfort, but too much is not necessarily a good thing, as many nurses told us during the pandemic. Weight gain and unhealthy eating were worrying them, and they wanted to find the best way to change those habits. We've heard from many people who stashed salty snacks in every cupboard and backpack, while chocolate seemed to be their sweet treat of choice. A number of studies have touted the benefits of dark chocolate. The Nielsen sales research group found that consumers bought nearly $3.7 billion in chocolate, up 6.7% from 2019 (Brown, 2020). There's even a chocolate meditation in the "Nourishing Well" chapter of this book. If you're going to eat chocolate, you might as well practice a meditation to accompany it!

And then there's alcohol. A glass of wine may help to relax us, but too much alcohol or alcohol consumed with greater frequency could be a harbinger of binging patterns, dependency issues, and increased health risks. The cultural myth that alcohol is a good way to solve problems can lead people in the wrong direction; it should not be a regular go-to solution. In fact, Nielsen (2020) reported that alcohol consumption and purchasing increased dramatically in the spring of 2020, finding that "alcohol sales in stores were up 54% in late March compared to the same period in 2019. Online sales were up almost 500% in April." Although self-monitoring is important, finding other wellness strategies is essential.

IN THEIR OWN WORDS

"Nursing guidance is like hand sanitizer for the soul."

During the pandemic, many of our nurses felt that caring was prioritized away. Physically, ethically, and morally, patients' rights had been affected to the point of injury. Nurses, no longer able to do the right thing due to prevailing conditions, felt that they were not enough. Daily measures of care for patients were not carried out, and when there was a shortage of nurses, there was a shortage of competence in different areas.

Nurses had to enter a new playing field. Frustrated patients, now in isolation due to the pandemic, missed their loved ones and were worried for them. The nurses had no opportunity to support and comfort with body contact and closeness, either physically or temporally.

There was always an obstacle through masks and visors and gloves. When caring for a patient at the end of her life who was lonely for her loved ones, a nurse told of surreptitiously taking off her glove to provide one last support by giving comfort and love through skin-to-skin contact.

Nurses' bodies were exposed to more fatigue by working with visors and masks. With long hours and little time for recovery, their mucous membranes became drier; neck and back problems arose. They had fewer days off, canceled holidays, were doing extralong shifts, and feared being ordered to another breeding ground for patients needing COVID care. Many nurses did not want to go to work. Several nurses reported being on sick leave. Thoughts grew increasingly heavier. Many nurses concluded during the pandemic that they had learned a lot, with the reflection, *I am an expert in corona nursing.*

When things are at their worst, nursing guidance is needed at its best.

During this time, it was important for nurses' groups to have supervision, as they were putting into words what had been spinning around in their heads about their experiences. They needed to be validated in their professional roles and in their nursing work, by understanding their own and others' situations. We worked with communication tools to manage nurses' anxiety, frustration, and perceived shortcomings. In groups, support and understanding came from colleagues and nursing supervisors, as nurses were allowed to talk about good things they had done. It was important to keep in mind that it was okay to do the best you can; you cannot do more. Also important was for the nurses to reflect over how they could relate to each other, remembering that priorities are always difficult, and that we had to be humble and not judge others or ourselves, especially now.

PRocess-Oriented Nursing Supervision (PRONS) is a pedagogical process model where clinical experiences are positioned in a professional context. The nursing theoretical perspective is the base, and it gives nurses the opportunity to become more aware and relate to different caring situations. A variety of reflection methods are used as a focus to clarify situations, articulate thoughts and feelings concretely, understand and analyze what happened, and critically formulate an action plan. Difficult situations may become more comprehensible, manageable, and meaningful through such reflection. PRONS is usually a process over 1.5 to 2 years, with a PRONS group consisting of between 5 and 8 participants who meet for 1.5 hours every second week. Each meeting is organized in the same way. The supervisor is a nurse with a specific education in supervision and is responsible for the supervision. In the supervision, the individual has the possibility for reflection using the model's three steps: purging, playing, and learning (PPL), in accord with Eriksson's Theory of Caring as Health (Eriksson, 1994; Carlson et al., 2020).

Communication tools we utilized in supervision included pedagogical symbols on a map, which corresponded to emotions. This tool supports the nurses' own empowerment to prevent burnout and to raise the quality of nursing in daily practice and reflections on nursing situations (Jenholt Nolbris et al., 2019). An empty body outline was a tool to encourage nurses to explain, as they drew on it, how their own bodies felt. The Bears (2022) is a set of 48 illustrated cards depicting bears with different expressions. The cards, developed in Australia, are a tool to help identify and talk about feelings and emotions (Deal and Wood, 2010).

These types of activities, with guidance and practice, may be useful tools to more fully understand and refine professional roles, or they can even lead to exploration of change and reevaluation of what nursing means in one's life. We must develop and increase support for nurses; strengthen, confirm, and protect their health and working environment; and improve their work situation and work environment.

October 6, 2021: Lotta Carlson, MS, RN, Department of Education, Research and Development, Sahlgrenska University, Molndal, Sweden; and Margaretha Jenholt Nolbris, PhD, RN, Institute of Health and Care Sciences, Sahlgrenska Academy, University of Gothenburg, Gothenburg, Sweden

GROUNDING DURING TIMES OF
INTENSE STRESS AND TRAUMA
◆

When the going gets really tough, of crisis proportions, then we need to have every available tool at our disposal. Often these moments occur when we are at work. Kristin Neff describes how to manage those

stressful or traumatic situations or when we feel triggered or experience flashbacks. She emphasizes that these are moments when you
want to be a "slow learner" and decelerate. Choose your self-compassion
strategies carefully.

Germer and Neff (2013) describe a unique and unexpected phenomenon that could occur during a crisis called backdraft. Yes, just
like the chemical flare-up that results when there is a sudden flood of
oxygen that fuels a fire. As they point out, the way many of us cope
with trauma is by "closing our hearts and minds" to protect ourselves.
Out of sight, out of mind. Sometimes, when we start to open our hearts
and practice coping strategies, the self-compassion and the self-love
rush in, and the traumatic pain rushes out. It's like fresh air feeding a
fire. While it's a good sign that you're doing the practice correctly, it can
also mean you need to go more slowly, because the backdraft can be
overwhelming, causing one to disconnect from the moment, become
anxious, or even panic.

In the midst of a crisis, you can take two "soft and slow" approaches:
a grounding mindfulness practice or a behavioral practice. Research
by Jones et al. (2017) shows that grounding techniques can be effective.
They help reduce the amygdala's reactivity, partly because our focus is
brought back to physical surroundings and not our emotions or racing
thoughts. You can do a grounding practice anywhere, any time and just
focus for a few moments on that feeling of connection of your feet to
the floor.

PUTTING IT INTO PRACTICE

Ground Yourself

Goal: To practice grounding by focusing on your physical surroundings

Time and Place: Approximately 1 minute or less, in any location

For this grounding practice, where you simply feel the soles of your
feet on the floor, you will literally ground or plant yourself into the
floor (or earth). During this practice, which takes only 30 seconds,
all of your awareness is directed to your feet. Feel your toes in your
shoe, the sides of your feet, and your heels, and then plant, imagining

roots reaching through the floor and into the earth. In chapter 3, we describe the steps for doing this exercise in private or in public.

And when you feel overwhelmed by difficult emotions, the most self-compassionate response may be to pull back temporarily—focus on the breath, the sensation of the soles of your feet on the ground, or engage in ordinary, behavioral acts of self-compassion such as having a cup of tea or petting the dog.

Using behavioral techniques is another way to ground yourself. Yes, it's good to be rested and eating well, but what if you need something right then and there, in the midst of a stressful moment? Neff uses the example of wanting a cup of tea, which calms and soothes. Although drinking the tea isn't possible at that moment, thinking about the cup of tea allows you to answer the question, what do I need right now? She points out that thinking about the cup of tea is associated with the intention of caring for yourself, and just the thought can prompt feelings of calm and self-compassion. Neff reminds us that perhaps "the best thing to do in that situation isn't putting your hand on your heart or saying something kind to yourself"; instead, maybe what you need to do to become calm is to have that cup of tea or take a walk. As soon as you can.

FAMILIES, FRIENDS, AND COLLEAGUES: STRESSORS OR STRESS RELIEF?

◆

Since late 2019, we've heard the word "stressed" more than we ever imagined. It is often embedded in the first statements heard from nurses in the field. Pre-pandemic, the effects of a stressor, such as being short-staffed, would be alleviated once the stressor was removed. In those pre-COVID days, nurses would leave work after a hectic day, head home, perhaps find respite among family and friends, eat a meal, and go to sleep. Not so during the pandemic.

For every nurse employed, there are partners, children, parents, or siblings who might not only be a source of support and comfort, but also a source of stress and worry. It is no secret that nurses were worried about bringing COVID home to their families, while they also worried about balancing their work-home responsibilities. In the early weeks of the pandemic, nurses stayed in hotels or even in their cars to protect their families, often not seeing them for months. And then there are the nurses' children.

IN THEIR OWN WORDS

My first time working COVID, I came home from work, and my husband told me he was sleeping downstairs with the kids. I would stay locked in our bedroom away from them, to be safe. My then-2-year-old was crying and banging on the door, screaming for me, and it just ripped my heart out. The tears rolled down my face, and all I could do was cry. I just sat on my bed in my room all alone, trying to process what was happening, and called my parents on FaceTime and cried. I said to them, if this is what life is, I do not want it! I thought about quitting because I was overcome with fear but knew nursing was something I wanted to do.

The more I worked COVID, the more I became comfortable knowing that I was doing everything I could to protect myself and my family. When I came home, I had a system and routine with my husband so that I wouldn't touch anything but just run into the shower and clean off.

The biggest challenge for me moving forward is making sure my kids are okay. I now have to help my family heal. My kids faced challenges due to the pandemic that I did not even realize because I was so consumed with what I was going through, I didn't see it. My kids have developed anxieties and fear over getting sick or making other people sick. We have sleepless nights from bad dreams that keep them up out of sheer terror.

My kids always beg me not to go to work. They are afraid I will get sick. I had an exposure to COVID and tested positive, but I was lucky enough to not have serious symptoms. Still, I was sent home from work when I found out. That day I will never forget. I came home to four little faces standing in the doorway looking at me scared and sad, asking me if I will be okay or will I die. That is something I could never prepare myself for.

The emotions are still raw.

The turning point for me and knowing how badly my kids were affected was when one of my children could not sleep at night because of all the fears that she had developed. It completely consumed her, and we had to just sit in her room and talk through how she was feeling. I realized then that avoiding the subject of COVID and not talking about it hurt my kids more than it helped. My husband and I knew then that we had to make a change. We had open communication with our kids to help lessen the fears and anxiety of the unknown, and to help them work through what they felt. We decided to not avoid talking about COVID but to face it head-on and be honest and reassuring that everything will be okay. We wanted them to feel like they could talk to us and ask us questions and feel comforted. When I asked my kids how they felt during COVID, they said, "Sad, scared, and depressed." That was eye-opening for me. They are such little kids to have such heavy emotions. That is a wow moment for me.

July 8, 2021: Kristen Bannister, BSN, RN-BC, Surgical-Orthopedic Unit, New Brunswick, New Jersey, United States

As painful as it is to read the words above, this nurse had improvised a solution to minimize her exposure and the exposure of the family to the virus. Children were brave and sometimes brutally honest when they talked to families and teachers. Their openness reminds us that they too struggled, and continue to struggle, with the chaos and losses in their lives. And they see and hear much more than we could ever imagine.

IN THEIR OWN WORDS

Looking back on this past year brings so much anxiety and sadness. Everything has changed. Nursing will forever be changed, and the appreciation for family and friends is so much stronger for me now. I do not ever want to take a day for granted again. My biggest support through the pandemic besides my husband and kids were my coworkers, specifically two of them. We would call each other at all hours of the day and night and just cry. We would be the support for each other when we were overcome with fear, anxiety, and sadness. My fellow coworkers and I developed team nursing, where we worked together and divided the shift. One of us was "dirty" in the morning, while the other stayed "clean" to run and grab what is needed to save on PPE and minimize our exposure. I would cry for no reason and just felt sad all the time. My kids would often ask me, "Mommy, why are you crying?" and it was something I could never explain to them.

August 12, 2021: Kristen Bannister, BSN, RN-BC, Surgical-Orthopedic Unit, New Brunswick, New Jersey, United States

But work colleagues knew exactly what she was talking about. Even nurses who are not working on the "front lines" or directly caring for patients with COVID-19 may experience collateral damage from this pandemic. Nurses in nearly every practice setting, not only intensive care units or emergency departments, have been directly and acutely affected by this public health crisis. A study by the International Council of Nurses (2021) found that almost 80% of their affiliated nursing associations have reported that nurses who are working in the COVID-19 response experience mental health distress. Nurses are not alone; in fact, they are experiencing collective stress and possibly collective trauma.

Collective stress refers to the psychological responses to an event that can affect an entire family, community, society, and in the case of the coronavirus pandemic, entire professions. The collective memory persists beyond the lives of individuals.

We are seeing our nursing colleagues come together—in many settings, among a variety of practices, and with a wide range of years of experience. Many nurses have referred to their colleagues as their "work family," who are every bit as important as their partners, children, parents, siblings, aunts, uncles, or cousins.

Since March 2020, we've heard many nurses describe how their work family has been there for them: "I'm in awe of my coworkers. We have each other's backs. They are my family. I've never felt closer." The shared experiences, both negative and positive, help unite us and protect us. Froma Walsh (2016) and other researchers and clinicians can attest to the value of the collective in building resilience.

THE SCIENCE OF COLLECTIVE RESILIENCE AND STRESS

We know that resilience is the capacity to overcome adversity; not only to bounce back but to bounce forward, to grow (Walsh, 2020). This dynamic, multilevel process is an indispensable approach in situations of collective trauma and stress. Because we are relational beings, we must recognize our interdependence on each other—it is necessary for our well-being and resilience. We share our pain, suffering, and stress with the people in our lives, whether we intend to or not.

Collective resilience, found in families and at work, is fostered by shared beliefs. Together we make meaning of the pandemic crisis and the challenges it presents to our personal and professional lives. Together we can gain or regain a positive, hopeful outlook that supports active efforts, and as a result, we rise above suffering and hardship through redefining our values, expressions of spirituality, and transforming our priorities, a sense of purpose, and deeper bonds (Walsh, 2020). As one nurse so clearly told us, "My work family is everything to me, but my family at home is my safety net."

Families can also be a source of anxiety and stress as nurses tried to balance work and home. So many struggled with the challenges of caring for elderly parents or children, sharing time with work-at-home partners or roommates, and their own work schedules. Many studies, such as that by Foli et al. (2021), revealed that nurses feared for their family's health, afraid to go home and bring the virus with them. Families had to adapt in the face of unfathomable threats to the mental and physical health of everyone.

While little is known about the long-term effects on nurses' families, future research will shed much needed light on this important topic. One new study may be paving the way. Kim et al. (2021) reported that nearly 80% of the nurses they studied in Southern California experienced high stress while caring for COVID patients. But for those nurses with high resilience, spirituality and family functioning appeared to be important coping mechanisms against stress, anxiety, and depression during the pandemic. Family functioning was measured using the Family APGAR tool with five indicators of family functioning: Adaptation, Partnership, Growth, Affection, and Resolve (Smilkstein, 1978). There is more to learn about how relationships and the mental health of family members fared during the pandemic and its aftermath.

(continued)

References

Foli, K. J., Forster, A., Cheng, C., Zhang, L., & Chiu, Y. C. (2021). Voices from the COVID-19 frontline: nurses' trauma and coping. *Journal of Advanced Nursing* 77: 3853–66.

Kim, S. C., Quiban, C., Sloan, C., & Montejano, A. (2021). Predictors of poor mental health among nurses during COVID-19 pandemic. *Nursing Open* 8(2): 900–907.

Smilkstein, G. (1978). The family APGAR: a proposal for a family function test and its use by physicians. *Journal of Family Practice* 6(6): 1231–39.

Walsh, F. (2020). Loss and resilience in the time of COVID-19: meaning making, hope, and transcendence. *Family Process* 59(3): 898–911.

A FEW FINAL THOUGHTS

◆

Remember that sustainable well-being practices include acknowledging the challenging times, situations, and emotions attached to them. Rather than masking these unsettling moments with food, alcohol, or other unhealthy habits, it is best to build up your health-promoting strategies now. Unlike behaviors that merely obscure our emotions, self-compassion and self-nurturing are investments that will grow and pay increasing dividends over time. This allows you to reach for them again and again, especially when bumps in the road inevitably appear.

REFERENCES

Brown, D. (2020). Americans are buying more chocolate as the pandemic rages on. *USA Today*, July 10, 2020. https://www.usatoday.com/story/money/2020/07/10/americans-buying-more-chocolate-during-pandemic/5412598002/

Carlson, L., Berg, L., & Jenholt Nolbris, M. (2020). Nurses' experiences of process-oriented supervision—acquiring new approaches to demanding situations. *Open Journal of Nursing* 10: 4.

Deal, R., & Wood, B. (2010). *The Bears.* Victoria, Australia: Innovative Resources.

Eriksson, K. (1994). Theories of caring as health. In: Gaul, A. D., & Boykin, A., eds. *Caring as Healing, Renewal through Hope.* New York: National League for Nursing, 3–20.

Freshwater, E. (2020). COVID 19: why we need to ditch the military terms. *Nursing Standard*, April 17, 2020. https://rcni.com/nursing-standard/opinion/comment/covid-19-why-we-need-to-ditch-military-terms-160071

Germer, C. K., & Neff, K. D. (2013). Self-compassion in clinical practice. *Journal of Clinical Psychology* 69(8): 856–67.

International Council of Nurses. (2021). The COVID-19 effect: World's nurses facing mass trauma, an immediate danger to the profession and future of our health systems. Accessed September 4, 2022. https://www.icn.ch/sites/default/files/inline-files/ICN%20COVID19%20update%20report%20FINAL.pdf

Jenholt Nolbris, M., Wigert, H., Carlson, L., & Berg, L. (2019). Using pedagogical symbols in a map in supervision. *International Journal of Nursing and Health Care Research* 4: 082.

Jones, L. K., Rybak, C., & Russell-Chapin, L. A. (2017). Neurophysiology of traumatic stress. In: Field, T. A., Jones, L. K., & Russell-Chapin, L. A., eds. *Neurocounseling: Brain-Based Clinical Approaches*. Alexandria, VA: American Counseling Association, 61–80.

Nielsen. (2020). Rebalancing the "COVID-19 effect" on alcohol sales. May 7, 2020, https://nielseniq.com/global/en/insights/analysis/2020/rebalancing-the-covid-19-effect-on-alcohol-sales/

O'Brien, T. (1991). *The Things They Carried*. New York: Harper Collins.

Prelutsky, J. (2009). *What a Day It Was at School!* New York: Greenwillow Books.

Ryff, C. D. (2014). Psychological well-being revisited: advances in the science and practice of eudaimonia. *Psychotherapy and Psychosomatics* 83(1): 10–28.

Sexton, J. D., & Pennebaker, J. W. (2009). The healing powers of expressive writing. In: Kaufman, S. B., & Kaufman, J. C., eds. THE *psychology of Creative Writing*. Cambridge: Cambridge University Press, 264–73.

Smith, L. (2006). *On Agate Hill*. Chapel Hill, NC: Algonquin.

The Bears. Innovative Resources, accessed July 22, 2022, innovativeresources.org/resources/card-sets/bears-cards.

Varvogli, L., & Darviri, C. (2011). Stress management techniques: evidence-based procedures that reduce stress and promote health. *Health Science Journal* 5(2): 74.

Walsh, F. (2016). *Strengthening Family Resilience*, 3rd ed. New York: Guilford Press.

CHAPTER 3

•

Exploring Mindfulness
and Meditation

*"I went from living in my head to living in my body.
It was the fastest way I could come back to myself."*

IN THEIR OWN WORDS

It's been a looooong two weeks. We moved houses, started an 11-year-old and a 13-year-old on virtual schooling, haven't been able to work, have presentations due, and have no Internet service. Don't get me wrong. I've been grateful for what we do have, but admittedly *cranky*.

And this was all pre-vaccine.

Let me start at the beginning. I was furloughed in March 2020, when the coronavirus pandemic took hold in the United States. I never got that job back. I had to transition to virtual work. The whole family discovered virtual learning. All of us were in the house online at the same time. Then we found out the landlord was raising our rent—and the lease was up in a few months. We had 60 days to find a new place to live. At the height of the pandemic. There was a massive exodus of people leaving the city—everyone thought they could run away from COVID. We joined the exodus.

We *had* to move, and it took a lot of strategic planning. It was such a stressful experience; we went from renters to first-time homeowners. We have two special needs kids who had to start school. And they needed to stay in the same school district.

Somehow, we did it.

On August 31st, six months into the pandemic, we moved to our house—unaware that we were about to go into a second surge. I couldn't get the weight of all we had been through off of me and move forward.

One morning a few weeks later, I got up earlier than everyone else. I walked into the backyard and looked around me. I had this longing to just touch the grass, take off my shoes, the way I did as a child. The earth was warm. The air was cool. I walked barefoot in the grass; it was instantaneous grounding, all at once.

I went from living in my head to living in my body. It was the fastest way I could come back to myself. The longer I walked in my backyard, the better I felt. Feeling the warm sunlight, listening to the birds. The earth was mothering me, welcoming me.

I thought to myself, *Everything is going to be okay*. The land was welcoming me; it was almost startling. And it was instantaneous, faster than yoga. The earth pulled me back into my body. I've walked in my backyard many times since then, but nothing could match that day in September of 2020. I had such an unexpected reaction.

It was like getting the warmest hug.

I'm doing part-time telehealth now. We'd been looking forward to the kids starting in-person school. But only days before the start of school, my community was hit by Tropical Storm Ida. So many basements were flooded, including ours. My husband is a high school teacher; his school is going back online while it repairs the damage from the storm.

Then this morning something happened that stopped me dead in my tracks and left me speechless. My boy was eating his breakfast, and we were chatting quietly about nothing in particular when we came to a pause in our conversation. After a quiet bit he suddenly said, "Thank you mommy." I looked up, surprised, and asked why he was thanking me.

He said, "Because you are... (he paused, searching for words)... a kind mother."

I couldn't find my own words right then. With so many emotions, I don't think my heart could swell up more than it did without bursting.

I love these kids.

Yes, I've been grateful for what we do have, and at times like this, I'm not cranky at all.

September 10, 2020: Milagros R. Elia, MA, APRN, ANP-BC,
Oncology Nursing, Putnam County, New York, United States

The origins of modern-day mindfulness and meditation began centuries ago, primarily in the Eastern part of the world, with ties in China, ancient Egypt, and India. Today, thanks to scientific inquiries of these ancient practices, mindfulness and meditation are often associated with well-being and stress management. On some occasions, the terms are used inconsistently or even interchangeably, but there are subtle yet specific differences. We've introduced you to mindfulness in earlier chapters, but let's look further at mindfulness and meditation and how you can enhance your well-being.

MINDFULNESS
◆

More than 40 years ago, physician Jon Kabat-Zinn studied with Zen Buddhist masters and founded Mindfulness-Based Stress Reduction (MBSR) and the Center for Mindfulness in Medicine, Healthcare, and Society. Kabat-Zinn (2013) defines mindfulness as "the awareness that emerges through paying attention on purpose, in the present moment, and non-judgmentally, to the unfolding of experience moment by moment" (145). It is a practice of finding acceptance and wisdom within the present moment that can expand into various realms of living. With awareness of the present moment at the center of mindfulness, this practice can take shape in many ways, depending on what works best for an individual's needs.

Meditation can be defined as a set of specific techniques, activities, or skills that enhance psychological and physical relaxation (Cardoso et al., 2004). In media portrayals, meditation is often misunderstood as a strict practice that requires perfect posture and the mental fortitude to clear one's mind on a moment's notice, but this is not entirely the case. Meditation practices are both informal and formal and include mindful breathing, compassion meditation, loving kindness–focused meditation, and the use of phrases or mantras as focal points for meditation (Behan, 2020).

In the context of mindfulness and meditation, the word "practice" is not defined as a rehearsal or refinement of a skill for the future. Kabat-Zinn (2013) adds that practice is a time of "being present on purpose" (29). Simply put, mindfulness is a state of mind, and meditation is the practice used to achieve that state of mind. The benefits of mindfulness interventions are many.

While the mental health benefits are enticing, sticking to meditation tends to be a challenge for most people. Even though meditation is a worldwide phenomenon with impressive scientific evidence, there are many misconceptions around mindfulness and meditation that leave people thinking they should be at monk-level status after their first meditation session, but that is not the case. It is, like most things, a practice, which in the words of Kabat-Zinn is time spent being present on purpose. As with any new skill, meditation requires time for refinement and honing this skill. Someday you can achieve the level of clear-headedness you've been dreaming of. Until then, it is in the challenge of the practice that these powerful benefits subtly unfold.

THE SCIENCE OF MINDFULNESS

In recent years, mindfulness and meditation have become more than just buzzwords or a wellness fad. Research has confirmed the benefits from mindfulness practices that aid in reducing stress, increasing emotion regulation, enhancing ability to deal with illness, decreasing depressive symptoms, improving overall health, and alleviating stress among health care professionals (Burton et al., 2017). Even as little as three minutes a day can reduce stress among nurses (Owens et al., 2020).

Mindfulness is closely tied to improvements in focus, attention, and cognitive flexibility, enhancing mental balance and well-being (Moore and Malinowski, 2009). A powerful meta-analysis by Goldberg et al. (2021) examined the effects of mindfulness-based interventions (MBIs) in 336 randomized clinical trials with 30,483 participants. The researchers found that interventions based on mindfulness meditation have significant potential for multiple mental health conditions, including depression and depressive episodes. When mindfulness-based interventions were compared to those on a wait list for other treatments, MBIs were superior for adults, children/adolescents, and health care professionals in treating depression, smoking, substance use, and psychiatric conditions, and on measures of mindfulness, stress, and psychiatric symptoms.

(continued)

Findings from randomized clinical trials and meta-analyses of MBIs have influenced organizational policies as well as national and international guidelines. Mindfulness-based cognitive therapy (Segal et al., 2013) is incorporated into the United Kingdom's National Institute for Health Care Excellence 2009 guidelines for depression treatment and identified as an evidence-based treatment for depression, with strong research support by the American Psychological Association Society of Clinical Psychology (Goldberg et al., 2021).

References
Burton, A., Burgess, C., Dean, S., Koutsopoulou, G. Z., & Hugh-Jones, S. (2017). How effective are mindfulness-based interventions for reducing stress among healthcare professionals? A systematic review and meta-analysis. *Stress and Health* 33(1): 3–13.

Goldberg, S. B., Riordan, K. M., Sun, S., & Davidson, R. J. (2021). The empirical status of mindfulness-based interventions: a systematic review of 44 meta-analyses of randomized controlled trials. *Perspectives on Psychological Science* 17(1): 108–30. https://doi.org/10.1177/1745691620968771

Moore, A., & Malinowski, P. (2009). Meditation, mindfulness and cognitive flexibility. *Consciousness and Cognition* 18(1): 176–86.

Owens, R. A., Alfes, C., Evans, S., Wyka, K., & Fitzpatrick, J. J. (2020). An exploratory study of a 3-minute mindfulness intervention on compassion fatigue in nurses. *Holistic Nursing Practice* 34(5): 274–81.

Segal, Z. V., Williams, J. M. G., & Teasdale, J. D. (2013). *Mindfulness-Based Cognitive Therapy for Depression*, 2nd ed. New York: Guilford Press.

THE SCIENCE OF MEDITATION

According to estimates (Esch, 2021), there are now 200–500 million people worldwide who regularly meditate. The specific number of those who meditate in different countries is not known, although a survey by Clarke et al. (2018) of the Centers for Disease Control and Prevention found that 14% of the adult population in the United States meditates, and in Germany, a nationally representative survey (Cramer, 2019) found that 16 million people, or almost 20% of the population, are currently meditating or interested in starting. Research on mindfulness and meditation has also grown. Looking at the evolution of mindfulness and meditation in publications for more than

100 years, a team of researchers from Korea and Australia (Lee et al., 2021) found a sharp increase in mindfulness research since 2000, an area that has increased exponentially and is likely to continue to grow for some time.

Yoga, meditation, and chiropractic treatment are some of the most commonly used holistic approaches (Clarke et al., 2018). Between 2012 and 2017, the use of meditation, especially mindfulness meditation, increased more than threefold in the United States (Clarke et al., 2018). Sedlemeier et al. (2012) found that people begin and continue to meditate for a variety of reasons. Beginning meditators say they frequently use these practices to seek calm, collect inner strength, and reduce negative experiences in their lives. Those who have mastered meditation or have practiced for a long time use it for deeper spiritual growth.

Studies (Van Gordon et al., 2014; Bach and Guse, 2015) have found that meditation practices enhance psychological well-being and can complement other therapies. A large body of research confirms that acute or chronic stress can cause changes in the hippocampus and the prefrontal cortex, areas of the brain that regulate mood and emotion (McEwen et al., 2016). Physiological markers of stress include alterations in blood pressure and heart rate, as well as changes in cortisol or cytokine levels, which affect stress and inflammatory responses. A team of researchers from Australia, Denmark, and Sweden reviewed various studies on the psychobiological effects of meditation (Pascoe et al., 2020). The research findings confirmed that meditation decreases reactivity at psychological, physiological, and neurobiological levels, decreasing stress and improving mood (Pascoe et al., 2020), and that meditation can modify psychological responses as well. This illustrates the strong connection between the body and the mind, with meditation as the driving force for improved well-being.

References

Bach, J. M., & Guse, T. (2015). The effect of contemplation and meditation on "great compassion" on the psychological well-being of adolescents. *Journal of Positive Psychology* 10(4): 359–69.

Clarke, T. C., Barnes, P. M., Black, L. I., Stussman, B. J., & Nahin, R. L. (2018). *Use of Yoga, Meditation, and Chiropractors among US Adults Aged 18 and Over.* Washington, DC: US Department of Health and Human Services, Centers for Disease Control and Prevention, National Center for Health Statistics.

(continued)

Cramer, H. (2019). Meditation in Deutschland: eine national repräsentative Umfrage. *Journal of Complementary Medicine Research* 26(6): 382–89.

Esch, T. (2021). Meditation in complementary and integrative medicine: taxonomy of effects and methods. *Complementary Medicine Research* 28(3): 183–87.

Lee, J., Kim, K. H., Webster, C. S., & Henning, M. A. (2021). The evolution of mindfulness from 1916 to 2019. *Mindfulness* 12: 1849–59. https://doi.org/10.1007/s12671-021-01603-x

McEwen, B. S., Nasca, C., & Gray, J. D. (2016). Stress effects on neuronal structure: hippocampus, amygdala, and prefrontal cortex. *Neuropsychopharmacology* 41(1): 3–23.

Pascoe, M. C., Thompson, D. R., & Ski, C. F. (2020). Meditation and endocrine health and wellbeing. *Trends in Endocrinology and Metabolism* 31(7): 469–77.

Sedlmeier, P., Eberth, J., Schwartz, M., Zimmermann, D., Haarig, F., Jaeger, S., & Kunze, S. (2012). The psychological effects of meditation: a meta-analysis. *Psychological Bulletin* 138(6): 1139–71.

Van Gordon, W., Shonin, E., Zangeneh, M., & Griffiths, M. D. (2014). Can mindfulness really improve work-related mental health and job performance? *International Journal of Mental Health and Addiction* 12: 129–37.

Lippelt et al. (2014) divide meditation practice into three categories: controlled focus meditation, open monitoring meditation, and loving-kindness meditation. The first involves focusing attention on an external object or sound, as well as an internal one, a sensation such as breathing, or movements such as yoga exercises. In the second type of meditation, the meditator also has to monitor their concentration, and if the mind wanders from the object of concentration, return attention to the object. Another meditation category is loving-kindness meditation, often called Metta (Lippelt et al., 2014).

PREPARING FOR MEDITATION

Much like the importance of sanctuary, finding a safe space to meditate or practice mindfulness is essential to cultivating an environment conducive to well-being. This might look like rolling out a yoga mat and sitting cross-legged on a blanket, or maybe it's propping yourself upright with pillows while sitting on your couch. However you decide to practice, it is important to *choose to be*. Allow yourself to find presence in the moment in a relaxed yet alert position, breathe deeply, and begin to let go of anything that is no longer serving you.

GRATITUDE
•

One of the core principles of mindfulness is to bring awareness to the present moment, which is just what a gratitude practice requires. One of positive psychology's better-known discoveries is validating the benefits of gratitude, which is both an attitude and a practice. While the research is current and compelling, many religions and cultures have practiced the concept of "counting your blessings" for centuries. It's a simple and effective way to boost well-being and train your brain to see the good.

Zahn et al. (2009) found that experiencing gratitude and its related emotions activates areas in the mesolimbic and basal forebrain, which are linked with feelings of reward and social bonds (Macfarlane, 2020). Gratitude also boosts subjective well-being (McCullough et al., 2008). There are positive outcomes for both the expresser and the recipient of gratitude, and they are related to increased life satisfaction and well-being (Lyubomirsky et al., 2011). Starkey et al. (2019) studied 146 acute care registered nurses and found that when the nurses received expressions of gratitude at work, not only were they more satisfied with the care they provided, but they also had improved psychological well-being as well as better physical health.

Regularly practicing gratitude has also been linked to health and wellness. In one study of people with chronic pain, patients who practiced gratitude had a decrease in pain as well as improved and longer sleep (Emmons and McCullough, 2003). Further studies have linked simple gratitude practices to improving what well-being theorist and researcher Carol Ryff embraces as "eudaimonic well-being": the sense that one's life has meaning, and that a person is living their life to the fullest (Watkins, 2013).

Expressing Gratitude

Goal: To develop a stronger sense of well-being

Time and place: 5 to 10 minutes, a quiet space

Take a few moments to think about three positive events or experiences that have happened within the past 48 hours and record them below. Consider using a journal exclusively for this practice.

1. _____

2. _____

3. _____

GRATITUDE IS #NOTCANCELED

♦

Dzung Vo (2020), a pediatrician who studied with Thich Nhat Hanh, suggests a short gratitude practice to help reframe older or current concerns, such as wearing masks, isolation, and missing activities as a result of the pandemic. This meditation can be adapted for your post-pandemic life, especially if there are children to consider. Ever-changing school rules, emerging vaccinations, and new policies will influence how families will be affected. This practice also helps one cope with the ongoing demands of a busy professional and personal life—when work crowds out the people, places, and activities that give us joy and pleasure. By reframing these "absences" and focusing on what we do have, we allow ourselves to feel gratitude.

Do this exercise when you first wake up, at the end of the day, or while sitting at the dinner table with your family. First, reflect on a few of the activities and events that have been canceled now or in the past—school, sports, graduations, parties. Acknowledge the grief of missing those things. Now, think about what has not been canceled. Simply ask yourself, "What has not been canceled today?" There *are* activities in our daily lives that are still present, bringing joy and peace—the sunshine in the summer, a blue sky, walks in your neighborhood. Share your thoughts with your colleagues, family, and friends, or post on social media. We invite you to share what is #NotCanceled in your life.

Take a Gratitude Inventory

Goal: To recognize people, events, and objects that give us comfort
Time and place: 5–10 minutes, any place

What are the top three events or experiences that are #NotCanceled?

1._____

2._____

3._____

Adapted with permission from Dzung Vo, Kelty Mental Health Resource Centre and Provincial Health Services Authority, British Columbia, Canada

---

MINDFULNESS AND BREATHWORK
•

One of the simplest ways to tap into a mindful space is to pay attention to the breath. Tuning into our breath, or *pranayama* as the yogis call it, helps to regulate our autonomic nervous system and bring our bodies into a relaxed state. Learn more about the categories of breathwork and the science that supports it below.

If you are new to breathwork, you may want to begin with this breathing practice.

- First, take a slow, deep breath in through your nostrils, and allow your belly to fill with air.
- You can hold this for a moment or so, whatever is comfortable for you.
- Then, exhale this air through your mouth.
- Try doing this for one minute straight, and notice what sensations you feel in the body.

Once you are comfortable with simply breathing for one minute, consider doing a formal breathwork practice like the ones suggested below. Dr. Andrew Weil calls this next exercise a natural tranquilizer for the nervous system. You can use it whenever something upsetting occurs, whenever you are aware of internal tension, or to help you fall asleep.

PUTTING IT INTO PRACTICE

Andrew Weil's 4-7-8 Breath Exercise

Goal: To regulate your breathing and relaxation response

Time and place: 3–5 minutes, in a quiet place

Sit in a comfortable position, with your back straight. Place the tip of your tongue against the ridge of tissue just behind your upper front teeth, and keep it there through the entire exercise. Exhale through your mouth around your tongue; try pursing your lips slightly if this seems awkward.

Next, follow these steps:

- Exhale completely through your mouth, making a "whoosh sound."
- Close your mouth and inhale quietly through your nose to a mental count of 4.
- Now hold your breath for a count of 7.
- Then exhale completely through your mouth, making a whoosh sound to a count of 8. These first four steps constitute one breath.
- Inhale again, and repeat the cycle three more times, for a total of four breaths.

The sequence 4-7-8 is important; try to keep the same count each time. At the minimum, do this practice twice a day to find the benefits of the exercise.

Do not do more than four breaths at one time for the first month of practice. Once you become more comfortable, you can extend it to eight breaths.

You can use the 4-7-8 exercise at work or at home, when you wake, or on your lunch break. It can be done somewhat quickly but will help keep stress levels down and allow you to take a moment.

Try this exercise any time, although it may be particularly useful following times of intense stress—perhaps after a code, when the team needs to take a moment to gather themselves, during huddles pre-shift, or while in a midday huddle.

Visit the links in the Resources section to read a downloadable handout for Weil's 4-7-8 breathing practice, watch a video demonstrating box breathing, or, when you're taking time for yourself at home, try the mindfulness of breathing practice with Amishi Jha at Mindful.org.

Used with permission from Dr. Andrew Weil and the Weil Foundation.

THE SCIENCE OF BREATHWORK

Clinicians identify broad categories of breathwork, among them: deep relaxation breathing, mindfulness breathwork, and yogic breathing (Aideyan et al., 2020). Each style is distinct in setting, context, the way breathwork is applied, and in the respiratory patterns that users are instructed to practice.

Deep relaxation breathing, or diaphragmatic breathing, has been found to be an effective way to decrease anxiety and train your mind to relax by engaging your attention on your breath. Deep breathing (Ma et al., 2017) is an efficient breathwork technique used by clinicians and practitioners in numerous disciplines. During diaphragmatic breathing, the diaphragm is contracted, the belly expands, and there is a deepening of inhalation and exhalation. As a result of these actions, respiration frequency decreases, lowering anxiety and stress. Varvogli and Darviri (2011) place diaphragmatic breathing among the most evidence-based interventions that can improve sustained attention, affect, and cortisol levels. Other studies using brain imaging have suggested that deep breathing inhibits amygdala overactivity and deactivates the limbic system (Brown et al., 2013). Decreased respiratory rate and oxygen consumption, decreased heart rate, and lowered blood pressure have been documented in multiple studies (Yau and Loke, 2021).

Mindfulness breathing interventions emphasize a strong focus on mindfulness and an awareness of one's breathing and its associated

(continued)

sensations. These practices, often called the backbone of mindfulness-based interventions (e.g., mindfulness-based stress reduction), can induce an altered state of conscious attention. Formal mindfulness breathing practices are structured to focus on the landscape of attention: noticing when your mind wanders, reorienting attention back to the focus area of the sensations of breathing, cultivating uninterrupted attention, and learning how to be more accepting and less judgmental of your own thoughts, emotions, or body sensations (Creswell, 2017). Mindful breathing has been used with veterans, secondary school students, and even younger children. Mindful breathing has positive effects that last beyond the breathing practice itself. In one study, participants spent 10 minutes practicing mindful breathing (Mrazek et al., 2013). When performing tasks after the practice, they experienced reduced mind-wandering.

Yogic breathing is an essential practice in the study of yoga. Yogic breathing, or pranayama, is defined as the "control of life force" and is aimed at increasing vital energy in the body and mind. It involves controlling the breath with specific patterns and variations in rates of respiration (Brown et al., 2013). Because yogic practices stimulate the vagus nerve (Streeter et al., 2012), there is a ripple effect on the body and brain, increasing neurotransmitter levels in the brain that reduce anxiety.

References

Aideyan, B., Martin, G. C., & Beeson, E. T. (2020). A practitioner's guide to breathwork in clinical mental health counseling. *Journal of Mental Health Counseling* 42(1): 78–94.

Brown, R. P., Gerbarg, P. L., & Muench, F. (2013). Breathing practices for treatment of psychiatric and stress-related medical conditions. *Psychiatric Clinics of North America* 36(1): 121–40. https://doi.org/10.1016/j.psc.2013.01.001

Creswell, J. D. (2017). Mindfulness interventions. *Annual Review of Psychology* 68: 491–516.

Ma, X., Yue, Z. Q., Gong, Z. Q., Zhang, H., Duan, N. Y., Shi, Y. T., Wei, G.X., & Li, Y. F. (2017). The effect of diaphragmatic breathing on attention, negative affect and stress in healthy adults. *Frontiers in Psychology* 8: 874.

Mrazek, M. D., Franklin, M. S., Phillips, D. T., Baird, B., & Schooler, J. W. (2013). Mindfulness training improves working memory capacity and GRE performance while reducing mind wandering. *Psychological Science* 24: 776–81. http://dx.doi.org/10.1177/0956797612459659

Streeter, C. C., Gerbarg, P. L., Saper, R. B., Ciraulo, D. A., & Brown, R. P. (2012). Effects of yoga on the autonomic nervous system, gamma-aminobutyric-acid, and allostasis in epilepsy, depression, and post-traumatic stress disorder. *Medical Hypotheses* 78(5): 571–79.

Varvogli, L., & Darviri, C. (2011). Stress management techniques: evidence-based procedures that reduce stress and promote health. *Health Science Journal* 5(2): 74.

Yau, K. K. Y., & Loke, A. Y. (2021). Effects of diaphragmatic deep breathing exercises on prehypertensive or hypertensive adults: a literature review. *Complementary Therapies in Clinical Practice* 43: 101315.

LOVING-KINDNESS MINDFULNESS MEDITATION

◆

Loving-kindness, or Metta, meditation is based in Buddhist tradition and has been touted in the present day as a "radical act of love." Similar to all forms of meditation, it is a practice that allows us to go within while at the same time bringing awareness and cultivating kindness and compassion toward the outside world. Research by Kok et al. (2013) and Fredrickson et al. (2017) has shown that with consistent practice, loving-kindness meditation can increase positive emotions, enhance connectedness, and lead to more positive and satisfying social interactions.

In its simplest form, loving-kindness is the repetition of personally meaningful phrases. Depending on your spiritual and religious background, this practice may be reminiscent of prayer. In loving-kindness, however, these personally meaningful phrases are wishes chosen by you to give to yourself and others. If you are new to loving-kindness meditation, the following phrases may be a promising start:

> May you be happy
> May you be healthy
> May you be safe
> May you be able to live in this world,
> peacefully, joyfully, and with ease

During the meditation, you repeat these phrases to yourself several times, pausing to notice what sensations arise within. Then, slowly and intentionally, you begin to wish them for others, being as general or specific as you would like.

_____

My journey as a nurse began in 2017, on a telemetry unit. In January 2020, I transitioned to the ICU, and completed my orientation in March 2020. I was so excited for this next chapter of my nursing career.

I started on the night shift in ICU, just as the pandemic was breaking. That was one of many challenges I was about to endure. I work in a 16-bed ICU that quickly turned into a full-blown COVID ICU by the end of March.

On April 5, 2020, I took care of an intubated patient. He was awake and alert; he was breathing on the ventilator in hopes that he would soon be extubated. I began my shift at 19:00, gathered and donned my PPE, and entered room 214. I introduced myself to my patient and began my routine assessment. Although he was intubated, I could tell he was trying to mouth something to me, which is not unexpected. He then began to try to spell it out, on the bed railing. On a normal night, this would be a simple fix, and I would give my patient a pen and a clipboard with a piece of paper so they could try to write out what they wanted to say, but I couldn't. I was in a COVID isolation room, and once you enter an isolation room, you don't leave. I looked around the room and found an IV butterfly needle package and a marker we use to write on our whiteboards. The only thing he wrote on the package was "casa." My heart immediately sank. I felt helpless. I assured him we were doing everything we could to make sure he got back home. That was all he wanted. This took place at a time where being a nurse during a pandemic wasn't understood by many. No one was taking the world's current situation seriously; my peers were still posting pictures on social media of them out and about, with groups of people. I decompressed with coworkers after I left my patient's room. We cheered the patient on throughout the night, encouraging him while he was on pressure support. It gave us hope.

Something changed for me on that drive home at 8:00 the next morning. I reflected on the night I had—unsure of how to relieve the doubts I had, and how helpless I felt at times, being in this profession.

I began to browse Spotify once I got home, flipping through multiple podcasts, searching for an answer. I finally came across one that made me feel some sort of relief. *Yoga Girl Daily*. I scrolled through and went to sleep.

I listened to my first *Yoga Girl Daily* podcast on April 7th, 2021. "I avoid feeling my feelings by . . ." was the title of the episode. Some of the highlights of this podcast were finding ways to process our feelings and acknowledging that we are doing the best that we can. This became my daily outlet. My access to self-healing. I got in my car each day and looked forward to each new podcast. A quote from *Yoga Girl Daily* that has stuck with me is, "The light you are seeking is within your own heart." There is a weekly intention every Monday, which allows you to check in with yourself and your needs. This encouraged me every week and helped create a path that I had longed for. I hope this resonates with other nurses and gives them assurance that there is some sort of outlet out there for everyone.

April 5, 2020: Brittni Palmer, BSN, RN, CCRN, NVRN-BC, Cardiac Care Unit / Cardiothoracic Intensive Care Unit, Paterson, New Jersey, United States

The nurse storyteller above found her way to meditating and continued to embrace intentions each day, creating a path to self-healing, one that she had been seeking for months. You can begin by practicing a loving-kindness meditation such as the one described below. To get started, go to some of the online videos below to help you become familiar with the words and rhythm of the meditation.

PUTTING IT INTO PRACTICE

A Loving-Kindness Meditation from Dzung Vo

Goal: To increase positive emotions and social connections

Time and place: 7–10 minutes, in a quiet space

This is a very old practice; it is called loving-kindness meditation. I'd like to invite everyone to find a comfortable position, wherever you

(continued)

are. It could be sitting, it could be standing, it could be lying down. You can have your eyes open; you can have your eyes closed.

I'm going to invite one sound of this meditation bell (or chime); this sound is an invitation from our friend to just be here right now. So, you can imagine that your best friend is here when you hear the bell. And the bell is just saying, "Hey, be here, right now."

[Bell]
There's nowhere else to go, there's nothing else to do.
Being here just as you are—is good enough.
There's nothing to prove.
Connecting with our breathing, knowing what it feels like to
    breathe.
Breathing in, I know that I'm breathing in.
Breathing out, I know that I'm breathing out.
In.
Out.
And now bringing to mind the image of someone you have warm
    feelings for,
Who it's easy to feel connected to,
So, this may be your child, but maybe it won't be.
Maybe it will be a pet, a friend, or a partner.
Maybe it will be a trusted colleague at work.
An ocean, a river, or a mountain.
Bringing this being to mind, the one you feel easily connected to.
You feel warmly. Seeing them in your mind's eye,
And inviting a wish of kindness.
Inviting this intention,
May you be well,
May you be at peace,
May you be at ease with any pain,
May you be well,
May you be at peace,
May you be at ease with any pain.
Just inviting that intention without forcing anything, simply asking if
    the heart is able to open right now.
Not expecting anything.
Not forcing anything.

Just inviting.

Just noticing.

[pause]

And then bringing to mind the image of the two of you together,

Your beloved person or being or place and yourself, next to each
    other, maybe holding hands. And inviting that same wish.

May we be well, together,

May we be at peace,

May we be at ease with any pain,

May we be well, may we be at peace,

May we be at ease with any pain.

Just noticing what happens, breathing in and out, inviting the hearts
    to open without forcing anything—just be curious.

And finally bringing the picture to mind of yourself letting the image
    of the beloved one fade away.

Holding your own image in your mind, considering that you deserve
    to be loved just as much as you love this being.

You deserve it just as much, no more, no less, and offering this same
    wish to yourself, May I be well, may I be at peace, may I be at
    ease with any pain.

Breathing with that.

We hear one sound of the bell to end.

Opening your eyes if they were closed,

Bringing your attention back to this room and community.

[Ring Bell]

This practice was adapted by Dzung Vo from Karen Bluth's interpretation of
the mindful self-compassion practice by Kristin Neff and Chris Germer, with
permission from Dzung Vo and the Dalai Lama Center, Vancouver, British
Columbia, Canada.

And there's more: Depending on the time you have available, you
can practice loving-kindness meditations using these videos on You-
Tube; links are listed in the Resources section at the end of the book.

Loving-Kindness Meditation with Dr. Dzung Vo (7 minutes)

University of New Hampshire Loving-Kindness Meditation
    (13 minutes)

Mindful Movement Loving-Kindness Meditation (25 minutes)
Loving-Kindness Meditation with Sharon Salzberg (45 minutes)

Choose the one that works best for you.

BECOMING GROUNDED

•

5-4-3-2-1. In times of panic and uncertainty, our minds can spiral out into worlds unknown and leave us feeling far from the present moment. If you've been to a yoga class or have any experience with mindfulness, you've likely heard of feeling grounded. This term means to find stability in being fully present, while mindfully engaging your awareness to get back into the moment and quiet your unsettled and thought-filled mind. Buddhists refer to this as your "monkey mind."

Grounding strategies and tools allow you to self-regulate in the face of sudden emotional distress. Grounding refocuses you in your present reality and diverts you from the anxious, chaotic negative thoughts that may spiral out of control. In other words, these are the tools you can have on hand and use, any time or any place. When you find one that works for you, make it your go-to skill.

Grounding strategies can take the form of an external distraction, such as smelling flowers, holding an object, or listening to music or even the hum of traffic. You can use visualization techniques or the sensory diffusers of physical or somatic experiences, such as clenching a fist and then letting go, visualizing turning down an "emotional dial," seeing your safe place, or as Kristin Neff suggests, imaging a cup of steaming tea waiting for you.

Take slow deep breaths, and remember that you are in a safe place in the present moment.

In the next simple mindfulness technique, awareness of the five senses allows us to focus our attention on the present, leading to a sensation of groundedness. This exercise is widely known for its ability to honor our mind-body connection, and it is often prescribed by mental health professionals to those experiencing anxiety and overwhelming experiences. Upon completing this exercise, you will feel the benefits yourself and will be able to use this tool whenever you need to calm your mind and become grounded.

The technique below uses the five senses in an easy to remember format. Give it a try. Look around you and ...

- *Search for five things you can see:* colors, objects, food, furnishings, or architectural characteristics of a room.
- *Search for four things you can touch:* your glasses, your shoes, your scrubs, the chair you're sitting on, the pen in your hand. Now focus on the sensation, the feeling of that object. Is it a light touch or intense? Does that sensation change over time?
- *Search for three things you can hear:* Pay attention to the sounds around you—traffic sounds, whispered conversations, whirring machines, voices singing, or instruments. Focus on any three of these sounds and hold your attention on them; fully accept and respect them.
- *Search for two things you can smell:* Identify two unique, unusual, or strong smells around you. Smells are known to trigger memories that are experienced during highly emotional events because the olfactory center in the brain is so close to the amygdala, the emotional bellwether. As a result, they can be paired in your memory. Try hunting for the smell of the outdoors or indoor plants and flowers. When this isn't possible, notice your own smell: the soap or shampoo you used in the shower, or the lotion you apply after you wash your hands. If necessary, move to a location where you can smell something pleasant.
- *Search for one thing you can taste:* Finding something you can taste while experiencing an intense emotional moment is difficult. If you have gum or hard candy in your pocket, place it in your mouth and move it around, under and over your tongue. Or take a small bite of something sweet; hold it in your mouth, and taste it mindfully. Notice how the food feels in your mouth. Soft and sticky, or crunchy and hard. Going forward, keep individually wrapped candies or dried fruit in your pocket. We have a wonderful chocolate meditation in chapter 5 if you want to practice this exercise with chocolate.

Finally, as we mentioned in chapter 2, grounding practices can be used whenever and wherever you might need them. The practice below is adapted from Kristin Neff at the Mindful Healthcare Summit.

Grounding and Planting

Goal: To boost psychological and physical support, especially during stressful situations

Time and place: 1–2 minutes, any place, at work or at home

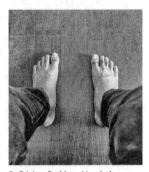

By Srinivas Reddy on Unsplash

1. Place both feet (in shoes or barefoot) uncrossed on the ground.
2. Simply feel the soles of your feet in your shoe or on the floor.
3. Direct all of your awareness to your feet.
4. Notice how the heel and sole of both feet make contact with the inside of your shoe or the floor.
5. Plant your feet, and imagine roots reaching through your shoe, the floor, and into the earth.
6. Now try to feel the ground underneath your shoes.
7. Press one foot firmly onto the ground, then the other, engaging your thighs and buttocks, then press both feet onto the floor at the same time.
8. Sense the effect on your spine and the rest of your body.
9. Keep doing this until you feel the connection with the ground. It may take as little as one minute.

Kristin Neff emphasizes the effectiveness of this particular grounding technique. It helps reduce the amygdala reactivity—partly because your attention is as far away from your brain as possible. So, ground your awareness in your feet. You can do this anywhere, any time. Just focus for a few moments on the feeling of connection between your feet to the floor.

And if you feel overwhelmed by difficult emotions, the most self-compassionate response may be to pull back temporarily—focus on your breath, the sensation of the soles of your feet on the ground. You can even think about ordinary, behavioral acts of calm, such as having a cup of tea or petting a puppy or kitten.

To conclude this chapter, we'd like to leave you with Dzung Vo's (2020) five suggestions for health care professionals, the people who struggled to cope with the pandemic in their personal and professional lives, and who continue to struggle today. These suggestions may be helpful in the many circumstances faced by nurses, in all kinds of settings.

1. *Stay in the present moment.* When uncertainty is a given, a simple way of coming back to the present is by using your breathing as an anchor.

2. *Show gratitude.* It's important to acknowledge and accept the loss of predictability and normalcy, and sadness of what has been changed or canceled during this time. See the gratitude inventory and practice earlier in this chapter.

3. *Do a walking meditation.* Walking has a powerful effect on us physically and emotionally, and it is deeply rewarding to spend some time outside. Noticing the world around you lets you "get out of your head."

4. *Be mindful of media consumption.* Although you may want to stay current on the changes happening in the world, in your community, and in the realm of health care, it is also important to know when you are taking in too much. Balance is the key. This is especially important for those of you with families. Children absorb not only the tone and information from the media messages, but also adult reactions to media reports.

5. *Practice daily formal meditation.* During uncertain, unpredictable, and stressful times, maintaining a daily routine is helpful. It can be a daily formal meditation practice, such as the ones you've seen in this chapter. Maybe you will begin your day with a practice, or do it after work, or maybe at the end of the day before you sleep. It is time to "just be."

Finally, remember to stay kind, calm, and safe. Please take good care of yourselves and each other during uncertain and challenging times.

Note: These five tips are presented here with permission from Dzung Vo, Kelty Mental Health, BC Children's Hospital Centre for Mindfulness, and the Provincial Health Services Authority, Vancouver, British Columbia, Canada.

REFERENCES

Behan, C. (2020). The benefits of meditation and mindfulness practices during times of crisis such as COVID-19. *Irish Journal of Psychological Medicine* 37(4): 256–58.

Cardoso, R., de Souza, E., Camano, L., & Leite, J. R. (2004). Meditation in health: an operational definition. *Brain Research Protocols* 14(1): 58–60.

Emmons, R. A., & McCullough, M. E. (2003). Counting blessings versus burdens: an experimental investigation of gratitude and subjective well-being in daily life. *Journal of Personality and Social Psychology* 84(2): 377–89.

Fredrickson, B. L., Boulton, A. J., Firestine, A. M., Van Cappellen, P., Algoe, S. B., Brantley, M. M., & Salzberg, S. (2017). Positive emotion correlates of meditation practice: a comparison of mindfulness meditation and loving-kindness meditation. *Mindfulness* 8(6): 1623–33.

Kabat-Zinn, J. (2013). *Full Catastrophe Living: Using the Wisdom of Your Body and Mind to Face Stress, Pain and Illness.* New York: Penguin Random House.

Kok, B. E., Coffey, K. A., Cohn, M. A., Catalino, L. I., Vacharkulksemsuk, T., Algoe, S. B., Brantley, M., & Fredrickson, B. L. (2013). How positive emotions build physical health: perceived positive social connections account for the upward spiral between positive emotions and vagal tone. *Psychological Science* 24(7): 1123–32.

Lippelt, D. P., Hommel, B., & Colzato, L. S. (2014). Focused attention, open monitoring and loving kindness meditation: effects on attention, conflict monitoring, and creativity—A review. *Frontiers in Psychology* 5(5): 1–5. https://doi.10.3389/fpsyg.2014.01083

Lyubomirsky, S., Dickerhoof, R., Boehm, J. K., & Sheldon, K. M. (2011). Becoming happier takes both a will and a proper way: an experimental longitudinal intervention to boost well-being. *Emotion* 11(2): 391–402.

Macfarlane, J. (2020). Positive psychology: gratitude and its role within mental health nursing. *British Journal of Mental Health Nursing* 9(1): 19–30.

McCullough, M. E., Kimeldorf, M. B., & Cohen, A. D. (2008). An adaptation for altruism? The social causes, social effects, and social evolution of gratitude. *Current Directions in Psychological Science* 17(4): 281–85.

Starkey, A. R., Mohr, C. D., Cadiz, D. M., & Sinclair, R. R. (2019). Gratitude reception and physical health: examining the mediating role of satisfaction with patient care in a sample of acute care nurses. *Journal of Positive Psychology* 14(6): 779–88.

Vo, D. (2020). Top 5 mindfulness tips for health care professionals during the COVID-19 pandemic. Kelty Mental Health Resource Centre, BC Children's Hospital, March 26, 2020. https://keltymentalhealth.ca/blog/2020/03/top-5-mindfulness-tips-health-care-professionals-during-covid-19-pandemic

Watkins, P. C. (2013). Gratitude interventions that have been shown to enhance well-being. In: *Gratitude and the Good Life: Toward a Psychology of Appreciation.* New York: Springer Science and Business Media, 225–30.

Zahn, R., Moll, J., Paiva, M., Garrido, G., Krueger, F., Huey, E. D., & Grafman, J. (2009). The neural basis of human social values: evidence from functional MRI. *Cerebral Cortex* 19(2): 276–83. https://doi.org/10.1093/cercor/bhn080

CHAPTER 4

•

Sleeping Well

*"The first good night's sleep was because I was out
on a tropical island far away from work."*

IN THEIR OWN WORDS

November rolled around; it was the second wave, and I was tired. There was no work-life balance, and I was just trying to survive. I gave up two vacation rounds to ensure that I would not fall too far behind with my work. The second wave eased up around February of 2021. I finally got my vacation booked for my 30th birthday. That was the time that I finally got to think and reevaluate what I was doing with my life. I was constantly being woken up for staffing challenges, issues to follow up on in the morning, or just general questions. This was a constant cycle from March of 2020 to April of 2021. For nearly a whole year, I was not getting any rest. The first good night's sleep was because I was out on a tropical island far away from work. I knew if this was going to continue once I arrived back, I would eventually get burnt out.

March 2020 to April 2021: Fredrick P. Apostadero, MSN, RN,
Resource Nurse, Coronary Care, Surgical, and Trauma
Intensive Care Units, Hackensack, New Jersey, United States

SLEEP AND WELL-BEING

•

Sleep is a crucial pillar of our well-being and longevity. When we don't get enough sleep, we feel it in every aspect of our lives—physically and emotionally. Our sleep and wake schedules are determined by the circadian rhythms that keep our bodies in sync with the environment. This complex body clock guides mental, physical, and behavioral changes every 24 hours. It is essential to follow these natural cues in order to maintain physical, mental, and emotional health. Ideally, the average adult (18–60 years old) should be getting at least seven hours of restful sleep, with the preferred range being seven to nine hours, according to the Centers for Disease Control and Prevention (CDC, 2017). It doesn't take much to disrupt our sleep—night shifts, irregular work schedules, and jet lag (Pang, 2016). A recent study revealed that on average, American nurses sleep just under seven hours per night (Stimpfel et al., 2020), especially on nights before workdays. While this difference may not seem significant, leading to a few extra yawns throughout the day, over time, this lack of sleep can be detrimental to your health and well-being.

Most people would agree that a good night's sleep is one of life's greatest pleasures, but getting that blissful rest can be hard to achieve. With this knowledge in mind, it's important to distinguish that even "good sleepers" can struggle with sleep deficiency. Sleep deficiency is a broader concept than sleep deprivation (not enough sleep), and it includes sleeping irregular hours (outside of circadian rhythms), not sleeping well or soundly (skipping cycles of sleep), and having a sleep disorder that affects sleep quality (National Heart, Lung, and Blood Institute, 2022). Considering the nature of nursing, with 12-hour-long shifts being the norm, most nurses likely fall into the category of being sleep deficient. According to the National Heart, Lung, and Blood Institute (2022), inadequate sleep, over time, has been linked to many chronic health problems, including heart disease, kidney disease, high blood pressure, diabetes, stroke, obesity, and depression. Sleep deficiency is also associated with an increased risk of injury in adults, which has led to tragic accidents at work, home, and on the road (National Heart, Lung, and Blood Institute, 2022).

Nurses and health care professionals often have hurdles to overcome when it comes to sleep, whether it is adjusting to night shifts or struggling to unwind after a chaotic day. Research findings from a New York University study (Stimpfel et al., 2020) revealed that nurses who have inadequate sleep may suffer deleterious effects in their performance at work and negative impacts on their health. Nursing is serious work that requires great skill, compassion, and attention to detail. Without adequate sleep, nurses cannot show up as their best selves for their families, colleagues, or their patients, and they risk negatively affecting their own health in the long run.

Unfortunately, we've heard from many stressed-out and busy nurses that sleep is on the bottom of their to-do list. Between their work lives, family and friends, and other obligations such as schooling, it might seem like getting the recommended seven to nine hours of sleep is a fantasy in itself. Add a pandemic on top of those stressors, and good sleep is nearly impossible. Myriad clinicians practicing across the health care spectrum experience sleep problems, anxiety, and stress, even under the best of circumstances.

The public health threat of the pandemic brought sleep problems into sharper focus. Many nurses were worried about caring for critically ill patients, or not knowing who tested positive for COVID-19, but many more feared bringing the virus home to their loved ones. One study by Jahrami et al. (2021) specifically evaluated the pandemic's impact on the lives of frontline workers. The findings confirmed that 75% of health care workers had poor sleep quality, and 84% had moderate to severe stress. Poor sleep quality, stress, and mental health problems among health care professionals could impair their cognitive abilities and their clinical decision-making.

Many nurses may find themselves looking for shortcuts to stave off sleepiness, adding coffee and other caffeinated drinks during their shifts to stay alert. While they may be quick fixes to beat drowsiness, they are not sustainable solutions.

A study that examined the relationship between Carol Ryff's model of psychological well-being and sleep behaviors found that women who reported higher levels of eudaimonic well-being (all dimensions except autonomy) had lower levels of disrupted sleep (Ryff, 2017). Mastery of one's environment and autonomy are two of Ryff's key elements of well-being that relate to sleep. Without a comfortable place to rest your head, a good night's sleep is nearly impossible to attain.

As we discuss later in this chapter, achieving quality sleep begins with what we do in our waking lives. Consider the impact of the foods we eat, the drinks we choose (alcohol and caffeine, anyone?), our physical activity, stress levels, and even screen time. In short, for many of us, how we choose to spend our days affects how our nights go. Nights filled with sleepless tossing and turning often lead to less-than-good days. Considering the importance of autonomy in achieving optimal well-being, restful sleep is necessary. In this chapter, we share science-backed ways to get a good night's rest while considering environmental impacts (i.e., family life) and structural systems (i.e., workplace management) that affect sleep so that you can achieve environmental mastery and autonomy to promote your well-being.

Disclaimer: The evidence-based sleep strategies and solutions in this chapter are not intended to replace guidance from your primary care provider (PCP) and/or medical team. Sleep disorders are serious conditions; please speak with your PCP if you are struggling with sleep on a regular basis, as it may be due to an underlying medical condition.

Before we talk about sleep strategies, let's explore some of the most important work done in the field, by Michael Grandner at the Behavioral Sleep Medicine Clinic at the University of Arizona, and his Social-Ecological Model of Sleep.

THE SCIENCE OF SLEEP

First, let's get to the science of why sleep is important. Sleep has a major impact on health and well-being. With the sleep industry forecasted to be worth $585 billion by 2024 (van Gelder, 2021), sleep "solutions" are appearing everywhere, from bedtime products you can purchase to apps you can download on your smartphone. While some people might be thrilled to see so many options, the choices can also be daunting and can lead to a classic case of "analysis paralysis." So, we've done the work for you and have found sleep solutions that are both accessible and based on evidence to save you time, money, and hours of sleeplessness all at once.

As a consumer, you can buy and try out all the white noise machines and cooling eye masks money can buy and still find yourself lying wide awake, counting sheep each night. That's because the process of attaining quality sleep doesn't start when our head hits the pillow, it actually begins when we are awake. Factors of our waking lives, such as how much activity we do daily, what we consume, our work hours, and screen time all affect sleep. Following a regimented schedule and having a healthy lifestyle is the ideal way to attain good-quality sleep on a regular basis.

While behavioral factors influence sleep, what we consciously do throughout the day is just one part of the equation. Dr. Michael Grandner, a psychologist and researcher at the University of Arizona Sleep and Research Program, developed the Social-Ecological Model of Sleep, which identifies the symbiotic relationship of sleep, health, and society (Grandner, 2017). This model illustrates that sleep is affected not only by what we do behaviorally but also by the systems and communities of which we are a part. The model consists of three overlapping levels.

At the societal level, sleep is influenced by factors such as technology, public policy, geography, and the environment. At a social level, home and work lives affect sleep along with factors such as the neighborhoods we live in, socioeconomic status, and our identity (race/ethnicity, religion, etc.). Finally, on the individual level, personal factors such as genetics, health, and behavior impact how well (or how poorly) one can expect to sleep (Grandner, 2017).

The Social-Ecological Model of Sleep illustrates how interconnected sleep is to our daily lives, acknowledging that the factors of a good night's rest are multifaceted. It also suggests that solutions to poor quality of sleep are not cured with a "one-size-fits-all" approach; instead, a restless sleeper may need to consider multiple methods and practices to achieve a good night's rest on a regular basis. Understanding the ways in which these levels overlap and identifying them in our own lives allows for greater awareness of what factors are in our control.

References

Grandner, M. A. (2017). Sleep, health, and society. *Sleep Medicine Clinics* 12(1): 1–22. https://doi.org/10.1016/j.jsmc.2016.10.012

van Gelder, K. (2021). Size of the sleep economy worldwide from 2019 to 2024. Statista. May 17, 2021. https://www.statista.com/statistics/1119471/size-of-the-sleep-economy-worldwide/

As we read about Grandner's work, the Hans Christian Andersen fairy tale "The Princess and the Pea" came to mind. Jo Byrne at See Your Words drew a lively interpretation of Grandner's theory, which appears below. The Social-Ecological Model of Sleep suggests that everyone is sensitive to sleep disruptions and interruptions from a variety of sources. No matter how deeply buried those factors might be, they can still affect our sleep.

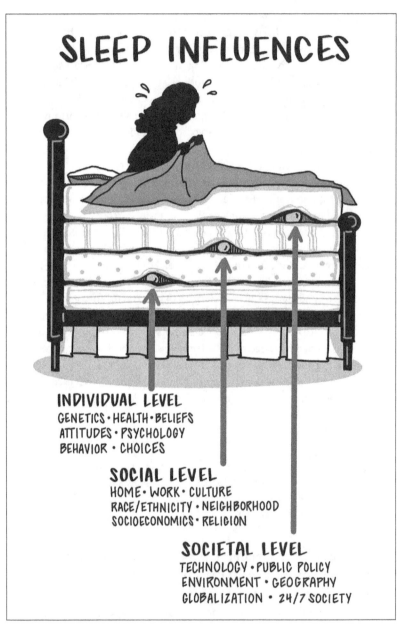

Nurses constitute one of the largest groups of the population affected by shift work. Across professions, shift work is associated with impaired alertness and performance owing to sleep loss and circadian misalignment, to which nurses and health care workers are particularly vulnerable (Ganesan et al., 2019). Researchers studying the impact of shift work on intensive care health care workers found that, compared to their performance during a day shift, workers who work subsequent night shifts had impaired outcomes of subjective sleepiness and psycho-motor vigilance test measures, based on shift time and sleep duration. This study's most noteworthy finding illustrates that although health care workers perceive themselves to be less alert on the first night shift compared to subsequent night shifts, objective performance is equally impaired on subsequent nights. While health care workers may believe they are adjusting to their night shift schedule each subsequent night, they actually aren't, and their performance at work may be affected. This finding raises concerns for the well-being of nurses, their colleagues, and their patients, potentially putting all parties at risk because of errors or oversights that may be made as a result of a lack of sleep.

PROVEN SLEEP STRATEGIES
◆

Now that we know the importance of adequate sleep on health and well-being, you might be asking yourself, "How can I possibly achieve that?" In this section, we will provide you with effective sleep strategies that can help you to wind down and prepare for a good night's sleep. As noted above, awareness and intention are crucial components to sleeping well. This means taking inventory of what factors are impairing your sleep; considering societal, social, and individual levels; and acknowledging what is in your control.

Our first recommendation for anyone is to establish a bedtime routine to get into the habit of utilizing these science-backed strategies on a regular basis and priming your body for rest. This routine can be as simple as turning off the television, computer, or phone an hour before bed and grabbing a book to read until your eyes are tired, but if that isn't enough to have you catching ZZZs, there's more that can be done. The sleep tools listed below include strategies and solutions that are science-backed alternatives to traditional sleep aids and prescriptions. These are not meant to replace prescriptions or medical advice; rather, they work best as a first-line defense to calm a restless sleeper and oftentimes can be used to complement any sleep aids that are used under the guidance of a medical professional. The science-backed sleep strategies listed below can be used by nearly anyone, with exceptions for allergies and age-restricted products, to create an effective bedtime routine that can help prepare you for a restful slumber.

Sleep Hygiene

The word "hygiene" may bring you back to squirming in your chair in grade-school health classes, but it so well encapsulates the importance of quality sleep. Hygiene is defined in the *Oxford English Dictionary* as "conditions or practices conducive to maintaining health and preventing disease, especially through cleanliness." Good sleep starts well before your head hits the pillow, and in many ways, your entire day prepares you for what kind of rest you will receive that night, whether you're aware of it or not. Everything you consume, be it food or beverages— especially alcohol and caffeine—affects your body and your ability to sleep soundly. So, if you want to set yourself up for success, consider these tips from the Sleep Foundation (Suni and Vyas, 2022), graphically represented by longtime sleep enthusiast Ethan Green (2022).

Controlled light exposure has been used successfully to treat sleep disorders associated with circadian system dysfunction. Zee and Goldstein (2010) report that to reduce circadian alignment disorders caused by night shift work, workers should get exposure to intense light during the night shift. In contrast, they recommended avoiding intense light in the final phase of the night shift until arriving at the house to sleep.

Aromatherapy and Essential Oils

Within the past few decades, the study of aromatherapy has grown from the botanical sciences to mainstream literature. In recent years, Eastern cultures have embraced essential oils as a healthier alternative to synthetic fragrances, and they appear in many household products, from laundry detergent to hand soap and lotions. One of the reasons essential oils are so revered is because of their almost immediate effect on the olfactory system. With a quick whiff, our bodies react to the

HEALTHY SLEEP HABITS

Improve your sleep with some positive lifestyle changes and consistent sleep habits

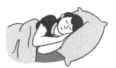

REGULAR SLEEP SCHEDULE
Try to maintain a consistent sleep pattern 7 days a week. Getting up at the same time every day can help.

RELAXING BEDTIME ROUTINE
Spend time before bed relaxing: read a book, stretch, do yoga, meditate, have a bath. Avoid difficult conversations, activities, or work.

AVOID STIMULANTS
Try not to consume caffeine or sugar in the evening. Avoid nicotine before bed. Only drink alcohol in moderation at night, if at all.

GOOD SLEEP ENVIRONMENT
Keep your bedroom clean and comfortable. Use a quality mattress and bedding. Keep the bedroom aired and between 60°F and 70°F.

BLOCK OUT NOISE AND LIGHT
Make sure the bedroom is dark and quiet. Use blackout curtains or a sleep mask. Use earplugs, white noise, or music to mask external noise.

EXERCISE AND DAYLIGHT
Try to do regular exercise, but not too intense, before bedtime. Even a short walk during the day can improve your sleep.

ONLY SLEEP AND INTIMACY
Only use the bed for sleep and intimacy. Avoid watching TV or using other devices in bed. That will help associate the bed with sleep.

EAT WELL
Try to eat a healthy diet. Avoid heavy, fatty, fried, or spicy food late in the evening if you get indigestion. Bananas, yogurt, or healthy cereal are good bedtime snacks.

Johnine Byrne, SeeYourWords.com, adapted from Ethan Green at No Sleepless Nights, with permission

scents we experience. When essential oils are used for a purpose or therapeutic effect (such as calming), it is considered to be aromatherapy. In studies of the therapeutic benefits of essential oils, lavender has been most frequently studied and found to be an effective, sweet-smelling natural sleep remedy.

THE SCIENCE OF ESSENTIAL OILS

Studies surrounding the use of essential oils for health benefits have been mixed, and there's not enough research to support evidence that human health is significantly improved by their usage. With regard to sleep, several notable studies found that using essential oils was beneficial for those experiencing mild sleep disturbances, with lavender oil being used most frequently (Lillehei and Halcon, 2014). In a study with elderly patients with dementia and sleep disturbances, essential oils were also found to be effective to promote sleep (Takeda et al., 2017).

References

Lillehei, A. S., & Halcon, L. L. (2014). A systematic review of the effect of inhaled essential oils on sleep. *Journal of Alternative and Complementary Medicine* 20(6): 441–51. https://doi.org/10.1089/acm.2013.0311

Takeda, A., Watanuki, E., & Koyama, S. (2017). Effects of inhalation aromatherapy on symptoms of sleep disturbance in the elderly with dementia. *Evidence-Based Complementary and Alternative Medicine* 2017: 1902807. https://doi.org/10.1155/2017/1902807

PUTTING IT INTO PRACTICE

Essential Oils

Goal: To learn how to use essential oils

Time and place: Any time, on the go, at home, or at work

- Essential Oil Diffusers
  - Essential oil diffusers typically use filtered water and any oil of your choosing to create a mist-like stream of air that allows the scent to fill the room. Diffusers are a great option to have at home or even at work in a break room, private office, or nurses station.
  - You can find good-quality diffusers online or at local health food stores, with price tags ranging from affordable to expensive, depending on the model.

> ► Essential Oil Roller Bottles
>   • Similar to perfume roller bottles, these are filled with either one essential oil or a blend of oils that is diluted with a carrier oil that is ready for topical use. Try rolling the oil onto your wrists, temples, behind your ears, or at the bottom of your feet.
>   • When using roller balls, take a few moments to breathe deeply and inhale the scent, allowing your body to fully appreciate this loving practice.
>   • You can find essential oil roller bottles at health food stores, local vendors, or online.

Herbal Tea

Drinking tea is commonly considered to be a therapeutic act in itself—brewing the hot water, letting the leaves steep in your favorite mug, and finally enjoying a warm sip. Its ritualistic origins date back to sixteenth-century Japanese tea ceremonies, which used green tea matcha and a highly skilled process involving the use of ceramic utensils. You can see artifacts and read more about this centuries-old tradition on the websites of the Metropolitan Museum of Art in New York City (Willmann, 2011) and the Genchō-an Tearoom in the Suntory Museum of Art in Tokyo, Japan.

Making tea does not need to include the traditional ceremony found in Japan, but the process of boiling water, steeping the herbs and leaves, and waiting for the tea to cool does allow for a calming nighttime ritual. Selecting an herbal tea or comparable cozy beverage that does not contain caffeine or added sugar can be the conduit to a good night's rest. Herbal teas do not come from the *Camellia sinensis* plant but from an infusion of leaves, roots, bark, seeds, or flowers from other plants. Examples of herbal tea infusions are peppermint, linden, chamomile, lemon balm, lemon pike, rosemary, sage, thyme, olive leaf, jasmine, rooibos, ginger, lemon peel, and orange. They are all caffeine-free.

Chamomile is derived from a floral plant found within the daisy family, and it is considered one of the oldest and most documented plants used for medicinal and healing purposes. As a tea, chamomile provides a calming sensation, and most people find it to be a palatable flavor that is light, earthy, and similar to its scent. Teas and infusions can interact with some medications and decrease the absorption of certain nutrients, so consumption must follow the indications and take into account possible adverse effects.

THE SCIENCE OF CHAMOMILE

While caffeine has been found to disrupt sleep, certain herbal teas have the opposite effect and could act as a beneficial sleep aid. Chamomile has been studied most extensively, and findings suggest it can be beneficial to health overall, notably improving cardiovascular conditions, stimulating the immune system, and providing some protection against cancer. Since ancient times, chamomile has been known for its calming and sleep-inducing effects. Scientists have found that chamomile extracts exhibit benzodiazepine-like hypnotic activity, which likely promotes sleep (Srivastava et al., 2010).

Reference
Srivastava, J. K., Shankar, E., & Gupta, S. (2010). Chamomile: a herbal medicine of the past with bright future. *Molecular Medicine Reports* 3(6): 895–901. https://doi .org/10.3892/mmr.2010.377

Supplements

While supplements do not have the oversight and approval of the US Food and Drug Administration (FDA), as pharmaceutical drugs do, certain supplements have been studied and found to have significant benefits on human health in regard to sleep. There are currently hundreds of supplements on the market that claim to help with sleep, but many of them have not been studied or tested by a third party to ensure their efficacy. Before spending money on a new supplement, it is wise to research whether any studies back the claims on their label. Below, we describe three popular supplements that have been extensively studied and shown to be effective in improving sleep, decreasing insomnia, and treating some sleep disorders.

Note: As always, speak with your primary care provider before starting any supplements. There may be drug interactions or side effects that these supplements can cause that are not listed in this section. Be mindful that the information below is for educational purposes and does not constitute medical advice.

Magnesium

Magnesium is one of the 24 essential minerals our bodies need to thrive and helps to facilitate many essential functions. It is common to have less-than-optimal magnesium levels, especially in women. This vital mineral is not naturally produced in the body, so it must be consumed in foods like dark leafy greens, seeds and nuts, and whole grains. The wide variety of magnesium supplements can be beneficial for general health and have been associated with improved quality and duration of sleep. But researchers suggest that more randomized clinical trials are indicated to confirm magnesium's causative role on sleep and how it facilitates many essential functions.

THE SCIENCE OF MAGNESIUM

Supplementing magnesium can help improve sleep time, sleep efficiency, sleep onset latency, and early-morning awakenings (Abbasi et al., 2012; Zhang et al., 2021). These effects occur in part because magnesium works to restore gabba-amniobutyric acid (GABA) levels, helping to regulate both mood and the ability to relax for sleep. The tolerable upper limit of magnesium supplements for adults is 350 mg daily but will vary widely depending on an individual's age and magnesium level (National Institutes of Health Office of Dietary Supplements, 2022). A good start is to eat a daily diet that includes some magnesium-rich foods and take a supplement, if directed by your health care provider, to correct a deficiency if your blood levels are low.

References

Abbasi, B., Kimiagar, M., Sadeghniiat, K., Shirazi, M. M., Hedayati, M., & Rashidkhani, B. (2012). The effect of magnesium supplementation on primary insomnia in elderly: a double-blind placebo-controlled clinical trial. *Journal of Research in Medical Sciences* 17(12): 1161–69.

National Institutes of Health Office of Dietary Supplements. (2022). Magnesium: fact sheet for health professionals. Last updated June 2, 2022. https://ods.od .nih.gov/factsheets/Magnesium-HealthProfessional/

Zhang, Y., Chen, C., Lu, L., Knutson, K. L., Carnethon, M. R., Fly, A. D., & Kahe, K. (2021). Association of magnesium intake with sleep duration and sleep quality: findings from the CARDIA study. *Sleep* 45(4): zsab276. https://doi.org/10.1093 /sleep/zsab276

CBD Oil

CBD, short for cannabidiol, is a household name, commonly known as a natural healing remedy for health issues ranging from joint pain to anxiety. Cannabidiol is one of many cannabinoid molecules found in cannabis plants, including marijuana and hemp. Unlike THC (tetrahydrocannabinol), CBD does not have psychoactive effects and is not an intoxicating substance. Consuming CBD works naturally within the body to attach to cannabinoid receptors, which can lead to numerous health benefits. Currently, the FDA has approved a prescription of CBD to treat two types of childhood epilepsy.

THE SCIENCE OF CBD (CANNABIDIOL)

CBD companies often claim that their products can help reduce anxiety, decrease pain, and improve sleep, but the data within scientific literature are still evolving in this arena. Preliminary studies have found that CBD is a promising sleep aid, as it addresses several of the root causes of insomnia, including anxiety and pain (Shannon et al., 2019). With CBD usage being so new, there is no universal dosage when used as a sleep aid. When looking for a CBD product to support sleep, examine the company's standards, ethics, and commitment to research before buying.

Disclaimer: While consuming full-spectrum CBD oil (meaning it contains legal trace amounts of tetrahydrocannabinol, or THC, the active ingredient in marijuana that causes a high) may be legal in your state, there are health concerns over the long-term use of CBD oil. Consuming a full-spectrum CBD oil can build THC levels in the body over time and may even show up in universal drug screening.

Reference
Shannon, S., Lewis, N., Lee, H., & Hughes, S. (2019). Cannabidiol in anxiety and sleep: a large case series. *Permanente Journal* 23: 18–41.

Environmental Accommodations

Creating a dark, cool, safe, relaxing, and comfortable sleep environment is one of the best ways to prepare for sleep and allow your body to rest. With hundreds of tools and gadgets on the market, it can be difficult to decipher what's going to be worth the investment. Below are several suggestions that are tried, true, and backed by research.

Weighted Blankets

- Feeling comfortable and safe is essential for a good night's rest, and weighted blankets can help facilitate this sensation, especially for people with anxiety. Being wrapped in the blanket or placing it over your body helps to calm the central nervous system by providing deep pressure stimulation, which has been linked to reducing pain, decreasing anxiety, and improving mood. Weighted blankets range between 5 and 30 pounds; select one that accounts for 10% of your body weight. Options include a removable cooling cover, for those who prefer to sleep in a cool environment.

- One study found that the added weight of this blanket may also provide a grounding sensation in the body, which helps to feel more centered while also reducing and resynchronizing cortisol levels in your body as you sleep (Ghaly and Teplitz, 2004).

THE SCIENCE OF WEIGHTED BLANKETS

A recent study from Swedish researchers found that people with depression and other mental health issues had improved quality of sleep through the night when using a weighted blanket (Ekholm et al., 2020). By the end of the trial, 42% of those who slept with an 18-pound blanket were considered to be in remission from their sleep troubles (based on their low Insomnia Severity Index scores), compared with 3.6% of the control group. The weighted blankets didn't have a significant effect on total sleep time, but they led to a significant decrease in nighttime waking, less daytime sleepiness, and fewer symptoms of depression and anxiety.

Reference

Ekholm, B., Spulber, S., & Adler, M. (2020). A randomized controlled study of weighted chain blankets for insomnia in psychiatric disorders. *Journal of Clinical Sleep Medicine* 16(9): 1567–77. https://doi.org/10.5664/jcsm.8636

Sound Therapy

Similar to touch, sound is a powerful sensory experience that can affect how well one sleeps. It is not uncommon to hear people share that they need background noise such as the television or music to fall asleep to. This background noise may give a sense of comfort or drown out startling or unfamiliar sounds. The sound therapy suggestions listed below have been studied and found to be effective in calming the nervous system and promoting more restful sleep.

Binaural Beats

Binaural beats work by simultaneously playing two different pulsing sounds (one in each ear), which encourages your brain to align with the brain waves of each beat, theoretically promoting relaxation and sleep. This method of sound therapy is created through the use of various types of audio frequencies. Beta, alpha, theta, and delta waves each have their own intended purpose (such as focus, sleep, or relaxation), and soundtracks are curated to address specific needs of listeners. In sleep research, theta waves are related to deep relaxation, daydreaming, and memory; delta waves are associated with deep sleep.

THE SCIENCE OF BRAIN WAVE ACTIVITY

In one study, 33 participants' brain wave activity was observed using an electroencephalogram, or EEG (On et al., 2013). Their baseline brain wave activity was recorded as well as their brain wave activity during binaural entrainment. Findings revealed that theta brain waves increased significantly after listening to binaural beats, and delta brain waves were incrementally affected but not significant. These results suggest that binaural beats can be used as a method of relaxation that may promote better sleep.

Reference

On, F. R., Jailani, R., Norhazman, H., & Zaini, N. M. (2013). Binaural beat effect on brainwaves based on EEG. Presented at the 2013 9th International Colloquium on Signal Processing and Its Applications. Institute of Electrical and Electronics Engineers, Kuala Lumpur, March 8–10, 2013. https://doi.org/10.1109/cspa .2013.6530068

White Noise

White noise machines are commonly associated with the sounds of an infant's nursery or a therapist's waiting room. This is because it provides a steady, ambient sound that blocks out other noises such as creaking home appliances or voices in another room. Based on data surrounding white noise and sleep arousal, it can be an effective option when curating an environment for better sleep.

THE SCIENCE OF WHITE NOISE

Stanchina et al. (2005) examined the sleep of ICU patients, and those who listened to white noise experienced less arousal from peak and background noises throughout the night compared to the control group. This suggests that the use of white noise can promote deeper states of sleep.

Reference

Stanchina, M. L., Abu-Hijleh, M., Chaudhry, B. K., Carlisle, C. C., & Millman, R. P. (2005). The influence of white noise on sleep in subjects exposed to ICU noise. Sleep Medicine 6(5): 423–28. https://doi.org/10.1016/j.sleep.2004.12.004

Mindfulness and Sleep

Difficulty sleeping is often associated with stress, anxiety, and racing thoughts. Switching gears into a state of mindfulness allows for thoughts to be rerouted to a given task that will aid in preparing your body for sleep. While mindfulness requires some degree of awareness, there are several exercises that use mindfulness to promote an easy and peaceful slumber.

THE SCIENCE OF MINDFULNESS AND SLEEP

Research surrounding the benefits related to mindfulness-meditation practices is growing, especially when examining their effect on sleep. In a 2015 randomized control trial (Black et al., 2015), participants

(continued)

met once a week for two hours, over a six-week duration. They were randomly assigned to one of two groups, a mindfulness meditation program or a sleep education program, and both had relevant home-work assignments. At the end of the six sessions, those in the mind-fulness group had less insomnia, fatigue, and depression compared with the people in the sleep education group. This illustrates that the use of mindfulness meditation practices may be more beneficial than merely education regarding sleep. It also suggests that nurses, with their extensive background and knowledge about health, including sleep, might be able to improve their sleep through nightly mindfulness meditation practices.

Most studies examining sleep health and mindfulness focus on how mindfulness affects sleep quality and behaviors. In a study of 61 full-time nurses, sleep health had an impact on next-day mindful attention (Lee et al., 2021). Over two weeks, nurses self-reported sleep characteristics and efficiency. Once the data were analyzed at the between-person level, participants with greater sleep sufficiency, higher sleep quality, and fewer insomnia symptoms reported greater mindful attention overall. These findings reveal that optimal sleep health is an antecedent of daily mindful attention in nurses. They suggest that when nurses improve their sleep, they have the potential to receive benefits to their well-being and to the quality of care they provide to patients.

Reference

Black, D. S., O'Reilly, G. A., Olmstead, R., Breen, E. C., & Irwin, M. R. (2015). Mind-fulness meditation and improvement in sleep quality and daytime impairment among older adults with sleep disturbances: a randomized clinical trial. *JAMA Internal Medicine* 175(4): 494–501. https://doi.org/10.1001/jamainternmed .2014.8081

Lee, S., Mu, C., Gonzalez, B. D., Vinci, C. E., & Small, B. J. (2021). Sleep health is associated with next-day mindful attention in healthcare workers. *Sleep Health* 7(1): 105–12.

Winding Down before Bed

JOURNALING

Goal: To release your thoughts and process your emotions

Time and place: 10–15 minutes, in a quiet space at home

▸ If your mind tends to race at night, it might be helpful to journal and/or set aside "worry time" before bed to allow yourself to get out all the thoughts and stories that are contained in the mind.

▸ Journaling an hour or two before going to sleep can be a mindful exercise of emptying the mind and preparing to be present for your next activity: sleep.

▸ Keep a journal or notepad by your bedside with a pen that lights, so you can write down any thoughts that may wake you in the middle of the night.

BODY SCAN MEDITATION

Goal: To release tension and promote sleep

Time and place: 10–30 minutes, in bed right before sleep

▸ Body scan meditation tends to be a favorite among those who are new to mindfulness. In this guided practice, one focuses on individual areas of the body by flexing or tensing muscles and then allowing them to relax. It is an effective way to release tension in places you may not even be aware of, and a newly relaxed body often eases the mind to sleep.

▸ There are a number of guided meditations that can help you sleep; see the Resources section at the end of the book for links to several guided practices.

FINDING YOUR OWN STRATEGIES

◆

Throughout this section on discovering the benefits of sleeping well, we provided a wealth of tips, tools, and strategies to help you get a better night's sleep. Whether you are someone who puts their head to their pillow and sleeps soundly for eight hours or a self-diagnosed insomniac, there is likely something in this section that can help you rest and restore.

Choose three of the strategies mentioned in this section that you can put into practice this week. Write them down and stick to them. In one week's time, notice if there are any changes or improvements, and decide if additional strategies are needed.

1. _____

2. _____

3. _____

In the field of health coaching and behavior change, coaches often use the acronym SMART with their clients in order to promote effective goal-setting (Moore et al., 2016). SMART goals are Specific, Measurable, Attainable, Realistic, and Time-bound. Using this formula promotes action-oriented steps that prompt behavior change and goal achievement.

As you consider incorporating some of these strategies to improve your sleep, what do you want to do, how will you know you're doing it, and how will you stick to this? Before creating your own plan, check out the example below.

Michelle is a 43-year-old nurse who is married, with two school-age children (7 and 4 years old). She works on an in-patient pediatric floor of her local hospital. Each week she has three 12-hour daytime shifts and struggles with getting enough sleep owing to her demanding job and role as a mother. When she has work, she sticks to a regimented 9:30 pm bedtime to be at the hospital by 7:00 am. On her days off, she stays up late watching television because she feels it's her only "quiet time" after the kids go to bed. When she does, she struggles to get up by 6:30 am the next morning and get her kids to school on time. She wants this sleep-deprived cycle to stop without sacrificing time for herself.

Here's the goal that worked for Michelle: *On my days off, I plan to give myself one hour of TV time each night by setting an alarm on my phone to remind me "lights out" by 10:00 pm. This way, I will get to sleep by 10:30 pm (one hour later than my "work bedtime"), and I will sleep a solid eight hours before waking up with the kids. I will try this out for four weeks and then check in to see how it's going.*

What's your SMART goal for improving your sleep? Remember, it should be

Specific...
Measurable...
Attainable...
Realistic...
Time-bound...

Share your sleep SMART goals with friends, families, and colleagues. You can all benefit from a good night's sleep.

REFERENCES

Centers for Disease Control and Prevention. (2017). How much sleep do I need? Last reviewed March 2, 2017. https://www.cdc.gov/sleep/about _sleep/how_much_sleep.html

Ganesan, S., Magee, M., Stone, J. E., Mulhall, M. D., Collins, A., Howard, M. E., Lockley, S. W., Rajaratnam, S. M. W., & Sletten, T. L. (2019). The impact of shift work on sleep, alertness and performance in healthcare workers. *Scientific Reports* 9: 4635. https://doi.org/10.1038/s41598-019-40914-x

Ghaly, M., & Teplitz, D. (2004). The biologic effects of grounding the human body during sleep as measured by cortisol levels and subjective reporting of sleep, pain, and stress. *Journal of Alternative and Complementary Medicine* 10(5): 767–76. https://doi.org/10.1089/acm.2004.10.767

Green, E. (2022). Sleep hygiene: healthy habits for better sleep. No Sleepless Nights. Last updated March 10, 2022. https://www.nosleeplessnights .com/sleep-hygiene/

Jahrami, H., BaHammam, A. S., AlGahtani, H., Ebrahim, A., Faris, M., AlEid, K., & Hasan, Z. (2021). The examination of sleep quality for frontline healthcare workers during the outbreak of COVID-19. *Sleep and Breathing* 25(1): 503–11.

Moore, M., Jackson, E., & Tschannen-Moran, B. (2016). *Coaching Psychology Manual*. Philadelphia, PA: Wolters Kluwer.

National Heart, Lung, and Blood Institute. (2022). What are sleep deprivation and deficiency? Last updated March 24, 2022. https://www.nhlbi.nih.gov /health/sleep-deprivation

Pang, A. S. K. (2016). *Rest: Why You Get More Done When You Work Less*. Greenwood Village, CO: Basic Books.

Ryff, C. D. (2017). Eudaimonic well-being, inequality, and health: recent findings and future directions. *International Review of Economics* 64(2): 159–78.

Stimpfel, A. W., Fatehi, F., & Kovner, C. (2020). Nurses' sleep, work hours, and patient care quality, and safety. *Sleep Health* 6(3): 314–20. https://doi.org /10.1016/j.sleh.2019.11.001

Suni, E., & Vyas, N. (2022). Sleep hygiene. Sleep Foundation. Last updated March 11, 2022. https://www.sleepfoundation.org/sleep-hygiene

Suntory Museum of Art. The Genchō-an Tearoom. Accessed September 6, 2022. https://www.suntory.com/sma/tearoom/

Willmann, A. (2011). The Japanese tea ceremony. Metropolitan Museum. April 2011. https://www.metmuseum.org/toah/hd/jtea/hd_jtea.htm

Zee, P. C., & Goldstein, C. A. (2010). Treatment of shift work disorder and jet lag. Current Treatment Options in Neurology 12(5): 396–411.

•

CHAPTER 5

Nourishing Well

"In those early days and weeks of the pandemic, what I
missed the most were Sunday dinners with my family.
Eating at a table with loved ones has always been a
love language of mine, so I decided to bring that weekly
ritual to work when we all needed it most."

IN THEIR OWN WORDS

As an ICU nurse in a busy East Coast hospital at the start of the pandemic, I was fearful and overwhelmed along with all of my colleagues.
We were thrown into a situation we never could have imagined—
intubating several patients per day and scrubbing down our bodies
in between patients. After a few weeks, the other staff members and
I decided we needed a program to de-stress. In the nicer weather, we
would do yoga instruction and meditation outside. These moments
were helpful in keeping calm and composed at work; we all felt like we
needed more connection.

Growing up with six siblings, I have always felt most content
around a table with my entire family. In those early days and weeks of
the pandemic, what I missed the most were Sunday dinners with my
family. Eating at a table with loved ones has always been a love language of mine, so I decided to bring that weekly ritual to work, when
we all needed it most. Although I was worried about people's reactions,
I proposed that the staff get together for a meal on the first Friday of
every month. Each month we chose a theme and shared food while
staying safe and socially distanced.

The most memorable meal we shared was in July of 2020. Cases were on the decline, and we finally felt like we could breathe—just a little bit. For this meal, we chose the Fourth of July to be our theme and decorated with red, white, and blue partyware. Since the Fourth of July is my nephew's birthday, this day holds a special place in my heart, so I wanted to bring something extra special. I ended up making blueberry muffins that were loved by my fellow staff—a small nod to my nephew's favorite fruit.

Summer 2020: Suong Nguyen, BSN, RN, Intensive Care Unit, Marlton, New Jersey, United States

NOURISHMENT AND WELL-BEING
◆

Nourishment and nutrition are fundamental components of well-being and health, and health care professionals often tell their patients to "eat well and exercise." Knowing the benefits of eating well is one thing, but taking action and following through is another. Implementing healthy habits and knowing how to make better choices can be overwhelming. This chapter will provide clarity on why it's important and how to make eating well a habit.

Across cultures and in different social settings, diet has affected how we interpret what is "healthy" and can potentially complicate how we nourish ourselves. Simply put, food is energy. Our daily choices affect how well we feel in our day-to-day life, which compounds over time in ways that prevent or contribute to disease. Finding the right balance is one of the greatest feats of living a healthy life, and diet is a significant component of this imperfect equation. For some, eating a regimented, "super-clean" diet might work for them, while for others, it is eating well most of the time but managing to indulge in desserts and sweets every now and then.

The media is awash with suggestions for the best diet to lose weight, maintain energy, build muscle, cure pain, and an endless list of other concerns. There are so many choices it can feel overwhelming, leading us to feel defeated and wonder how one chooses. Nutrition science indicates that many foods can convey health benefits, and for this reason there is no "one-size-fits-all" approach or strict meal plan that can guarantee everyone the results they are looking for. Generally speaking, certain foods and their natural nutritional properties do have an impact on various different aspects of our health, from healing inflammation and easing pain to boosting our cognitive capacity and brain health.

You can drive yourself mad trying to keep up with the latest trends, ranging from keto to juicing to intermittent fasting and "doctor-formulated meal replacements." It's essential that you determine what works for you and your lifestyle—ask yourself what's realistic and what is likely to never happen. What tiny changes can you make today that will get you toward your end goal? If there are areas of your health you're looking to improve, according to the American College of Lifestyle Medicine (2022), adapting your diet is one approach that may help.

Although eating healthy may seem to be simple, it's not necessarily easy or accessible in most places in the world. Many areas of the United States and around the world are food deserts, or places with limited access to affordable and nutritious food. It's estimated that 13.5 million people in the United States experience this disadvantage to healthful living (Wright, 2021). Additionally, societal, health, and financial crises influence the way we eat. An Icelandic study of the financial crisis of 2008–10 found that the intake of fruit increased steadily in the decade before the crisis and decreased slightly during the crisis (Asgeirsdottir et al., 2016). The intake of sweets continued at a high level during the crisis but began to decrease as soon as it was over.

Accessibility to healthy produce can be determined by what are best described as the social determinants of health. These factors include economic stability, education, health and health care, neighborhood and built environment, and social and community context (Healthy People, 2022). Adding to these existing barriers is the coronavirus pandemic, which has also affected people's access to healthy foods and produce. Food retailers noted that during the pandemic, the production of fruit and vegetables in Europe was at risk for decreasing supplies owing to a lack of seasonal labor in agriculture from outside the European Union. The result? Increased prices of fruit and vegetables, with a disproportionate impact on groups on low incomes or people without jobs. Members of these populations are already at risk for the lowest intake of fruit and vegetables. This was not unique to Europe and continues to be a concern around the globe as a result of other crises, such as the Russian invasion of Ukraine. Unfortunately, there is no solution we can offer to resolve these issues. But becoming aware of the inequalities of health can bring us greater compassion for ourselves and our neighbors around the world. What's most important is nourishing ourselves in the best ways that we can, and making healthy choices that are accessible and affordable. Expensive supplements and fancy powders likely aren't going to be transformational in the ways marketing teams would like us to believe, so we encourage you to eat simply and locally whenever you can.

As we discuss later in the chapter, food is more than a way to keep us alive and moving. Choosing to nourish well affects various areas of one's life, and with that, well-being follows suit. In Carol Ryff's model of psychological well-being, nourishing well through food relates to the key components of environmental mastery, self-acceptance, autonomy, and positive relations with others (Echeverría et al., 2020). Sharing food allows for opportunities to gather with loved ones, but you don't need to plan an elaborate meal to try new recipes, test out new cooking skills, or immerse yourself in the vibrant colors, flavors, and scents of a single moment. These are all vital experiences that contribute to improving our well-being. Being confident and capable in the kitchen, whether that means throwing together a quick salad or working hard to create a five-course meal, can be transformative in harnessing self-acceptance and autonomy. Unlike the societal pressures of diet culture and fear-mongering, we want you to feel empowered and content by the choices you make in nourishing well, and this chapter outlines ways you can make that dream a reality.

THE EMERGENCE OF NUTRITIONAL PSYCHIATRY

◆

What we eat affects our mood; we know this anecdotally and through research (Jacka et al., 2017). Studies have found dietary interventions are a promising way to reduce symptoms of depression across the population (Firth et al., 2019). Uma Naidoo, author of *This Is Your Brain on Food* (2020), points out how what we eat affects our mood. In fact, food can be an important part of an overall treatment plan, including recommendations for how we can eat to beat stress. Naidoo describes how to use food as medicine for mental health. Nutritional psychiatrists describe key guidelines that can nourish our mental health: eat whole foods (80% of your diet), eat the rainbow (more on that later), avoid refined sugar and sweets, and stay away from foods that trigger anxiety. Even journalists who write for popular magazines, such as *Bon Appetite*, have introduced their readers to nutritional psychiatry:

> Nutritional psychiatrists, unlike regular psychiatrists, incorporate food into their overall treatment plans. Nutritional psychiatry leans on certain nutrient-packed foods—those filled with vitamins, minerals, antioxidants, fiber, pro-and prebiotics, and protein—while cutting way back on nutritionally "empty" foods (sorry, sugar). These adjustments are designed to reduce brain inflammation, better regulate serotonin and dopamine, and influence a host of other mood-boosting reactions. (Ruland, 2021)

Eating to reduce stress is a plan we can all take to heart. Naidoo (2021) suggests that consuming less caffeine, alcohol, and artificial sweeteners can reduce stress, while increasing our intake of fiber, Omega-3 fatty acids, and aged, cultured, and fermented foods may play an important role in decreasing anxiety.

THE RELATIONSHIP BETWEEN
STRESS AND NOURISHMENT
♦

After a long, hard day, most of us reach for comfort foods. The choices that may remind us of our childhoods are meals that are rich and soothing in the simplest of ways. We seek comfort from food, assuming that it will make us feel better or dull the pain of the challenges we faced that day. As self-soothing as it may seem, research suggests that these comfortable indulgences are not any more beneficial for our mood than other food or no food at all (Wagner et al., 2014). Does that mean you should erase them from your diet altogether? Absolutely not. In addition to nourishment through micro- and macronutrients, food is meant to be an experience that is enjoyable. We don't want to deprive ourselves of things that bring us joy, but rather find a realistic balance of what nourishes our bodies and minds from a cellular level while filling up our souls at the same time.

When we are under immense amounts of stress, we tend to make choices that affect our health in negative ways—we reach for something fast and easy that we can grab out of a cabinet, our refrigerator, or even our coat pocket. The coronavirus pandemic magnified the way our habits can change while under stress and the implications of these choices. Changes in eating and movement habits as a result of the pandemic and society's measures can increase the risk of overweight and obesity, as well as reduce muscle mass, leading to more falls among the elderly.

The impacts of stress and eating habits are a global problem. Nurses around the world have reported having a difficult time with weight gain and poor nutritional habits owing to the stress of the pandemic. This is especially concerning because there are clear signs that chronic diseases such as obesity, cardiovascular disease, Type 2 diabetes, and cancer can increase the risk of dying from COVID-19 (Rawshani et al., 2021). In Sweden, researchers have found that obesity continues to increase and has been linked to developing low-grade chronic inflammation, causing a disrupted immune system (Alsiö et al., 2021). Not only is this a concern for the individuals affected by it, but increased rates of obesity could be problematic during public health crises (Childs et al., 2019). Unhealthy eating habits are a major contributor to these chronic diseases (Knudsen et al., 2019). Our general health and nutritional condition thus affect our ability to tackle this viral disease. Conversely, the virus's entry into society likely affected our eating habits, both directly and indirectly in the short and long term.

At this point, you might be wondering, "What can I do to avoid this?" First, it is important to acknowledge which habits are least helpful and most healthful for you, right now. Then, in the following pages, as you gain more insight into science-backed ways of how to eat, you can begin to adapt your habits to fall more in line with what is recommended by the research. With the right support, eating habits can be improved with the knowledge that unhealthy eating habits increase the risk of developing chronic diseases. Ensuring healthy functioning of the immune system can be a motivator to improve eating habits as well (Eustachio Colombo et al., 2020). But it is important to take into account that groups with low socioeconomic status may need other types of support in addition to the knowledge required to improve their eating habits. These supports can include structural changes in the environment, a healthy and affordable range of food and meals, and joint efforts among leaders and organizations in our local community. Getting involved in these efforts is one way to advocate for those who are food insecure.

In the following pages, you'll learn all about brain foods that promote the prevention of disease and illness, both physical and mental. Importantly, some foods should be avoided to aid in stress reduction and other mental and emotional health conditions. As you continue reading, keep in mind that this information is not a replacement for nutritional advice from your primary care provider or nutritionist. These are general recommendations that do not factor in your unique nutritional needs or health status.

THE SCIENCE OF NUTRITIONAL PSYCHIATRY

We say to children that they must eat all their fruits and vegetables to grow big and strong. This sentiment is well informed, and researchers continue to discover just how important certain foods are to healthy development and aging. How we choose to nourish ourselves affects physical health along with cognitive functioning and mental health. That's why "brain foods" can benefit both your mind and body.

Brain foods are foods that are linked to improving your mental health and well-being. They are not meant to be a substitute for traditional physical or mental health care, but knowing what brain foods are and consuming them regularly can be good for your health. Nutritional psychiatrist Uma Naidoo explains that the mechanism through which this occurs is the mind-gut connection (Naidoo, 2019). The gut-brain axis (GBA) is a bidirectional communication system between the central and enteric nervous systems. It links the brain's emotional and cognitive centers to peripheral intestinal functions. Gut microbiota, the microorganisms that live in the intestinal track, can influence this complex relationship between the brain and the gut (Carabotti et al., 2015).

(continued)

In a *New York Times* article, health and wellness journalist Tara Parker-Pope (2022) brought these concerns to the general public when she presented a host of recent research studies on the way our brain and gut work in sync with one another: "The connection between the stomach and the brain is strong, and it starts in the womb. The gut and brain originate from the same cells in the embryo. One of the main ways the brain and gut remain connected is through the vagus nerve, a two-way chemical messaging system that explains why stress can trigger feelings of anxiety in your mind and butterflies in your stomach."

Dietary interventions can have a powerful effect on our mental health by nourishing our brains with nutrients, instead of depriving them. Australian researchers Mujcic and Oswald (2016) examined food diaries of 12,385 randomly sampled adults from an ongoing government survey. Findings suggest that higher fruit and vegetable intake predicted increased happiness, life satisfaction, and well-being. The psychological gains were equivalent to moving from unemployment to employment. Additionally, people who changed their diet to include more vegetables saw mood improvements within two years.

References

Carabotti, M., Scirocco, A., Maselli, M. A., & Severi, C. (2015). The gut-brain axis: interactions between enteric microbiota, central and enteric nervous systems. *Annals of Gastroenterology: Quarterly Publication of the Hellenic Society of Gastroenterology* 28(2): 203–9.

Mujcic, R., & Oswald, A. J. (2016). Evolution of well-being and happiness after increases in consumption of fruit and vegetables. *American Journal of Public Health* 106(8): 1504–10. https://doi.org/10.2105/AJPH.2016.303260

Naidoo, U. (2019). Nutritional psychiatry: the gut-brain connection. *Psychiatric Times* 36(1): 11A.

Parker-Pope, T. (2022). The best brain foods you're not eating. *New York Times*, January 24, 2022. https://www.nytimes.com/2022/01/24/well/eat/brain-food.html

BENEFICIAL BRAIN FOODS

It's time we all start thinking about food choices we make, not for the way they will help us fit into our jeans, but instead how they will benefit our daily lives. Some days, mood and cognitive functioning may seem like they are beyond our control, but with a few dietary changes, we may find our brain power is amplified.

If you're wondering how you'll ever remember what foods are best for your brain, it's in the name. Nutritional psychiatrist Uma Naidoo, author of *This Is Your Brain on Food*, uses the acronym BRAINFOODS:

B: Berries and beans
R: Rainbow colors of fruits and vegetables
A: Antioxidants
I: Include lean protein and plant-based protein sources
N: Nuts (almonds, walnuts, Brazil nuts, and cashews)
F: Fiber-rich foods, fish, and fermented foods
O: Oils (unrefined)
O: Omega-3-rich foods like fish and seafood, nuts and seeds, dark leafy vegetables, and plant-based oils
D: Dairy (yogurt and kefir, certain cheeses)
S: Spices

BRAINFOODS are foods that nourish and fuel your mind and body. You'll notice that there aren't hard-to-find niche ingredients or superfoods that are promised to pack a punch. These brain foods are all identifiable, everyday ingredients that may remind you of home-cooked meals as a kid, prepared fresh and made with love.

BRAIN FOOD BREAKDOWN

Later in this chapter are several recipes approved by our nursing colleagues that show you how to incorporate brain foods in tasty and time-efficient ways. Now, let's get an understanding of these foods and their unique benefits.

Leafy Greens

Leafy greens can be rotated seasonally, depending on what is locally grown near you. These include greens like kale, spinach, collards, and broccoli that are rich in brain-promoting nutrients like vitamin K, lutein, folate, and beta carotene. Research suggests that these plant-based foods may help slow cognitive decline and protect against dementia (Yeh et al., 2021).

Rainbow of Colorful Fruits and Vegetables

The colorful message of "eating the rainbow" promoted in school cafeterias around the globe is not just for kids. Studies suggest that the compounds in brightly colored fruits and vegetables like red peppers, blueberries, broccoli, and eggplant can affect inflammation, memory, sleep, and mood. In fact, reddish-purplish foods are "power players" in this category, meaning they hold even more potential to benefit these areas of our health.

Nuts, Beans, and Seeds

Nuts and seeds are high in healthy fats that enhance the absorption of phytonutrients from other vegetables. Beans are high in fiber and a great plant-based source of protein.

Omega-3s

Omega-3-rich foods promote brain health by lowering inflammatory markers and protecting neurons from excessive inflammation (Naidoo, 2021). Consumed in moderation, foods like fish and seafood, nuts and seeds, dark leafy vegetables, and plant-based oils are all great sources of Omega-3s and are ultimately beneficial for brain health.

Herbs and Spices

Aromatic herbs and spices add flavor, depth, and character to any meal. Plus, a little can go a long way to improve health. Studies suggest certain spices may lead to a better balance of gut microbes, reduce inflammation, and even improve memory. Most notably is turmeric, a spice often found in Indian and Southeast Asian cuisines. Studies suggest that its active ingredient, curcumin, may help improve attention and overall cognition, and is best absorbed with black pepper.

Fermented Foods

As mentioned above, the gut-brain connection is powerful, and the health of our microbiome is linked to our mental health. Fermentation is an ancient technique for preserving food that enables the breakdown of carbs like starch and sugar by bacteria and yeast. Common fermented foods include sauerkraut, kimchi, miso, kombucha, tempeh, yogurt, and kefir.

Dark Chocolate

Dark chocolate is a rich source of antioxidants; just be sure to choose a chocolate with a high percentage of cacao and lower sugar content. One study found that consumption of chocolate, particularly dark chocolate, may be associated with reduced odds of clinically relevant depressive symptoms (Jackson et al., 2019).

FOODS THAT CAUSE "BRAIN BUFFERING"

•

We hope that you're learning how much power we gain when we make choices that nourish us. Of course, not all foods have the same benefits, and some even can be detrimental to our health and well-being even if they are naturally derived. Too much of a good thing can still be too much.

You may have heard the term "buffering" before, reminding you of endless minutes of waiting in front of a computer screen. Buffering refers to downloading a certain amount of data before being able to engage with it. Eventually, the data will load, but buffering can feel painstakingly slow and ineffective.

We can apply this concept to the impact certain foods have on our physical and mental health. Brain-buffering foods are those that aren't optimal for our brains and bodies, leaving us lagging. The more we consume, the greater the harm done. Depending on our unique sensitivity, we may consume the food, drink, or substance and feel the sensation almost immediately—just like the little loading circle keeps going round and round while nothing happens. There just isn't any meaningful link to connect to (Hansen, 2013).

The effects of brain-buffering foods aren't all negative—in fact, we are drawn to them by their tempting, quick fixes for energy—like caffeine and sugar. But the research is clear that there are risks to frequent consumption, and they will more than likely make your brain "buffer" in the moment and over time.

THE SCIENCE OF SUGAR, CAFFEINE, AND ALCOHOL

Sugar has been a hot topic for the past few decades, as processed foods have increased sugar consumption in the United States and around the world. In 2019, researchers completed a meta-analysis of 10 observational studies, including more than 37,000 people with depression. Findings revealed that consuming sugar-sweetened beverages put people at a higher risk for depression. Drinking just over a 12-ounce can of soda per day (which contains 45 grams of sugar) increased their risk by 5%. For those who drank two-and-a-half cans of soda a day (98 grams), their risk jumped to 25%. This means that the more sugar one consumes, the higher the likelihood of experiencing depression (Hu et al., 2019).

Caffeine is a stimulant to the central nervous system, making you feel perkier and peppier after that first cup of coffee you enjoy each morning. Caffeine has obvious benefits—such as feeling more alert and energized—but there are common unwanted side effects that affect mood, including heightened anxiety (Fiani et al., 2021).

A recent study out of Basel University in Switzerland examined the relationship between daily caffeine intake, sleep quality, and neuroplasticity. The results indicated that caffeine consumed as part of the study did not result in poor sleep as anticipated; however, the researchers observed changes in gray matter (Lin et al., 2021). Gray matter refers to the parts of the central nervous system made up primarily of the cell bodies of nerve cells. Gray matter allows us to control our movements, retain memories, and regulate our emotions, among other functions. Although researchers found the changes in gray matter to be temporary, there is cause for concern when it comes to monitoring your caffeine consumption.

Alcohol may have some carefree effects ("liquid courage"), but despite its stimulating qualities, alcohol is a depressant to the central nervous system. It affects your mood, cognition, thoughts, and consciousness. Alcohol is known as a social lubricant, a way to make interacting with other people easier and more enjoyable. While these effects are enticing, people with social anxiety are four times more likely to develop an alcohol use disorder (Terlecki et al., 2014.) The harms of alcohol use can happen moments after consumption, but most notice the effects the next day. It is not uncommon to wake up jittery, on edge, and anxious, symptoms associated with mild alcohol withdrawal. One study found that people who are anxious have poor sleep with regular alcohol consumption (Becker, 2012.)

References

Becker, H. C. (2012). Effects of alcohol dependence and withdrawal on stress responsiveness and alcohol consumption. *Alcohol Research: Current Reviews* 34(4): 448–58.

Fiani, B., Zhu, L., Musch, B. L., Briceno, S., Andel, R., Sadeq, N., & Ansari, A. Z. (2021). The neurophysiology of caffeine as a central nervous system stimulant and the resultant effects on cognitive function. *Cureus* 13(5): e15032. https://doi.org/10.7759/cureus.15032

Hu, D., Cheng, L., & Jiang, W. (2019). Sugar-sweetened beverages consumption and the risk of depression: a meta-analysis of observational studies. *Journal of Affective Disorders* 245: 348–55. https://doi.org/10.1016/j.jad.2018.11.015

Lin, Y. S., Weibel, J., Landolt, H. P., Santini, F., Meyer, M., et al. (2021). Daily caffeine intake induces concentration-dependent medial temporal plasticity in humans: a multimodal double-blind randomized controlled trial. *Cerebral Cortex* 31(6): 3096–106. https://doi.org/10.1093/cercor/bhab005

Terlecki, M. A., Ecker, A. H., & Buckner, J. D. (2014). College drinking problems and social anxiety: the importance of drinking context. *Psychology of Addictive Behaviors* 28(2): 545–52. https://doi.org/10.1037/a0035770

Drinking is often used as a crutch to deal with challenging times, assumed to relieve the stress of the situations ailing us. Drinking regularly can quickly become a slippery slope, gaining momentum until the habit is out of control and negatively affecting both your mental and physical health. If you suspect your alcohol use is having an impact on your well-being, please seek the support of a health care professional and search the international services listed in the Resources section.

When consumed in moderate amounts (which can vary from person to person), sugar, caffeine, and alcohol can all be enjoyed and celebrated. We share this research in an effort to empower you to make the best decisions for your health and well-being. Acknowledging the potential harms of certain foods and nutrients is not to instill shame or fear of consuming them. As always, ask your primary care provider (PCP), mental health professional, or nutritionist to help determine what is right for you.

And now, here is something that will make your mouth water. Take a few minutes to mindfully think about food.

Chocolate Mindfulness Meditation

Goal: To use the multisensory experience of chocolate as a meditation prompt

Time and place: 5–15 minutes, any place but better if a quiet space

Chocolate increases the level of endorphins in the brain, lessening pain and decreasing stress. One of the chemicals that causes the release of serotonin is tryptophan, which is found in chocolate. And that's not all. Tryptophan is good for your heart and keeps your blood pressure low. The following chocolate meditation is one of the most pleasurable, "delicious" forms of mindfulness meditation. It's convenient and simple enough for beginners, but effective enough to interest those who are experienced with meditation. The chocolate meditation brings similar benefits, stress relief and centering, and it has a built-in reward—chocolate! Here's how to do it.

1. Take a small piece of chocolate (or raisins if you are sensitive to chocolate). You'll need a bite-sized piece of chocolate. Dark chocolate with a high cocoa content contains the most benefits, but you can use whatever kind of chocolate you'd like. But try to make it special, perhaps from a favorite store or manufacturer.
2. Breathe and relax. Sit comfortably, take a few deep breaths and work on releasing tension from your muscles. You want to start your chocolate meditation as physically relaxed as possible. If you are comfortable, you can close your eyes too.
3. Hold the chocolate for closer inspection. Look at it as if you have never seen it before. And you haven't, at least not this piece. If it is wrapped, unwrap it. Now look at the naked chocolate and take it all in, its surface features, color and shape, heft and weight. Are you fighting the urge to pop it in your mouth? Be conscious of your emotions.
4. Smell the chocolate and enjoy the aroma. Does the smell stimulate other senses, taste or touch?
5. Taste. You can finally take a small bite of your chocolate. Notice how your hand feels as you raise the chocolate to your lips, holding it between your fingers, placing it in your mouth. Let it sit on your tongue and melt in your mouth. Notice the flavors, and how the

melting chocolate affects your tongue, teeth, and lips, becoming completely absorbed in the experience, *right now*. Continue your deep breathing, and concentrate on the sensations in your mouth.

6. Focus on the sensations of eating. Swallow. Focus on how the chocolate feels as it slides down your throat. Does your mouth feel empty, or is there a lingering taste? Now take a second bite, try to even notice how your arm feels as you raise the chocolate to your mouth, how it feels between your fingers, and then in your mouth. Again, focus on the sensations you are feeling in the present moment.

7. Refocus on the present. If other thoughts come into your mind during your chocolate meditation, gently refocus your attention to the flavors and sensations associated with the chocolate. The idea is to stay in the present moment as much as you can.

8. Savor the sensations. When you're done savoring your chocolate, revisit the feeling throughout your day and recall the relaxation. You may choose to continue your meditation after the chocolate is gone, or simply resume your day immediately afterward.

9. If you want, ring Tibetan meditation bells to signal the end of the meditation.

This exercise is adapted with permission from Mindfulness and the Art of Chocolate Eating by Adam Dacey at https://www.mindspace.org.uk/.

PLANT-BASED FOOD PHILOSOPHY
•

In this chapter, each recipe or meal idea is curated with an emphasis on plant-based foods. It's important to gain an understanding of what a healthy plant-based diet looks like and why it's beneficial. Nutrition science has evolved tremendously over the past 50 years, moving away from the idea that all meals must have a diet centered around animal-based protein and by-products in order to be considered health-promoting.

Consuming plant-based foods daily and in high quantities is one way to ensure you're getting in as many nutrients as you can. As you can likely gather from the name, plant-based diets are composed primarily of plants, including vegetables, fruits, leafy greens, nuts, seeds, legumes, beans, whole grains, and even sea vegetables. Following a plant-based diet does not necessarily mean you are "vegan" or "vegetarian" (which can be ethical labels built upon a belief system of not harming other living beings), but it does mean that your plate is filled primarily with plants. Depending on your preferences and dietary needs, a plant-based diet can include other animal-based foods, in moderation.

As with any way of eating, nourishing yourself on a plant-based diet requires a healthy balance of fats, carbohydrates, and protein. Your plate will vary depending on what your individual needs and goals are, but most experts agree that vegetables and whole grains should be the stars, followed by protein, fruit, and fat. And don't forget to hydrate with plenty of water. In the following pages, you'll gain a deeper understanding of the benefits of a plant-based diet through the research.

HARVARD HEALTHY EATING PLATE

Depending on your age and cultural background, you might remember reviewing what a healthy diet is in grade-school health classes. For Americans, this was the Food Pyramid created by the US Department of Agriculture, which promoted a low-fat, grain-heavy diet. This visual guide gave little education about why it was considered healthy to eat this way and how these foods fueled our bodies. It led to confusion and ultimately was ineffective in promoting a healthy lifestyle.

Currently, public health and nutrition experts along with other medical researchers have acknowledged the mistakes of the past when promoting healthy diets. What was once confusing and subject to interpretation is now clarified by the Harvard Healthy Eating Plate (Harvard T. H. Chan School of Public Health, 2021). This visual aid translates across cultures in both content and accessibility, and it is available in 25 different languages. While certain regions and cultures have their own ways of eating and preparing foods, this healthy eating plate aims to be inclusive of these differences while emphasizing the importance of portion sizes and ratios of produce (vegetables and fruit) to healthy proteins, whole grains, and healthy oils. You'll notice that in this guide, only one-quarter of the plate is filled with healthy proteins, which is

THE SCIENCE OF A PLANT-BASED DIET

There are currently five locations in the world, known as Blue Zones, where people are the healthiest and have longer life spans. The five Blue Zones include Okinawa, Japan; Sardinia, Italy; Nicoya, Costa Rica; Ikaria, Greece, and Loma Linda, California. While they are located on different points of the globe, they all have commonalities in their lifestyles that promote health and vitality. Buettner and Skemp (2016) from Harvard studied these areas and the factors that contribute to the longevity of their communities, with many residents exceeding 100 years of age. They have identified nine common elements between them, including a "plant-slant," meaning they eat primarily plant-based diets. Their findings suggest that eating a diet high in plant-based foods may help you live longer and stay healthy as you age.

Research shows that adopting a plant-based diet is a lifestyle change that can have significant impacts on health. In a review of the literature, researchers have found eating this way to be a cost-effective, low-risk intervention that may lower body mass index, blood pressure, HbA1C, and cholesterol (Tuso et al., 2013). In some cases, these diets may also reduce the number of medications needed to treat chronic diseases and lower ischemic heart disease mortality rates.

References

Buettner, D., & Skemp, S. (2016). Blue Zones: lessons from the world's longest lived. *American Journal of Lifestyle Medicine* 10(5): 318–21. https://doi.org/10.1177/1559827616637066

Tuso, P. J., Ismail, M. H., Ha, B. P., & Bartolotto, C. (2013). Nutritional update for physicians: plant-based diets. *Permanente Journal* 17(2): 61–66. https://doi.org/10.7812/TPP/12-085

different from the norms of many Western cultures. Not all animal-based diets are created equal, and this guide recommends choosing fish, poultry, beans, and nuts over red and processed meats. Another notable difference is that the Harvard Healthy Eating Plate does not promote dairy as a part of a healthy plate. Instead, they recommend limiting dairy to one to two servings per day at most. These changes emphasize the plant-powered direction nutrition science and public health are embracing, utilizing diet as a lifestyle tool to prevent disease and promote improved health outcomes.

While this visual aid is representative of what a healthy plate should look like, it's merely a suggestion and is not meant to restrict how much a person eats, since nutritional requirements vary from person to person. The main message of the Harvard Healthy Eating Plate is to focus on the quality of your diet by choosing the most nourishing foods possible. This can be done by implementing small tweaks like adding in veggies to your weekly pasta dinner and swapping your normal refined pasta for a whole-grain variety. "Healthy food" is not something to be feared or dreaded; instead, it should be just as fun and enjoyable as traditional meals on the not-as-healthy side of the spectrum. With a bit of creativity and an open mind to trying new things, you'll be gaining the benefits of eating with a "plant-slant" and maximizing your health, one bite at a time.

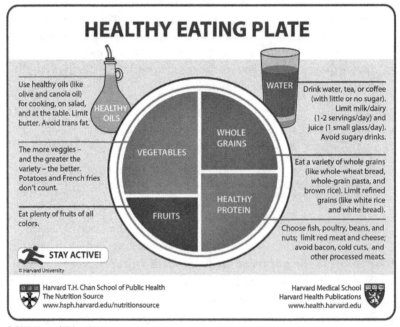

© 2011, Harvard University

GETTING THE GOODS

•

Thanks to the World Wide Web, buying healthy foods no longer requires special stops at health food stores or searching high and low for the best organic produce and niche ingredients. Now, there are dozens of websites that can have healthy food sent to your door with just the click of a few buttons, and it is more affordable than you may think.

Supporting Local Farmers with CSAs

If you're looking for the freshest, locally grown food, local community-supported agriculture (CSA) is the best way to get your hands on the ripest seasonal fruits and vegetables. Depending on where you live, CSAs typically last from late spring to early fall and provide weekly boxes of the latest harvest, usually spanning 20 weeks. Most times, you pay in advance for the "share" you are purchasing, and once the CSA season has started, you can pick up your weekly box at the farm or location near you, depending on how your chosen program works.

Although the upfront cost is usually a few hundred dollars (depending on the size box you would like), CSAs are a cost-effective way to get access to the freshest, most nutrient-dense produce that's always in season. A quick Web search of "your location + CSA" will likely generate a few options to choose from, and some might even include other agricultural products, like grains, dairy, eggs, and even poultry and meat.

Online Delivery Options

If you are interested in trying out a CSA-like option without the commitment of an entire season, there are some other food delivery services listed in the Resources section. Note that these services are not available everywhere, and you may need to find what is local to you in your country or community. Web-based produce delivery services not only provide healthy food but also save you time. They are just as affordable as they are fresh and nourishing for your body.

PLANT-POWERED RECIPES FOR NURSES, THEIR FAMILIES, AND FRIENDS

•

In the following pages, we provide plant-powered recipes that have been tested and tried by practicing nurses just like you. The reality of nursing often means that time is limited, but that does not mean healthy options need to be. The recipes included in this chapter have either been created by nurses or tested by them and given a seal of approval that they are both delicious and easy to prepare. When curating these recipes, in addition to flavorful favorite reviews, we looked for three things: simple and accessible ingredients, preparation in 30 minutes or less, and transportability. Just like all the other chapters in this book, we encourage you to take what you need from these recipes and make them your own. They are meant to inspire you to make simple swaps to include more nourishing foods in your daily life as a nurse.

Balanced Buddha Bowls

If you've been to any new, hip restaurants lately, odds are they have a Buddha bowl on the menu. These bowls are named after Buddha, who each morning carried around a bowl that he filled with food donations from locals and ate what he was given (Sacks, 2017). Just like Buddha's original bowl, which included a variety of healthy, unprocessed foods, the modern Buddha bowl does the same.

The beauty of this bowl is that it is fully customizable and never has to follow a traditional recipe; you can use what you have on hand or prepare in advance. It's a great dinner or late-lunch option and can easily be transported to work in a reusable glass or stainless-steel container. With several components, including hearty, crunchy, sweet, and salty elements, Buddha bowls have limitless possibilities of deliciousness.

Essential Elements of a Buddha Bowl
- Greens
  - At its foundation, include some type of green—whether it's raw, steamed, or sauteed, this is where the nutrient density begins.
  - Options include marinated kale, sauteed spinach, chard, and mixed spring greens.

- Grains
  - Grains provide satiety with their fiber content and help to make bowls more filling and satisfying.
  - Options include quinoa, steamed brown rice, millet, farro, and amaranth.
- Protein
  - Protein provides long-lasting nourishment to keep you full and focused, while your body uses it for cellular repair and regeneration.
  - Plant-based options include tofu, tempeh, lentils, edamame, roasted chickpeas, and warm black beans.
  - Animal-based options include hard-boiled eggs, fresh fish, free-range chicken, and grass-fed beef.
- Vegetables
  - Vegetables can be steamed, roasted, or sauteed to give this bowl more nutrient power, fiber, and density.
  - Options include roasted broccoli, roasted red pepper, roasted sweet potato, sauteed mushrooms, cucumber, carrots, tomatoes, and red onion.
- Dressing
  - Any dressing gives a meal like this its flare and brings together all the elements of your bowl. Most dressings provide healthy fat from either nuts and seeds or a healthy oil like olive or avocado as a base.
  - Options include lemon tahini, hummus, balsamic vinaigrette, vegan ranch, and avocado lime.
- Toppings
  - Toppings on this bowl can range from microgreens to sunflower seeds, and everything in between. Much like dressings, their presence brings all the bowl's elements together, plus they add an element of crunchy, chewy, or flavor-filled fun.
  - Options include microgreens, roasted nuts, sunflower seeds, fresh berries, apple slices, craisins, and sauerkraut.

Balanced Buddha Bowls to Try at Home

Many food bloggers provide daily inspiration for Buddha bowls, leading to endless options of greens, grains, and extras to choose from. Social media can also be a wonderful tool to discover new recipes and learn how to prepare them. The Resources section at the back of this book provides links to some of our favorite bloggers that make Buddha bowls anything but boring, including Cookie + Kate, Minimalist Baker, The Kitchen Girl, and The Simple Veganista.

Plant-Based Bento Boxes

Sometimes salads go from a quintessential work lunch to a less-than-exciting meal, and the days of hospital buffets being top choice are long behind most of us. Although the daily special in the cafeteria might be tempting to dig into instead of planning ahead, odds are it's not as satiating and nourishing as it could be. If you're eager to switch it up by adding variety without sacrificing health benefits, these bento boxes are for you.

Bento boxes originated in Japan as single-serving to-go containers with multiple sections. They have become a popular way to bring small meals wherever you go in an efficient way that sparks creative combos. Using containers that are already portioned out is an effective way to include all the elements of a balanced meal with adequate amounts of carbs, protein, and fat.

Planning your combinations at the beginning of the week can help you prepare healthy portions for the entire week. If you're eager to get your greens in as well, add a simple side salad to any of these combinations.

Combo #1
- Quinoa salad with beets and pepitas
- Sugar snap peas
- Whole strawberries and dark chocolate

Combo #2
- Avocado, cherry tomatoes, black bean, lime, cilantro salad
- Brown rice with lime
- Orange slices

Combo #3
- Greek yogurt or coconut yogurt with vegan protein powder
- Gluten-free, refined-sugar-free granola
- Fresh-sliced peaches

These recipes were adapted from food bloggers The Edgy Veg (2019) and Gathering Dreams (2021).

Protein-Packed Quinoa Salad with Beets and Pepitas

If you think it's impossible to have a delicious homemade salad without spending hours chopping and prepping in the kitchen, you're about to be proven wrong. This quinoa salad is not only jam-packed with nutritiously dense ingredients like quinoa, edamame, and spinach, it is also incredibly easy to make. Within 30 minutes, you'll have a scrumptious salad ready to eat or prepped for the days ahead. This recipe was adapted from the raw beet salad with carrot quinoa spinach recipe from Cookie + Kate (2021).

Ingredients

Salad
- ½ cup uncooked quinoa, rinsed
- 1 cup frozen organic edamame (optional)
- ⅓ cup pepitas (green pumpkin seeds)
- 1 medium raw beet, peeled and grated
- 1 medium-to-large carrot, peeled and grated
- 2 cups packed baby spinach, roughly chopped
- 1 avocado, cubed

Vinaigrette
- 3 tablespoons apple cider vinegar
- 2 tablespoons lime juice
- 2 tablespoons olive oil
- 1 tablespoon chopped fresh mint or cilantro
- 2 tablespoons honey or maple syrup or agave nectar
- ½ to 1 teaspoon Dijon mustard, to taste
- ¼ teaspoon salt
- freshly ground black pepper, to taste

Instructions

1. Prepare quinoa according to package instructions; be sure to rinse before boiling.
2. Prepare edamame according to package instructions.
3. While the quinoa and edamame are cooking, peel and grate the beets and carrots. Once completed, chop the spinach, and cube one avocado.
4. To prepare the vinaigrette, whisk together all ingredients until emulsified. Adjust ingredients to desired taste.
5. Assemble the salad: In a large bowl, combine the pepitas, cooked edamame, prepared beet(s) and/or carrot, roughly chopped spinach, cubed avocado, and cooked quinoa.
6. Finally, drizzle dressing over the mixture, and gently toss to combine. As you do so, you'll notice the quinoa turning pink from the beets. Season to taste with salt (up to an additional ¼ teaspoon) and black pepper. Serve immediately or store in the fridge for later use.

Sweet and Savory Toasts

Toast and butter—what was once a childhood classic has been reimagined into simple and satisfying meals with many more flavor combinations. Yes, you can have your bread and eat it too. You just might have to swap out your old favorite for one that's more filling to get you through your day. Choose from sweet or savory toppings, and you've got yourself a quick, easy, and often transportable meal.

Tasty Toast Combos

Combo #1
- Almond butter
- Strawberries
- Cacao nibs
- Shredded coconut

Combo #2
- Cow-milk or non-dairy ricotta (see recipe below)
- Juice and zest from one lemon

- Sea salt
- Olive oil

Combo #3
- Avocado
- Lime juice
- Salt and pepper, to taste
- Red pepper flakes (optional)

Tofu Ricotta
This is a simple plant-based, protein-packed alternative to traditional cow's milk ricotta. You can use this on toasts, in pasta dishes, or however you'd like.

Ingredients
- 1 block (14 oz.) tofu (firm or extra firm works best)
- 1–2 tablespoons nutritional yeast
- 2 teaspoons white miso paste
- ½ teaspoon garlic powder
- ½ teaspoon onion powder
- Salt and pepper, to taste
- Juice of one lemon

Equipment Needed
- Food processor or blender

Instructions
To make tofu ricotta, add crumbled tofu, miso, nutritional yeast, garlic powder, onion powder, salt, pepper, and lemon to the bowl of a food processor or blender, and blend until creamy. You may need to stop to scrape down the sides to ensure a consistency in the texture. Adjust the spices and lemon juice to your desired taste. Makes about 2 cups.

This recipe was adapted from The Simple Veganista (2022).

NOT ALL BREAD IS CREATED EQUAL

♦

White, refined flours found in your childhood loaves are not the best choice if you want to feel full, satisfied, and balance your blood sugar. For a smarter choice, choose a bread that is made with whole grains, whole wheat, sprouted grains, or a fermented variety like sourdough. Always be sure to check the nutrition labels, and avoid any added refined sugars (like cane sugar, fructose, corn syrup, etc.) or preservatives.

The best bread is made fresh daily at your local bakery or bread-maker's storefront. If you have access to fresh bread straight from the baker's oven, we recommend supporting them. Choosing a bread that is less refined and made with whole wheat, whole grains, or fermented dough will keep you fuller longer, and has more nutritional benefits like protein and fiber. If you're looking for a go-to bread that you can find at your local grocery or health food store, experiment, read the labels, and look for brands you and friends and family like. Stick to these tried-and-true brands, making sure they are packed with high-quality ingredients.

EMBRACING THE POWER OF PLANTS
ON YOUR PLATE

♦

If you have one takeaway from this chapter, we hope it's that plants have power. They fuel us, nourish us, and even have the ability to enhance our brain's functioning. Ideally, we would love for you to incorporate all of the tips and knowledge gained from this chapter but realize that this might involve drastic changes to your diet. Whenever you are ready, we encourage you to take sustainable steps toward your goals. Start simple and small. If your goal is to feel more energy, start out by eating more of the brain foods you already know and love. Want to get in a few servings of greens every day? Make it happen by adding a handful of spinach into your morning smoothie, or eating your protein of choice over a bed of greens. Looking to make healthier swaps? Determine what foods you eat daily that you can switch out with healthier options; perhaps this means exchanging your less nutritious chocolate for a higher-quality one. Whatever your long-term goals are for healthy eating, make them granular, and decide how you can work toward them on a daily basis.

The information and recipes included in this chapter are a select few out of endless options to choose from. If you are creative in the kitchen, take a leap of faith and try some of the BRAINFOOD recommendations. Or, if you're cooking-averse, consider what quick, healthy options are local to you that you can rely on in a pinch. As we noted earlier in this chapter, food should be an enjoyable experience. We know not all of our readers will opt for a plant-based diet, whether it's a matter of preference or dietary restrictions. When considering adapting your diet to be healthier and longevity-promoting, we suggest you check out Harvard's Healthy Eating Guidelines, the Mediterranean diet, and Blue Zones Food Guidelines. You might even want to try mindful eating in the spirit of the great Thich Nhat Hanh (2015). Balance is achieved when we can embrace the connection and culture that food brings while choosing healthful foods that nourish our bodies.

REFERENCES
Alsiö, Å., Nasic, S., Ljungström, L., & Jacobsson, G. (2021). Impact of obesity on outcome of severe bacterial infections. PLoS One 16(5): e0251887.
American College of Lifestyle Medicine. (2022) What is lifestyle medicine? Accessed July 25, 2022. https://www.lifestylemedicine.org/ACLM /About/What_is_Lifestyle_Medicine/ACLM/About/What_is_Lifestyle _Medicine_/Lifestyle_Medicine.aspx?hkey=26f3eb6b-8294-4a63 -83de-35d429c3bb88
Asgeirsdottir, T. L., Corman, H., Noonan, K., & Reichman, N. E. (2016). Lifecycle effects of a recession on health behaviors: boom, bust, and recovery in Iceland. Economics and Human Biology 20: 90–107.
Childs, C. E., Calder, P. C., & Miles, E. A. (2019). Diet and immune function. Nutrients 11(8): 1933.
Cookie + Kate. (2021). Build-your-own buddha bowl. Accessed April 8, 2021. https://cookieandkate.com/buddha-bowl-recipe/
Echeverría, G., Tiboni, O., Berkowitz, L., Pinto, V., Samith, B., et al. (2020). Mediterranean lifestyle to promote physical, mental, and environmental health: the case of Chile. International Journal of Environmental Research and Public Health 17(22): 8482.
Eustachio Colombo, P., Patterson, E., Lindroos, A. K., Parlesak, A., & Elinder, L. S. (2020). Sustainable and acceptable school meals through optimization analysis: an intervention study. Nutrition Journal 19(1): 1–15.
Firth, J., Marx, W., Dash, S., Carney, R., Teasdale, et al. (2019). The effects of dietary improvement on symptoms of depression and anxiety. Psychosomatic Medicine 81(3): 265–80.
Gathering Dreams. (2021). 5 awesome lunch box ideas for adults (perfect for work!). Accessed March 8, 2021. https://gatheringdreams.com/lunch-box -ideas-for-adults/

Hanh, T. N. (2015). *Mindful Eating, Mindful Life*. London: Hay House.

Hansen, J. (2013). Have you ever caught your brain buffering? Money Women and Brains, November 11, 2013. http://www.moneywomenandbrains.com/ever-caught-brain-buffering/

Harvard T. H. Chan School of Public Health. (2021). Healthy Eating Plate, March 16, 2021. https://www.hsph.harvard.edu/nutritionsource/healthy-eating-plate/

Healthy People. (2022). Access to foods that support healthy eating patterns. Office of Disease Prevention and Health Promotion Website. Last updated February 6, 2022. https://health.gov/healthypeople/priority-areas/social-determinants-health/literature-summaries/access-foods-support-healthy-dietary-patterns

Jacka, F. N., O'Neil, A., Opie, R., Itsiopoulos, C., Cotton, S., et al. (2017). A randomised controlled trial of dietary improvement for adults with major depression (the "SMILES" trial). *BMC Medicine* 15: 23. https://doi.org/10.1186/s12916-017-0791-y

Jackson, S. E., Smith, L., Firth, J., Grabovac, I., Soysal, P., et al. (2019). Is there a relationship between chocolate consumption and symptoms of depression? A cross-sectional survey of 13,626 US adults. *Depression and Anxiety* 36(10): 987–95.

Knudsen, A. K., Allebeck, P., Tollånes, M. C., Skogen, J. C., Iburg, K. M. et al. (2019). Life expectancy and disease burden in the Nordic countries: results from the Global Burden of Diseases, Injuries, and Risk Factors Study 2017. *The Lancet Public Health* 4(12): e658–e669.

Naidoo, U. (2020). *This Is Your Brain on Food: An Indispensable Guide to the Surprising Foods that Fight Depression, Anxiety, PTSD, OCD, ADHD, and More*. London: Hachette UK.

Naidoo, U. (2021). Eat to beat stress. *American Journal of Lifestyle Medicine* 15(1): 39–42.

Rawshani, A., Kjölhede, E. A., Rawshani, A., Sattar, N., Eeg-Olofsson, K., et al. (2021). Severe COVID-19 in people with type 1 and type 2 diabetes in Sweden: a nationwide retrospective cohort study. *The Lancet Regional Health–Europe* 4, 100105.

Ruland, L. (2021). What is nutritional psychiatry? For starters, it's delicious. *Bon Appétit*, June 9, 2021, https://www.bonappetit.com/story/nutritional-psychiatry

Sacks, K. (2017). The truth about all those Buddha bowls you see on Pinterest: how the Buddha bowl got its name. Epicurious, April 25, 2017. https://www.epicurious.com/expert-advice/buddha-bowl-history-recipe-article

The Edgy Veg. (2019). Easy vegan bento box ideas for lunch. August 29, 2019. https://www.theedgyveg.com/2019/08/29/easy-vegan-bento-box-ideas-for-lunch/

The Simple Veganista. (2022). Tofu ricotta. Accessed July 25, 2022. https://simple-veganista.com/tofu-ricotta/

Wagner, H. S., Ahlstrom, B., Redden, J. P., Vickers, Z., & Mann, T. (2014). The myth of comfort food. *Health Psychology* 33(12): 1552–57.

Wright, A. (2021). Interactive web tool maps food deserts. US Department of Agriculture, April 30, 2021. https://www.usda.gov/media/blog/2011/05/03/interactive-web-tool-maps-food-deserts-provides-key-data

Yeh, T. S., Yuan, C., Ascherio, A., Rosner, B. A., Willett, W. C., & Blacker, D. (2021). Long-term dietary flavonoid intake and subjective cognitive decline in US men and women. *Neurology* 97(10): e1041–e1056.

CHAPTER 6

•

Implementing Daily
Movement and Exercise

*"One day, I wasn't running late, but after I parked the car, I ran.
I ran with my heavy pink backpack and my mask on. I ran through
the eerily empty streets of New York City, and I chanted in my head,
'you can do this, you are brave.' I felt silly, ridiculous actually. I don't
know why I started running at that moment, but it helped me."*

IN THEIR OWN WORDS

I was paralyzed with fear, overcome with worry, and filled with
uncertainty. It felt like all of the security I am normally accustomed
to was gone. Like it was all crashing down around me. It was a global
pandemic, and here I was caring for COVID-19 patients, trying to learn
everything I could, and trying desperately not to bring this new devastating illness home to my family. I was trying to survive mentally and
physically.

Even though I had my husband, my friends, and my coworkers,
I somehow felt completely alone. I certainly couldn't relate to people
binge-watching *Tiger King* or having Zoom happy hours. I was scared
to get physically close to my colleagues . . . the hugs, support, laughter,
even the groans . . . it was all put on hold. I avoided the nursing station,
wheeling a computer into the hallway to chart—who knows how many
of us were infected. We needed to keep our distance. At times, I slept in
the guest room at home, terrified I was going to infect my husband. At
least one of us needed to survive to care for our children.

I was petrified, but someone had to do it. Someone had to take care of the patients; I couldn't possibly just walk away. I was needed. I am a nurse. So I kept going, even though I felt paralyzed.

Somehow I kept moving, compartmentalized, faked it . . . not just at work but at home too. I didn't want my kids to worry—there were enough changes they were going through, so I needed to be completely present for them. It was exhausting. But then, I started to learn how to cope. I began driving to work instead of taking the train because of the pandemic. I parked where I felt comfortable, but it wasn't very close to the hospital. One day, I wasn't running late, but after I parked the car, I ran. I ran with my heavy pink backpack and my mask on. I ran through the eerily empty streets of New York City, and I chanted in my head, "you can do this, you are brave." I felt silly, ridiculous actually. I don't know why I started running at that moment, but it helped me. I reminded myself that I am strong and capable and I got my blood moving. I felt a glimmer of hope and a sense of calm.

It just came about naturally; I went where I always go to feel healthy and take care of myself. I ran. Because when I run, at that moment all I am committed to is moving my body. It is so incredibly simple. I have been a runner for over 20 years. I prefer to run alone; there is no obligation to hold a conversation. I can run fast and transfer stress, anger, worry, grief, right into the pavement. I can run at a comfortable pace and just let my mind wander completely uninterrupted. I can even focus on my breathing or the beat of my music and try to be mindless.

Running is time just for me—it becomes whatever I need at that moment. I always finish with a clearer head and renewed energy. I was so overwhelmed by the flood of emotions and added tasks on my to-do list that I hadn't considered taking a run before that spontaneous dash through the streets. I was more focused on seeking information about COVID-19, disinfecting everything, planning out meaningful school activities for my children who were now home full-time from preschool, and figuring out how to get groceries and toilet paper. There were new challenges in multiple aspects of my life. Running and exercise were on a pause, now a nonessential category in my mind. There was no time for me to figure out how to manage my stress; I was just trying to survive and fulfill all of my responsibilities. But after that day, I got to work early and ran along the East River before every shift.

I realized I needed to do it for myself, to cope, to feel prepared, and to help me face the challenging day ahead. Taking care of myself made me better equipped to take care of others. I am so grateful that somehow when I forgot to turn to my main coping mechanism that somehow my body magically reminded me—just run!

Summer 2020: Alison Glorioso, BSN, BA, RN, RNC-OB, Antepartum and Labor and Delivery, New York, New York, United States

This story illustrates the power of movement and how innate it is for us as humans. Our bodies know what we need, even if we miss the first few dozen clues it gives us. Eventually, we will get the hint. In this case, running was this nurse's outlet and coping mechanism in the midst of working in America's initial epicenter of pandemic. Running allowed her to release worries, fears, and stress for however many miles, and then show up better for herself, her family, and her patients.

In this chapter, we discuss how movement is more than just a way to be fit and manage weight—it is "nature's antidepressant" and can improve mental health by way of boosting the production of neurotransmitters like serotonin. Physical activity promotes well-being through positive biological and psychological effects that affect the brain and cognitive functioning. It also plays a significant role in counteracting normal and pathological aging (Mandolesi et al., 2018). It's a way to be in our bodies and out of our heads. Unlike competitive sports, it is not about being the best player or athlete on a team. It is simply about being the best self you can be—your body and your mind in all the ways that work for you. In the words of Zen Master Thich Nhat Hanh and Lilian Cheung (2011), "When it comes to health and well-being, regular exercise is about as close to a magic potion as you can get" (149).

THE BENEFITS OF MOVEMENT
♦

The human body's capability of movement has been celebrated for thousands of years, from gladiators training in ancient Rome and Greece to monasteries teaching Tai Chi in China and the beginnings of

THE SCIENCE OF EXERCISE AND MENTAL HEALTH

Researchers are now noticing that movement is important not only for physical health and longevity, but it also can promote improved mental health. In a 2020 study of more than 150,000 participants, researchers at University College in London examined the important benefits of exercise for mental health. Findings revealed that people with low aerobic and muscular fitness were roughly twice as likely to experience depression. They were also predicted to be 60% more likely to suffer anxiety seven years after the fitness tests (Kandola et al.).

Reference
Kandola, A. A., Osborn, D., Stubbs, B., Choi, K. W., & Hayes, J. F. (2020). Individual and combined associations between cardiorespiratory fitness and grip strength with common mental disorders: a prospective cohort study in the UK Biobank. BMC Medicine 18(1): 303. https://doi.org/10.1186/s12916-020-01782-9

yoga in northern India. Since the beginning, intentional movement and physical activity have been known to benefit one's well-being. Though some forms of movement began with competitive origins, many were focused on improving the mind and body consistently over time in the form of a practice. Today, movement continues to be celebrated in the form of televised national sports league games, the Olympics, and city-wide marathon races. While witnessing movement is a beloved pastime for many, more than a quarter of the world's adult population (1.4 billion adults) are insufficiently active (World Health Organization, 2020). This is a result of a variety of factors and social determinants, from the prevalence of sedentary work to income disparities and unsafe neighborhoods.

Simply put, participating in regular exercise can improve almost every dimension of health. When moving mindfully, with considerations of injuries and health conditions, the benefits of physical exercise can be noted, literally, from head to toe. The majority of exercise research suggests that dedicating time for regular, moderately challenging physical activity, for about 30 minutes per day, will create lasting benefits to both physical and mental health. There is substantial evidence of the multifaceted benefits of physical activity, including its potential to improve health-related factors such as cardiorespiratory fitness, muscular fitness, and bone health, while reducing the risk of noncommunicable diseases such as coronary heart disease and Type 2 diabetes mellitus (Reiner et al., 2013; Ding et al., 2020).

The nature of nursing, especially bedside nursing, requires flexibility and agility—running from room to room and patient to patient—which in itself is physically laborious and elevates the heart rate in the moment. This can lead many of you to feel that a day's work is exhausting enough, and the motivation to exercise can fall to the wayside. Surveys have shown that a significant proportion of nurses are not getting enough physical activity (Kumbrija et al., 2007; Owusu-Sekyere, 2020). Some studies have found that as many as 50% to 70% of nurses were not sufficiently active (Nahm et al., 2012; Blake and Harrison, 2013). In many cases, nurses have a health-promotion role recommending the benefits of physical activity to their patients; however, the research suggests they may not be walking the talk themselves.

Physical activity and exercise are also associated with psychological and social well-being, specifically the key components of environmental mastery, self-acceptance, and autonomy. In a South African study, participants who consistently engaged in physical activity perceived themselves as more autonomous, felt a greater purpose in life, had positive relations with others, and increased their environmental mastery. They also experienced greater self-acceptance, sport competence, and conditioning than non-exercisers (Edwards et al., 2005). Using a Spanish translation of Ryff's psychological well-being scale, researchers in a recent study found that physical activity clearly influenced the psychological well-being of young adults (Granero-Jiménez et al., 2022).

Movement can be done virtually anywhere, and making the most of your physical space in pursuit of movement is a form of environmental mastery. This can be as simple as a walk around the block or doing a full yoga flow with colleagues on your unit's floor. Engaging in movement that you and your body enjoy allows self-acceptance to take place and provides a greater sense of autonomy, two crucial components of Ryff's model. In a world where broadcast and online media, distorting camera filters, and Photoshop dominate, bodies are sculpted to fit unrealistic ideals rather than societal norms. Accepting the body you live in can be challenging. Choosing to move your body out of love, gratitude, and acceptance is a radical act that deserves to be celebrated. Unlike the common association between movement and body shape and size, we want you to feel empowered and content by the choices you make in choosing the movement that best suits you. This chapter identifies various forms of movement that are beneficial and will get you up on your feet to reach the finish line of a 5K or onto a mat in a downward-facing dog pose.

Typically, the question people ask surrounding exercise is not *why* to do it, but rather *how* to get started and stay committed. The answer depends on you—your physical limitations, likes, dislikes, as well as how much time you are able to commit and when. We will discuss a few methods of goal-setting and behavior change later on in this chapter in order to help you get (and stay) moving.

EXPLORING THE MODES OF MOVEMENT

◆

Maintaining a regular exercise regime is probably simpler than you think. It does not require expensive private gyms or personal trainers—unless that works best for you—and most activities can be done at home or in your neighborhood. Whether you live alone, with family, or roommates, these can all be done solo or as a group activity. Read below to learn more about the benefits of different types of exercise.

THE SCIENCE OF ENDURANCE, STRENGTH, BALANCE, AND FLEXIBILITY

Researchers in the area of exercise science and physiology have taken an interest in determining which movements are best for human health and why. They've found that not all exercise has the same function and benefits; as a result, it may be important to move in a variety of ways. The four types of exercise that experts in the field recommend are endurance, strength, balance, and flexibility (National Institute on Aging, 2021).

Endurance activities, also known as aerobic exercise, increase breathing and heart rate and are typically done for durations longer than two minutes at a time. They are done to exert energy at a steady rate and help your body function optimally in daily activities.

(continued)

Researchers have long studied how these exercises improve heart health, lung capacity, and circulatory function (Miller et al., 1997).

Strength exercises help to build muscles for improved fitness and can improve functionality for daily activities, such as moving furniture and carrying groceries. These are also known as strength training or resistance activities. They can be done with weights or using body-weight, at home, in a gym, or outdoors.

Of the four types of exercise recommended, balance and flexibility may be the most overlooked when it comes to choices made by the novice gym-goer or road runner. Both balance and flexibility exercises are beneficial for long-term health and daily tasks, and they can even help prevent injuries (Emilio et al., 2014). Balance and flexibility tend to be lower impact, but that doesn't mean they come easily. Flexibility describes the range of motion available at a joint or group of joints. Balance describes your body's ability to navigate obstacles and resist forces that can cause injury, like falls. These movements complement endurance and strength-based workouts, giving the body the proper foundation to recover and repeat over time.

References

Emilio, E. J. M. L., Hita-Contreras, F., Jiménez-Lara, P. M., Latorre-Román, P., & Martínez-Amat, A. (2014). The association of flexibility, balance, and lumbar strength with balance ability: risk of falls in older adults. *Journal of Sports Science and Medicine* 13(2): 349.

Miller, T. D., Balady, G. J., & Fletcher, G. F. (1997). Exercise and its role in the prevention and rehabilitation of cardiovascular disease. *Annals of Behavioral Medicine* 19(3): 220–29.

National Institute on Aging. (2021). Four types of exercise can improve your health and physical ability. Last reviewed January 29, 2021. https://www.nia.nih.gov/health/four-types-exercise-can-improve-your-health-and-physical-ability.

ENDURANCE AND AEROBIC ACTIVITIES
◆

Walking

Walking is likely the easiest way possible to get around and get your body moving, and it requires nothing more than a safe path and a pair of sneakers. Whether you're making laps around a local high school track or leisurely strolling through your neighborhood, each step you take is one toward improving your health. Another perk of walking is that you can customize this time. It can be filled with mindful moments, a time to connect and be social with others, shared with an accountability partner, or an opportunity to learn something new by putting on headphones with an audiobook or podcast.

- Walking has been shown to boost immunity during flu season. People who walked at a moderate pace for 30–45 minutes a day had 43% fewer sick days and fewer upper respiratory tract infections compared to those who don't walk daily (Nieman et al., 2011).
- The benefits of walking go beyond exercise, as it can also be a way to cultivate mindfulness. A 2020 study from the University of California, San Francisco, coined the term "awe walks," referring to people's conscious awareness of the vistas and objects around them on a walk. Those who engaged in this behavior reported being more hopeful and upbeat than walkers who did not. Ultimately, researchers concluded that being mindful during exercise seems to improve their mental health (Sturm et al., 2020).

Running and Jogging

A good pair of sneakers, a plan, and a favorite playlist are all you need to be a runner. Running is the most basic form of cardiovascular activity, which means it elevates your heart with every step.

Studies have shown that running as little as 5 to 10 minutes per day at a pace of 6 miles per hour (this equates to running a 10-minute mile) can reduce the risk of a heart attack and cardiovascular diseases, while also lowering the risk of developing cancer and neurological diseases (Lee et al., 2017).

Biking

While biking does require equipment (either an outdoor or stationary bike), the benefits can be well worth the investment. Biking or cycling is considered a low-impact exercise, meaning its smooth movements are great for strengthening joints and building muscle. If running or other high-impact activity doesn't feel great for your body, especially your knees, biking may be a better bet for you and your joints.

- A recent study found that repeated maximal effort cycling with short exercise time (i.e., 4 seconds) and short recovery time (15–30 seconds) has a powerful impact on metabolic health (Satiroglu et al., 2021). Simply put, this means it's possible to work out more efficiently for a shorter period and still achieve the metabolic benefits of traditional exercise.

Dancing

One of the many perks of dancing is that it can be done anywhere, and all you need is a beat. Since the beginning of humankind, dancing has been a natural form of movement and expression across cultures. Today, we can appreciate the history of dancing and find joy sweating to songs you know and love. If freestyling isn't for you, consider joining a local dance studio or trying a Zumba class. If you'd rather not dance in person, there are many resources online, from YouTube to videos from private studios.

- Dance is an effective form of cardiovascular activity and is beneficial for balance, strength, and cognitive functioning. Neuroscience researchers believe that engaging in dance regularly may actually slow down the aging process.
- A 2017 study at the German Center for Neurodegenerative Diseases compared the impact of two types of exercise on older people: a traditional endurance training program (cycling, Nordic walking, etc.) and a mix of dance classes (jazz, line dancing, etc.). They found that both forms of exercise increased the areas of the brain that decline with age, but only dancing led to significant behavioral changes, like improved balance (Rehfeld et al., 2017).
- Dance movement therapy (DMT) is the psychotherapeutic use of movement to promote emotional, social, cognitive, and physical integration of the individual, for the purpose of improving health and well-being (American Dance Therapy Association, 2022). It has been utilized since the 1940s, when experienced dancers began to notice that this form of movement led to increased well-being and healing.
  - In a systematic review of studies, researchers at Edge Hill University in the United Kingdom found that DMT was

cited as an effective therapy for the treatment of adults with depression (Karkou et al., 2019).

- DMT might even reduce psychiatric symptoms. Latest research suggests it has significant potential as a treatment for a range of conditions and symptoms (Millman et al., 2021).

Strength-Based Movement

HIIT

High-intensity interval training, also known as HIIT, is a type of workout that packs a punch by providing many benefits in a short amount of time. It's a structured workout that consists of short periods of intense movement followed by a shorter recovery time, then back to intense movement again.

HIIT workouts are 10–30 minutes in duration and can be done with or without equipment. It is most touted for its ability to burn lots of calories and increase metabolic rate for hours after you exercise (Wingfield et al., 2015).

Strength Training and Weightlifting

If cardio is your go-to, there is increasing evidence to support the need for strength training in your weekly workout routine. Strength training is especially important for aging adults, and implementing this form of movement can help with functionality and continued independence.

- Strength training, also known as resistance training, has been linked to building lean body mass, reducing body fat, increasing bone density and bone health, as well as improving posture, strength, and stability (National Institute on Aging, 2020).
- Some examples of strength training include:
  - Bodyweight exercises like planks, push-ups, squats, and crunches
  - Resistance bands
  - Free weights (i.e., dumbbells and kettlebells)
  - Resistance machines (such as those found at your local gym)

Balance and Flexibility
Yoga

Depending on the type of yoga you choose to practice, the benefits can range from reducing stress to decreasing chronic pain. Yoga provides the opportunity to explore your body and all that it carries with it day to day by easing into asanas (postures) and releasing tension while building strength and flexibility.

- Studies have assessed the physiological impacts of yoga by measuring cortisol of participants before and after a two-week yoga intervention. Researchers found that those who practiced yoga regularly had lower serum cortisol levels, indicating reduced stress (Katuri et al., 2016).
- Types of yoga include:
  - *Vinyasa:* These yoga classes follow a sequence of poses that are moderately paced and are often considered to be "flows," with little to no stillness in the practice. Expect to be challenged and work on your strength and flexibility.
  - *Hatha:* Hatha yoga typically contains a blend of postures, breathing, and meditation, which makes it an ideal class for beginner yogis.
  - *Yin:* A slower style of yoga that is often used for active recovery from traditional yoga practice or other types of movement. Poses are held from one to five minutes to increase joint circulation and improve flexibility.
  - *Power:* Much like vinyasa, this type of class is done at a quicker pace and is meant to strengthen muscles and increase flexibility.

Disclaimer: Before beginning any new movement or exercise routine, consult your primary care provider or specialist to determine whether it is right for you. Always be sure to hydrate before and after vigorous exercise. Stop exercising immediately if you are lightheaded or feel unwell.

PAIRING MOVEMENT TO MUSIC
♦

Motivation to exercise and exercise sessions themselves are heightened and enhanced by the music that accompanies your physical activity. If you've ever taken a studio or group fitness class with loud, energizing music, bodies to your right and left, front and back, the enthusiasm is palpable and spreads through the room. No doubt, music and songs motivate you to take on your workout.

Tips for Creating a Playlist

1. *Match the music to the mood:* Include songs that go with the mood you are looking to set. Are you trying to be calm or get energized? Which songs will play best with the exercises you are doing?
2. *Consider beat-based workouts:* Popular music apps such as Apple Music or Spotify have curated playlists with songs that follow certain beats per minute. This information can be helpful in cardiovascular activities such as running or spinning, where being on the beat is one component of the work.
3. *Save the best for last:* If you tend to fatigue during the end of a workout, try to include one of your favorite songs toward the end. Saving the best for last can help give you an extra burst of energy for a strong finish to your workout.

WORLD HEALTH ORGANIZATION GUIDELINES
FOR PHYSICAL ACTIVITY
♦

The World Health Organization has issued the following guidelines for individuals aged 18–64.

1. Complete at least 150 minutes of moderate-intensity aerobic physical activity or at least 75 minutes of vigorous-intensity aerobic physical activity throughout the week. Another alternative is to do an equivalent combination of moderate- and vigorous-intensity activity.
2. Aerobic activity should be performed in bursts of at least 10 minutes' duration.

3. For additional health benefits, adults should increase their moderate-intensity aerobic physical activity to 300 minutes per week, or engage in 150 minutes of vigorous-intensity aerobic physical activity per week. Another alternative is to do an equivalent combination of moderate- and vigorous-intensity activity.
4. Muscle-strengthening activities should be done involving major muscle groups on two or more days a week.

HOW TO GET MOVING
◆

Right now, you might be wondering, "How do I get going?" In the field of behavior change, breaking down goals into small, actionable steps is best—just like we did with SMART goals in chapter 4.

When it comes to movement, there are several considerations to make before taking the first step:

1. Consider what's motivating you to move. Is it maintaining fitness, improving mental health, finding inner strength, or something else?
2. Visualize movement in your life. What does it look like? When will it happen?
3. Invite a friend, partner, family member, or coworker to be your accountability partner.

Nurses and their colleagues embraced physical activity throughout the pandemic. One group of nurses made it a point to take their lunchbreak outside, in the parking lot. Before lunch, however, they held a dance class that brought smiles and laughter. They took turns planning and leading the session and selecting the music. Even when the weather turned cold, they had their dance class outside—layered in jackets and sweaters.

REFERENCES
American Dance Therapy Association. (2022). What is dance/movement therapy? Accessed July 26, 2022. https://adta.memberclicks.net/what-is-dancemovement-therapy
Blake, H., & Harrison, C. (2013). Health behaviours and attitudes towards being role models. British Journal of Nursing 22(2): 86–94.

Ding, D., Mutrie, N., Bauman, A., Pratt, M., Hallal, P. R., & Powell, K. E. (2020). Physical activity guidelines 2020: comprehensive and inclusive recommendations to activate populations. *The Lancet* 396(10265): 1780–82.

Edwards, S. D., Ngcobo, H. S., Edwards, D. J., & Palavar, K. (2005). Exploring the relationship between physical activity, psychological well-being and physical self-perception in different exercise groups. *South African Journal for Research in Sport, Physical Education and Recreation* 27(1): 59–74.

Granero-Jiménez, J., López-Rodríguez, M. M., Dobarrio-Sanz, I., & Cortés-Rodríguez, A. E. (2022). Influence of physical exercise on psychological well-being of young adults: a quantitative study. *International Journal of Environmental Research and Public Health* 19(7): 4282.

Karkou, V., Aithal, S., Zubala, A., & Meekums, B. (2019). Effectiveness of dance movement therapy in the treatment of adults with depression: a systematic review with meta-analyses. *Frontiers in Psychology* 10: 936. https://doi.org/10.3389/fpsyg.2019.00936

Katuri, K. K., Dasari, A. B., Kurapati, S., Vinnakota, N. R., Bollepalli, A. C., & Dhulipalla, R. (2016). Association of yoga practice and serum cortisol levels in chronic periodontitis patients with stress-related anxiety and depression. *Journal of International Society of Preventive and Community Dentistry* 6(1): 7–14. https://doi.org/10.4103/2231-0762.175404

Kumbrija, S., Milaković, S. B., Jelinić, J. D., Matanić, D., Marković, B. B., & Simunović, R. (2007). Health care professionals—attitudes towards their own health. *Acta Medica Croatica: Casopis Hrvatske Akademije Medicinskih Znanosti* 61(1): 105–10.

Lee, D. C., Brellenthin, A. G., Thompson, P. D., Sui, X., Lee, I. M., & Lavie, C. J. (2017). Running as a key lifestyle medicine for longevity. *Progress in Cardiovascular Diseases* 60(1): 45–55. https://doi.org/10.1016/j.pcad.2017.03.005

Mandolesi, L., Polverino, A., Montuori, S., Foti, F., Ferraioli, G., Sorrentino, P., & Sorrentino, G. (2018). Effects of physical exercise on cognitive functioning and wellbeing: biological and psychological benefits. *Frontiers in Psychology* 9: 509.

Millman, L. M., Terhune, D. B., Hunter, E. C., & Orgs, G. (2021). Towards a neurocognitive approach to dance movement therapy for mental health: a systematic review. *Clinical Psychology and Psychotherapy* 28(1): 24–38.

Hanh, T. N., and Cheung, L. (2011). *Savor, Mindful Eating, Mindful Life*. New York: HarperOne, 149.

Nahm, E. S., Warren, J., Zhu, S., An, M., & Brown, J. (2012). Nurses' self-care behaviors related to weight and stress. *Nursing Outlook* 60(5): e23–e31.

National Institute on Aging. (2020). Real life benefits of exercise and physical activity. Accessed March 4, 2021. https://www.nia.nih.gov/health/real-life-benefits-exercise-and-physical-activity

Nieman, D. C., Henson, D. A., & Austin, M. D., & Sha, W. (2011). Upper respiratory tract infection is reduced in physically fit and active adults. *British Journal of Sports Medicine* 45: 987–92.

Owusu-Sekyere, F. (2020). Assessing the effect of physical activity and exercise on nurses' well-being. *Nursing Standard* 35(4): 45–50.

Rehfeld, K., Müller, P., Aye, N., Schmicker, M., Dordevic, M., Kaufmann, J., Hökelmann, A., & Müller, N. G. (2017). Dancing or fitness sport? The effects of two training programs on hippocampal plasticity and balance abilities in healthy seniors. *Frontiers in Human Neuroscience* 11: 305. https://doi.org /10.3389/fnhum.2017.00305

Reiner, M., Niermann, C., Jekauc, D., & Woll, A. (2013). Long-term health benefits of physical activity—a systematic review of longitudinal studies. BMC *Public Health* 13 (1): 1–9.

Satiroglu, R., Lalande, S., Hong, S., Nagel, M. J., & Coyle, E. F. (2021). Four-second power cycling training increases maximal anaerobic power, peak oxygen consumption, and total blood volume. *Medicine and Science in Sports and Exercise* 53 (12): 2536–42. https://doi.org/10.1249/ MSS.0000000000002748

Sturm, V. E., Datta, S., Roy, A., Sible, I. J., Kosik, E. L., et al. (2020). Big smile, small self: awe walks promote prosocial positive emotions in older adults. *Emotion* 22 (5): 1044–58. https://doi.org/10.1037/emo0000876

Wingfield, H. L., Smith-Ryan, A. E., Melvin, M. N., Roelofs, E. J., Trexler, E. T., Hackney, A. C., Weaver, M. A., & Ryan, E. D. (2015). The acute effect of exercise modality and nutrition manipulations on post-exercise resting energy expenditure and respiratory exchange ratio in women: a randomized trial. *Sports Medicine—Open* 1 (1): 11. https://doi.org/10.1186/s40798-015-0010-3

World Health Organization. (2020). *WHO Guidelines on Physical Activity and Sedentary Behaviour*. Geneva: World Health Organization.

CHAPTER 7

•

Embracing Nature and the Outdoors

"Group and solo riding is therapy for me. Each ride is different.
In a funeral escort, I will bring mountain smoke and share it
with other riders. Riding makes me think of my cheii [maternal
grandfather], and I pray for safety in every journey."

IN THEIR OWN WORDS

I am a member of the Navajo Nation. I am Bįįh Bitoodnii (Deer Springs Clan), born for Tábąąhá (Edge Water People); my maternal grandfather is Tł'ááshchí'i (Red Bottom People), and my paternal grandfather is Kinyaa'áanii (Towering House Clan).

I've had a busy few years—work, graduate school for my family nurse practitioner (FNP), and my FNP clinicals. I had surgery on September 23. It's definitely been a continual challenge over the past two years. I lost my mom to pancreatic cancer January 3, 2021, and then my uncle four weeks later, along with a few cousins and extended family members to COVID and, most recently, another uncle in June.

The Navajo Nation has been ravaged by COVID-19. In May 2020, it reported the highest per capita infection rate in the United States. Since the beginning of the pandemic, the Navajo Nation has seen more than 74,000 cases and more than 1,500 deaths. Experts attribute the spread to the prevalence of multigenerational housing and poor sanitation infrastructure—many homes lack running water. Like medical centers across the country, local hospitals across the Navajo Nation experienced shortages of personal protective gear.

My coworkers and friends, Cheryl and Corrina, were two members of the Navajo Nation who died after contracting the coronavirus. They were almost joined at the hip. They lived together with their mother and helped raise each other's children. The sisters shared an office at Tuba City Regional Health Care in Arizona. Cheryl conducted reviews to make sure patients were receiving adequate care. Corrina was a social worker. Their desks were just inches apart.

The sisters succumbed to COVID-19 a few weeks apart, at ages 40 and 44. We were coworkers and close friends. I used to sit in Cheryl's chair. Corrina and I would just start talking, catch up on what we did during our time off, laugh and joke. It's been difficult to visit their old office area. Healing takes time.

Cheryl and Corrina are among hundreds of frontline health care workers who have died of COVID-19. *The Guardian* and *Kaiser Health News* are investigating more than 1,000 of these workers' deaths in the Lost on the Frontline Project.

Many times, during school, I thought about stopping, but then I looked back at what I'd already put into it. I told myself, "You've already invested so much. You've got to want it." Then I got COVID, in July of 2020, and was in the hospital for a few days. I withdrew from my classes; I was worried I wouldn't be able to finish my work. That night, still in the hospital, I looked at my assignments and told myself, "I'm going to beat COVID." I called the school and got reinstated. I got my assignments done after they gave me extra time, and I was able to finish everything by the time the semester ended.

The last two and a half years in FNP school have been hard, especially trying to complete clinicals during a pandemic. My family and friends who became family helped me out; my mother helped me until she got sick. I miss my mom, but I try to stay focused on school and my work. My clinicals and assignments keep me busy. Nursing is a passion; you have to want to do it, and it will be harder than you think. Passion carries you through the good and bad, especially the bad.

My other passion is riding my motorcycle on Diné Bikéyah (the Navajo lands). I am not only a founding member of Riders4Warriors, but I also ride. We ride for veterans and first responders; there are many honor riders on the reservation. As honor riders, we ride for different events like benefits, welcoming veterans home, and funeral escorts. My *cheii* [maternal grandfather] was an army veteran of the invasion of Normandy during World War II, and my father was a Korean War army veteran as well as a retired Navajo Nation police officer. Many of my family members are in the service now. Recently Riders4Warriors organized a fundraising ride for a young boy with leukemia, son of a Navajo Nation police officer. Last month, that 10-year-old rang the bell at Phoenix Children's Hospital, symbolic of what he and those who love and cared for him accomplished. He is now cancer-free.

Group riding is therapy for me. Each ride is different. In a funeral escort, I will bring mountain smoke and share it with other riders. Riding makes me think of my *cheii* and many more veterans and first responders. I pray for safety in every journey.

Sometimes I go alone. It gives me peace and tranquility. I just ride until...

You go as far as you can go.

Sometimes I'm gone for one or two days. It allows me to think about things. I ask myself, "Are my goals working out? Maybe I need to do this better. How can I do this better?" I have a Siberian husky. He's a form of therapy for me too.

Hunting and fishing are therapies as well. I enjoy getting out in the woods with family and friends to embrace the serenity, elements, and nature. Tossing a line and enjoying the scenic view is priceless. Identifying ways for therapy is essential to have a life-long career as a nurse.

October 11, 2021, Indigenous People's Day: Lynette Goldtooth, MSN, NREMT-P, RN, SANE, Family Nurse Practitioner, Navajo Nation, Tuba City, Arizona, United States

Consider for a moment how modern-day luxuries and necessities make our lives safer and more comfortable. Air conditioning, computers, even plumbing, while convenient, also make it easy to stay indoors. Depending where you live or work, whether hospitals, schools, or high-rise buildings, opening windows for a breath of fresh air may be a rarity or even impossible. Is there a price we might pay for spending most of our days and nights within four walls? The COVID-19 pandemic gave us the answer, loud and clear. A wake-up call was broadcast all over the world through a new vocabulary—lockdown, self-isolation, quarantine, stay at home. Buzzwords we wished we'd never heard. No one knows this reality better than nurses. Many of you, depending on where you worked, were cordoned off from other units in your hospital, and most of you were isolated from friends and family. In some ways, going outside became your salvation—walking or running to work, lunch in the parking lot with friends, and standing on a patch of grass, or anything green, became your goal. You felt better. Embracing nature and being outdoors became the new prescriptions for health and well-being.

Nature, green spaces, blue spaces, biophilia, ecopsychology, and ecotherapy. Words that once seemed unfamiliar and intriguing are now commonplace in a field that is growing by leaps and bounds. A field that has relevance for our health and well-being. This chapter will open your eyes to the many dimensions of nature and ecopsychology. By the end of this chapter, you will ultimately learn more about your relationship with nature and yourself, as we prescribe a daily dose of nature for your health.

But first, let's go over some definitions. While we all have a clear understanding of nature, or the flora and fauna of the earth, green spaces are a bit more challenging to define. Taylor and Hochuli (2017) confirm there is a lack of consensus on the definition of green spaces. Most authors agree that forests, landscapes, wilderness areas, farms, and gardens are green spaces, as are vegetation in cities, parks, and even backyards. Blue spaces are defined as visible water such as coastal waters, rivers, ponds, lakes, canals, and even fountains. These bodies of water can be natural or human-made. They are accessible to human beings, either to be in, on, or near the water, or being able to see or hear it. The term "biophilia," from a Greek word meaning "love of life and the living world," was first proposed by the American biologist E. O. Wilson. His theory states that there is a genetically based, fundamental human need to affiliate with life and lifelike processes. According to Sempik and Bragg (2013), green care centers are interventions that use plants, animals, and natural environments with the goal of improving health and well-being. Green care is not an informal encounter with nature but a structured and planned treatment approach. Some organizations emphasize that green care is for those with defined social or medical needs, and treatment is tailored to each client's unique situation.

The definition and scope of ecopsychology have evolved over the past 50 years, with Robert Greenway (1995) first defining ecopsychology as a search for language to describe the human–nature relationship. Ecopsychology allows us the opportunity to better understand that relationship from the vantage point of multiple disciplines, such as ecology, psychology, anthropology, and philosophy. He also explores the role that humanity has in the degradation of planet earth. Years later, in his book *The Voice of the Earth*, Roszak broadly defined ecopsychology as the blending of ecology and psychology as well as the skillful integration of ecological theories to the practice of psychotherapy.

Clinicians Buzzell and Chalquist (2009) describe ecotherapy as an umbrella term for nature-based interventions that promote physical and psychological healing. Ecotherapy is a relatively new concept in this field but recognizes the essential role of nature and the human–nature relationship in our lives. Built on current scientific evidence as well as Indigenous insights, ecotherapy reinforces the idea that people are intimately connected to and surrounded by nature; we cannot separate the two.

Some authors suggest that we divide ecotherapy into two types: (1) ecotherapy as "applied ecopsychology," and (2) ecotherapy as "green care" (Hasbach, 2012). Applied ecopsychology explores the intimate relationship between humans and nature, a theory pioneered through Cohen's (2003) research on people and natural systems more than 50 years ago. Applied ecopsychology proposes that both the degradation of the earth's environment and the human conditions of isolation, stress, and dysfunction emanate from our fundamental denial of our relationship to nature. When we reconnect with nature, authentic nature, we have the potential of reversing those disorders.

Trigwell et al. (2014) suggest that those who feel more connected with nature experience greater psychological functioning, specifically the dimensions of well-being modeled by Carol Ryff (2021). In one study of more than 600 students, those who scored high on nature connectedness also measured high on subjective well-being. Other researchers (Cervinka et al., 2012; Zelenski and Nisbet, 2014) have found similar results with a positive relationship between nature connectedness and Ryff's well-being dimensions of personal growth, autonomy, and purpose in life. Research in this area points to a consensus that being emotionally connected to nature is meaningful and promotes a sense of well-being (Ryff, 2022).

The Center for Greater Good at the University of California, Berkeley, reports that hundreds of studies have shown that living in or near a natural setting can have a positive impact on our thinking, well-being, emotions, and social relationships. Even looking at photographs of nature or watching nature documentaries can release emotions that are positive, rewarding, and calming. These in turn help us build increased openness and connections with others, and ultimately resilience. Let's take a look at the research that supports nature-based therapies.

THE SCIENCE OF NATURE'S EFFECT ON WELL-BEING

In her book *The Nature Fix* (2017), Florence Williams describes how nature makes us happier, healthier, and even more creative. Hundreds of studies support her premise that nature has an impact on our health and well-being.

Exposure to nature has distinctive benefits. Early researchers found that natural settings allowed escape from closed indoor environments and the state of human exhaustion (Kaplan, 2001). Beaches, mountains, lakes, and forests became ideal places to restore attention, allowing focus and concentration upon returning to daily lives. Research continues to grow, confirming that finding respite in nature can help you be much more effective in your day-to-day job. Natural environments not only help to relieve stress but can also prevent it.

Ming Kuo (2015) has identified 21 "pathways" that link nature and human health. The pathways include environmental factors, physiological and psychological states, and behaviors or conditions, each of which has been empirically tied to nature and has implications for specific physical and mental health outcomes. Enhanced immune function, according to Kuo (2015), is the central/key pathway.

Dutch environmental psychologist Agnes Van den Berg (2017) suggests that the natural environment is a central component of interacting with nature, and that green space may promote health. The available evidence suggests three main pathways that explain how interacting with nature can promote health and well-being. The first regulates immunological and physiological (stress) responses; the second enhances psychological states like mood, self-esteem, vitality, and attention; and the third facilitates health-promoting behaviors such as exercise and social contacts.

Living near green spaces has its own set of rewards (Wood et al., 2017). A four-year study of Australian city dwellers found that there was a lower cumulative incidence of loneliness among those who had green space within 1,600 meters, or about a mile, of their homes (Astell-Burt et al., 2022). This correlation was especially significant for people who lived alone.

Williams and Harvey (2001) also studied wilderness programs and settings and found that forests and mountains can generate a moment of transcendence. The fascination and novelty that these places instill in people ultimately adds to spiritual fulfillment.

References

Astell-Burt, T., Hartig, T., Eckermann, S., Nieuwenhuijsen, M., McMunn, A., Frumkin, H., & Feng, X. (2022). More green, less lonely? A longitudinal cohort study. *International Journal of Epidemiology* 51(1): 99–110.

Kaplan, S. (2001). Meditation, restoration, and the management of mental fatigue. *Environment and Behavior* 33(4): 480–506.

Kuo, M. (2015). How might contact with nature promote human health? Promising mechanisms and a possible central pathway. *Frontiers in Psychology* 6: 1093.

Van den Berg, A. E. (2017). From green space to green prescriptions: challenges and opportunities for research and practice. *Frontiers in Psychology* 8: 268.

Williams, F. (2017). *The Nature Fix: Why Nature Makes Us Happier, Healthier, and More Creative.* New York: W. W. Norton.

Williams, K., & Harvey, D. (2001). Transcendent experience in forest environments. *Journal of Environmental Psychology* 21(3): 249–60.

Wood, L., Hooper, P., Foster, S., & Bull, F. (2017). Public green spaces and positive mental health–investigating the relationship between access, quantity and types of parks and mental wellbeing. *Health and Place* 48: 63–71.

Since the early 1800s, park and landscape designers have known that these green spaces are restorative to the human spirit, often citing their refreshing rest and reinvigorating nature (Olmsted, 1881). Restorative environments (Kaplan, 1995) take us away from the stresses of our daily lives, fascinate us, take us to a new world, and surround us with a sense of belonging. American president Theodore Roosevelt inspired the creation of the US National Park System after the deaths of his mother and wife, when he found that the only way he could heal from his loss was by spending time in nature. Why do we respond to nature and natural settings with a sense of calm and relaxation? There is a large body of research that supports several theories. The first, stress reduction theory, contends that the first reaction people have when in a natural environment is not cognitive, but emotional.

Even urban settings and gardens have an impact on one's functioning. A cross-cultural study of Canada and Japan found that different garden styles, such as a natural landscape or a Japanese garden, could have significant psychological, emotional, and healing values for people (Elsadek et al., 2018). A garden can bring relaxation and calm or increase one's visual attention. Viewing green spaces from a window can significantly lead to better mental health and psychological well-being for urban-dwellers (Elsadek et al., 2020). There was a significant increase in the words the participants used to describe their experience, such as "comfortable," as well as an improvement in their moods.

The healing power of nature and the outdoors has been documented for decades in poetry and prose alike, and just now is beginning to receive some real attention in the health care field, particularly in the years following the coronavirus pandemic. Embracing the outdoors has been found to positively affect human health in major ways. Researchers and experts use the term "green spaces" to describe any area with trees, parks, and gardens. Biophilic design and added green spaces are beginning to be applied to hospital campuses (Totaforti, 2018), providing patients and providers with a natural space that is free from illness.

THE SCIENCE OF GREEN SPACES

Green spaces can be beneficial to health in various contexts. In hospital settings, patients in rooms with views of nature or green space, rather than a painting or blank wall, had significantly improved health outcomes, including hospital costs. In a study examining cortisol, a marker for stress in the body, results indicated that people living in neighborhoods with tree canopy, gardens, and parks had less cortisol in their saliva than those who did not, which remained significant with controls for socioeconomic conditions (Beyer et al., 2014).

Evidence supporting the beneficial effects of nature continues to mount. When people spend time in forests, there is a positive effect on their blood pressure and immune function (Peterfalvi et al., 2021). We feel less pain when we are outside (Diette et al., 2003). People who live in communities closer to green spaces have a lower prevalence of disease, after controlling for a range of socioeconomic factors (Maas et al., 2009). Walking and exercising in a garden or park revitalize us (Thompson Coon et al., 2011), relieve our stress (Van den Berg and Custers, 2011), and restore our attention (Berman et al., 2012).

These studies indicate what most of us innately know—getting outside is a good thing, and being a witness to nature has significant positive effects on our health outcomes and stress levels.

References

Berman, M. G., Kross, E., Krpan, K. M., Askren, M. K., Burson, A., Deldin, P. J., Kapla, S., Sherdell, L., Gotlib, I. H., & Jonides, J. (2012). Interacting with nature improves cognition and affect for individuals with depression. *Journal of Affective Disorders* 140(3): 300–305.

Beyer, K. M., Kaltenbach, A., Szabo, A., Bogar, S., Nieto, F. J., & Malecki, K. M. (2014). Exposure to neighborhood green space and mental health: evidence from the survey of the health of Wisconsin. *International Journal of Environmental Research and Public Health* 11(3): 3453–72.

Diette, G. B., Lechtzin, N., Haponik, E., Devrotes, A., & Rubin, H. R. (2003). Distraction therapy with nature sights and sounds reduces pain during flexible bronchoscopy: a complementary approach to routine analgesia. *Chest* 123(3): 941–48.

Maas, J., Verheij, R. A., de Vries, S., Spreeuwenberg, P., Schellevis, F. G., & Groenewegen, P. P. (2009). Morbidity is related to a green living environment. *Journal of Epidemiology and Community Health* 63(12): 967–73.

Peterfalvi, A., Meggyes, M., Makszin, L., Farkas, N., Miko, E., Miseta, A., & Szereday, L. (2021). Forest bathing always makes sense: blood pressure-lowering and immune system-balancing effects in late spring and winter in central Europe. *International Journal of Environmental Research and Public Health*. 18(4): 2067.

Thompson Coon, J., Boddy, K., Stein, K., Whear, R., Barton, J., & Depledge, M. H. (2011). Does participating in physical activity in outdoor natural environments have a greater effect on physical and mental wellbeing than physical activity indoors? A systematic review. *Environmental Science and Technology* 45(5): 1761–72.

Van den Berg, A. E., & Custers, M. H. (2011). Gardening promotes neuroendocrine and affective restoration from stress. *Journal of Health Psychology* 16(1): 3–11.

WHAT WE CAN LEARN FROM LEADERS
IN THIS MOVEMENT
•

Now, let's take a look at the wide range of nature therapies and interventions based in natural settings. Holistic health care highlights treating individuals as a whole by meeting the full spectrum of their emotional, social, and spiritual needs. Naturopathy is based on the theory that human beings can be healed without medication and treats disease with natural healing modalities such as diet, exercise, massage, and herbs. Shinrin-yoku, or forest bathing, enhances physical and psychological well-being by taking in and absorbing the sensory experience of the forest atmosphere. Other therapies can include animals. Equine-assisted therapy or therapy dogs are especially helpful for people with anxiety disorders or depression. Nature meditation, or restoration skills training, and mindful awareness focus on the sensory experience of the natural world through sight, sound, touch, and smell. Social and therapeutic horticulture is based on the propagation of plants and plant-related activities such as gardening. Agrotherapy, or care farming, has its foundation in agriculture and provides opportunities for optimizing healing, mental health, grieving, and social relationships. Wilderness programs have long been used for adolescents and veterans struggling to transcend barriers to successful and healthy transitions in their lives.

Organizations that emphasize the importance of prescribing a dose of nature or prescribe physical activity in parks can be found worldwide. Program goals include the prevention and treatment of chronic disease by promoting wellness strategies in the natural world. In the United Kingdom, a dose of nature prescription is a 10-week program that introduces participants to the mental health benefits of nature. And there are many more (Chatterjee et al., 2018).

Perceiving and utilizing nature as medicine is a growing movement, and many experts are on board with these initiatives, merging collaborations between industries and roles, including the outdoor industry, health care, policy makers, and conservation advocates. Park Rx is an organization based in the United States that is spearheading the initiative to have health care providers prescribe going to parks, and their website includes a tool to find one near you. Growing research links being outdoors to improved mental health, better cognitive development, more regulated blood sugar control in diabetics, and decreases in hypertension. Plus, spending time outdoors is linked to being more physically active, which can lower rates of obesity and subsequent health issues.

Researchers and leaders in the field of nature-based interventions suggest that we look at the human-nature-based approach as an alternative treatment, not as an add-on to existing, perhaps more traditional treatment methods (Lord and Coffey, 2021). Health care organizations and institutions may be well served to incorporate the nature connection and not rely solely on the medical model as the dominant treatment framework. As nurses, such interventions will serve us and our patients well.

We must look beyond simply inserting or adding nature into health and well-being interventions. Instead, we can learn and practice new and essential approaches learned from non-Western narratives, cultures, and communities (Wilson, 1996).

FOREST BATHING

◆

If you've ever gone for a leisurely stroll with fresh blossoms and bright green foliage all around you, you've likely felt a sense of bliss from this sensory experience in nature. Immersing yourself in the sights, scents, and sounds of nature in this way is called Shinrin-yoku, or forest bathing. This term emerged in the 1980s in Japan, once the physiological and psychological benefits of this practice began to be more widely recognized. Its popularity is growing, along with research, to be a form of ecotherapy. Studies that have examined benefits of this practice all point to similar findings, including a reduction of stress (Carrus et al., 2017). Further studies (Li, 2018) have revealed that the color green alone promotes calmness and relaxation, further adding to the sensory experience that is forest bathing.

IN THEIR OWN WORDS

"For various reasons, I tended to ride my bike to the morning nursing shift for a 7 am clock-in; a beautiful experience on a sunny June morning,

quite the opposite in a damp Welsh January... I studied a map and decided
I would seek the daydream wilderness feeling during this space between,
this transit space; I would re-wild my commute."

The image of a vast wilderness frequently fills my daydreams; I imagine wandering for days, seeing what is behind the next ridge or forest, following serendipity and impulse rather than a schedule. It's fair to say this is hard to reconcile with the life of a nurse. The duty rota (roster of tasks) fills my diary for months into the future; and anyway, it is rarely compatible with the responsibilities of family life. This is before I even start unpacking the logic of the masculine colonizer implicit in these notions of wilderness; ideas that no doubt rooted in my formative boyhood mind many years ago.

So, this impasse left me to work out how those feelings of wild wandering (because it is all about feelings isn't it... let's park up the cognition for now) could be satiated in the space between the ward and the school gate (pickup typically followed the early shift). I reflected on this space between, this transit space, this time of movement. What was the purpose of this frequent, but brief, episode in my working week? It could be about unhelpful rumination on the shift to come, or the shift just completed. On reflection, it often was: We nurses carry some complex and conflicted things in our heads!

For various reasons, I tended to ride my bike to the morning nursing shift for a 7 am clock-in; a beautiful experience on a sunny June morning, quite the opposite in a damp Welsh January. The temptation was to put something distracting on my headphones and stare at my front wheel while I grinded up the hill to my shift. I should say, the hospital in question is on a big hill about 400 feet above sea level; the views are great, but the leg burn on a bike is not so!

I studied a map and decided I would seek the daydream wilderness feeling during this space between, this transit space; I would re-wild my commute.

This led to a daily detour and frequently a mud-splattered nurse at clock-in.

My detour was through a local woodland that this edge of the town is blessed with. I swapped to a mountain bike, left the straight tarmac roads, and found uneven trails winding between the trees. Due to the

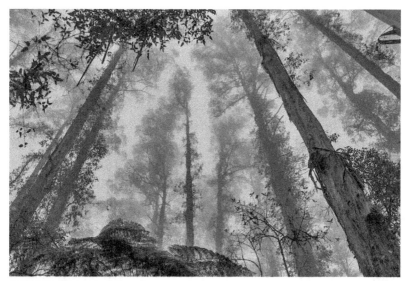

By Phoebe Strafford on Unsplash

topography, there are spaces in these woods where the sounds of the city are lost, and all that can be heard is the birdsong and the river racing its way from the moor at the top of the woods to the sea at the bottom. A hundred years ago, this area was a hive of industrial activity; I love the trees growing out of the abandoned brick factory, the wooded ridges made by a quarry, the gated-over mine shafts: in these woods, it feels like clock time is mocked as nature slowly takes over again. Perspective.

Time was tight on these commutes, and the clock-in machine was taunting me at the top of the hill (or the school bell at the bottom), but I would try to stop momentarily in one of these secluded spaces, take my helmet off, breathe deeply, watch, smell, listen. A moment of mindfulness. There was also refuge in the movement; no headphones needed here, the trail would hold my concentration as I furiously pedaled, zig-zagged between trees, jumped obstacles, ducked under low branches, mud-splattered in winter, dusty in summer. There was no rumination possible on this re-wilding commute, but there was definitely a visceral reflective practice.

October 7, 2021: Ed Lord, RMN BA(Hons), MSc, PhD, Lecturer in Mental Health Nursing, Swansea University, Swansea, Wales, United Kingdom

WAYS TO CONNECT WITH NATURE
♦

Suzi Tarrant, a clinical psychologist and ecotherapist in Wales, United Kingdom, incorporates nature and the outdoors into her practice. In addition to her work as director of Reconnect in Nature in Wales, she is head of the Staff Psychological Wellbeing Service for Hywel Dda University Health Board, National Health Service in West Wales; she promotes organizational health and staff well-being. Here she shares some of her strategies with us. Be sure to visit her website (www.suzi tarrant.com) and follow her on Instagram (@ecotherapy_wales) for a daily dose of the great outdoors. Tarrant notes that many suggestions are likely to be outside of working hours, affording a much-needed break. But she emphasizes that clinicians must also take rest and recovery breaks *during* their working hours. This is essential to maintain engagement, support well-being, and ensure effective performance and patient care. Supporting the culture of taking breaks, which she describes as a "massive and ongoing project," as well as the provision of appropriate indoor and outdoor spaces in which breaks can happen is essential for a healthy workplace. She notes that competing priorities alongside limited physical space requires much work and a creative approach. You'll notice that these strategies are not focused on or tasked to a single individual, the nurse, but require a system-wide commitment and effort to change the culture of the workplace at all levels. Here are some of her suggestions:

- Facilitate/urge/encourage administrations and systems to release staff for necessary breaks, considering coverage during shifts and accommodating changing staffing numbers. Because many of the wards are below minimal staffing levels already, Tarrant is focused on coming together to bring even a small amount of capacity within teams, so that each can take a break in turn.

- Support the culture of taking breaks during each working shift, and raise awareness of how this promotes patient and staff safety, outcomes, and experience as well as helps to sustain staff engagement and well-being. This work can take place in different ways, including leadership development, briefings and discussion at senior levels, consistent messaging for staff, role modeling, and more.

- Evaluate existing staff rest areas and accessible outdoor spaces for rest and recovery. Build a program for improving the quality of these areas and creating more, with a focus on collaboration and co-design, and for bringing in as many biophilic elements as possible.
- Raise awareness of how to connect with nature and the natural environment as an important way of restoring attention and having restorative breaks, and how we can do this during working hours.
- Provide guidance for staff around taking mini nature breaks:
  - Identify where in the working environment there may be a good view of nature through a window, or where there might be a lovely piece of nature-based art or a photograph of a landscape or natural environment. Spend a few moments to take in and absorb that view, do some deep breathing or grounding exercises, appreciating the beauty of what you see, noticing what you enjoy.
  - Make use of television and computer screens with nature films, views, and sounds where views of or access to nature is limited or not possible. Such strategies have already been shown to have significant impacts on patients and staff in intensive treatment units and intensive care units.
  - Provide resources and/or brief training sessions for staff to be confident to undertake their own guided nature-based relaxation break—whether 30 seconds or 3 minutes—drawing attention to the research on micro-breaks, short and informal respite activities, and the impact on directed attention fatigue (Kim et al., 2017; Wang et al., 2021).
  - Use all the senses for nature-based recovery—sound, smell, and touch—and advertise and demonstrate these resources so that staff can choose what best suits their interests and needs.
  - Encourage staff to share their experiences with each other of successfully using the resources to help create a culture in which it is seen as beneficial to stop and pause and to support nature connectedness.

Below are more strategies that you can use as an individual or in small groups outside of work. Consider making these nature stops on your way home, or maybe even before work.

- Go for a walk in a nearby park or forest. Use your senses to guide you—take in the sights, sounds, and smells of your surroundings. Sit in the grass with a book, listen to music, or plan a picnic (or even a meeting) with friends or colleagues.
- Forest bathe. Get out into your local woods and soak up all the green foliage you can get.
- Garden, even if it means tending a few herb plants on your windowsill. Working in nature in this way takes time and patience, but the outcome is twofold: you harvest a crop of your own and nurture yourself as well.
- Plan a trip, a short excursion, or even a quick stop after work at a green or blue space—a park, stream, or farm. Whether you're taking a day hike or planning an entire cross-country road trip, choose to make witnessing and embracing nature the main attraction.
- Create a green space inside and outside the walls of your home. Inside, you can gather potted plants that not only clean the air but also add beauty to your space. Carve out space for growing your own green—a backyard, balcony, or windowsill—and get your hands dirty, dig deep, and plant whatever flowers, trees, and shrubs make your space feel like an oasis.
- Follow a guided meditation that can be practiced outdoors or includes nature imagery, allowing your mind to find nature within you.

PUTTING IT INTO PRACTICE

A Chill in the Air and Gratitude in Your Heart

Goal: To bring a mindfulness practice to the outdoors

Time: As long as you need, as short as a 5-minute walk during a break, a longer walk on a day off, or walking home after work

This is a wonderful mindfulness practice for outdoors ... even when it's cold! You may be heading home from work and decide to walk, or you might need a bit of time after work to process the day or release stress. Perhaps it's a bit colder than usual; maybe snowflakes are beginning to drift from the sky. But you have a scarf, mittens, and a heavy jacket. First, make sure you are zipped, buttoned, and ready to go. Then take a moment to pause before opening the door and stepping outside.

This practice focuses on colder weather, but it can be adapted for any season, sun or rain. Try this when you walk home from work or during your lunch break. Yes, even a break. Put the meditation on your phone, written or recorded. Record yourself saying the words below, and keep the audio track on your phone.

- Turn your attention from the parts of your body that are cold (perhaps your hands, the top of your head, or your feet if your socks aren't thick enough) to an area that feels warm.
- If you're wearing layers, a cozy sweater, turtleneck, or a warm jacket, focus your attention here.
- What does this warmth feel like? Examine the sensations of your body as the warmth emanates from within you. How does the warmth feel? What do you notice about it? Really study the sensations of this area of your body that is warm.
- Now take a moment to be grateful for your warm shirt, sweater, or jacket and to be grateful for yourself for putting it on this morning.
- Now look up and ignite your sense of sight. What do you notice about the trees in your field of vision? If it's still fall, are the leaves turning colors? Do you see decorations around you, or architectural details like stone carvings or ornate balconies you might normally overlook? Can you admire the beauty of any and all nature around you and the craftsmanship of the buildings in your field of vision?
- Look down for a moment. Are you walking on leaves just fallen from trees around you? Or snow and ice? Or do you see footprints in the snow or on patches of ice?
- What are all the colors you see around you? Are there different shades of green or brown, white, or gray? Notice how light affects the details of a building or a tree near you. Take a moment to be

(continued)

grateful for all the colors in your environment and for your good fortune to notice and admire all the shades of the colors around you.

▸ Now turn on your sense of smell. Can you detect the aroma of logs burning in a fireplace from a nearby home? Pretzels or chestnuts for sale on a street corner? Coffee from a cafe you're passing by? Take a moment to be grateful for all the delicious smells in your environment.

▸ Now go back to your sense of feeling. What does your warm clothing feel like on your body? What does the ground feel like under your shoes? What do your shoes feel like on your feet? Let gratitude rise within you for sidewalks that are smooth and safe to walk on, for gravity, and for everything that makes it possible for us to easily walk down the street.

▸ Continue lighting up your senses and circling between these and the feeling of warmth wherever you feel it in your body.

You can do this practice for 5 minutes or 30—and as you continue to practice it, you will find it shifts your mindset toward gratitude for what you have, rather than disappointment for what you don't, or the feeling of anger after a difficult day at work. Enjoy and be grateful that you can shift your attention so easily—and whenever you need to.

This exercise is adapted from a meditation by Dina Kaplan (2017), with permission. See Kaplan's The Path website at https://www.thepath.com.

Finally, meditating in nature will double the benefit. The Insight Timer app has a number of guided practices that center on the ocean, fields, and mountains (https://insighttimer.com/meditation-topics/naturalenvironment). And think about the words of John Muir (1909), as meaningful today as they were more than 100 years ago:

Walk away quietly in any direction and taste the freedom of the mountaineer. Camp out among the grasses and gentians of glacial meadows, in craggy garden nooks full of nature's darlings. Climb the mountains and get their good tidings, Nature's peace will flow into you as sunshine flows into trees. The winds will blow their own freshness into you and the storms their energy, while cares will drop off like autumn leaves. As age comes on, one source of enjoyment after another is closed, but nature's sources never fail. (56)

REFERENCES

Buzzell, L., & Chalquist, C. (2009). *Ecotherapy: Healing with Nature in Mind*. San Francisco: Sierra Club.

Carrus, G., Dadvand, P., & Sanesi, G. (2017). The role and value of urban forests and green infrastructure in promoting human health and wellbeing. In: Pearlmutter D., et al., eds. *The Urban Forest: Cultivating Green Infrastructure for People and the Environment*. Cham, Switzerland: Springer, 217–30.

Cervinka, R., Roderer, K., & Hefler, E. (2012). Are nature lovers happy? On various indicators of well-being and connectedness with nature. *Journal of Health Psychology* 17: 379–88.

Chatterjee, H. J., Camic, P. M., Lockyer, B., & Thomson, L. J. (2018). Non-clinical community interventions: a systematised review of social prescribing schemes. *Arts and Health* 10(2): 97–123.

Cohen, M. J. (2003). *The Web of Life Imperative: Regenerative Ecopsychology Techniques That Help People Think in Balance with Natural Systems*. Bloomington, IN: Trafford.

Elsadek, M., Sun, M., Sugiyama, R., & Fujii E. (2018). Cross-cultural comparison of physiological and psychological responses to different garden styles. *Urban Forestry and Urban Greening* 38: 74–83. https://doi.org/10.1016/j.ufug .2018.11.007

Elsadek, M., Liu, B., & Xie, J. (2020). Window view and relaxation: viewing green space from a high-rise estate improves urban dwellers' wellbeing. *Urban Forestry and Urban Greening* 55: 126846.

Greenway, R. (1995). The wilderness effect and ecopsychology. In: T. Roszak, M. E. Gomes, & A. D. Kanner. *Ecopsychology: Restoring the Earth, Healing the Mind*. San Francisco: Sierra Club, 122–35.

Hasbach, P. H. (2012). Ecotherapy. In: P. H. Kahn Jr. & P. H. Hasbach, eds. *Ecopsychology: Science, Totems, and the Technological Species*. Boston: Massachusetts Institute of Technology Press, 115–40.

Kaplan, D. (2017). Meditation for gratitude (and cold weather). *ForbesWomen*, November 26, 2017. https://www.forbes.com/sites/dinakaplan/2017/11/26 /meditation-for-gratitude-and-cold-weather/?sh=795a7c4270db

Kaplan, S. (1995). The restorative benefits of nature: toward an integrative framework. *Journal of Environmental Psychology* 15(3): 169–82.

Kim, S., Park, Y., & Niu, Q. (2017). Micro-break activities at work to recover from daily work demands. *Journal of Organizational Behavior* 38(1): 28–44. https://doi.org/10.1002/job.2109

Li, Q. (2018). *Forest Bathing: How Trees Can Help You Find Health and Happiness*. London: Penguin.

Lord, E., & Coffey, M. (2021). Identifying and resisting the technological drift: green space, blue space and ecotherapy. *Social Theory and Health*, 19(1): 110–25.

Muir, J. (1909). *Our National Parks*. Boston: Houghton Mifflin.

Olmsted, F. L. (1881). *A Consideration of the Justifying Value of a Public Park*. Boston: Tolman & White.

Roszak, T. (2001). *The Voice of the Earth: An Exploration of Ecopsychology*. Newburyport, MA: Red Wheel / Weiser.

Ryff, C. D. (2021). Spirituality and well-being: theory, science, and the nature connection. *Religions* 12(11): 914.

Ryff, C. D. (2022). Positive psychology: looking back and looking forward. *Frontiers in Psychology* 13: 1–17.

Sempik, J., and Bragg, R. (2013). "Green care: origins and activities." In: Gallis, C., ed. *Green Care: For Human Therapy, Social Innovation, Rural Economy, and Education*. New York: NOVA Science, 11–32.

Sempik, J., & Bragg, R. (2016). Green care: nature-based interventions for vulnerable people. In: J. Barton, R. Bragg, C. Wood, J. Pretty, eds. *Green Exercise*. Boca Raton, FL: Routledge, 116–29.

Taylor, L., and Hochuli, D. F. (2017). Defining greenspace: multiple uses across multiple disciplines. *Landscape and Urban Planning* 158: 25–38.

Totaforti, S. (2018). Applying the benefits of biophilic theory to hospital design. *City, Territory and Architecture* 5(1): 1–9.

Trigwell, J. L., Francis, A. J., & Bagot, K. L. (2014). Nature connectedness and eudaimonic well-being: spirituality as a potential mediator. *Ecopsychology* 6(4): 241–51.

Wang, H., Xu, G., Liang, C., & Li, Z. (2021). Coping with job stress for hospital nurses during the COVID-19 crisis: the joint roles of micro-breaks and psychological detachment. *Journal of Nursing Management*. https://doi.org/10.1111/jonm.13431

Wilson, E. O. (1996). *In Search of Nature*. Washington, DC: Island Press.

Zelenski, J. M., & Nisbet, E. K. (2014). Happiness and feeling connected: the distinct role of nature relatedness. *Environment and Behavior* 46: 3–23.

CHAPTER 8

Finding Sanctuary in Words, Images, and Sounds

"Photography for me was like my salvation. I would get home at night and download my photographs and process what had happened that day. A bit like processing images in a dark room, the images would reveal themselves and my emotions would run wild, sometimes I would cry, but mostly I'd pray and reflect in the moment and ask for strength and guidance."

IN THEIR OWN WORDS AND IMAGES

I never realized that I had an eye for taking photographs until I met these two amazing photographers who taught me how to use a Gowlandflex 4 × 5 camera and gave me my first Nikon to shoot with. I love taking photos, but I also love being part of saving lives, and, strangely, the pandemic has merged these two passions for me.

In March 2020, I realized that COVID-19 was here, and most likely here to stay. When I say stay, I thought it would be for a few months. Our pediatric ward was converted to an adult COVID ward. Patients were admitted to my ward, one after another, a lot of whom were, sadly, palliative patients. I'd never experienced this level of sickness and death before, and at times it was completely overwhelming.

I was now the supervisor, or matron, for the new adult ward and the adjacent children's ward, and I was working in ICU. I felt a huge sense of responsibility, for not just patients and families, but also for the staff, especially the junior members of the team who had not experienced death before. Most of the time I kept my emotions and fears to myself and processed my feelings through my photography. Photography for me was like my salvation. I would get home at night and download my photographs and process what had happened that day. A bit like processing images in a darkroom, the images would reveal themselves, and my emotions would run wild. Sometimes I would cry, but mostly I'd pray and reflect in the moment and ask for strength and guidance.

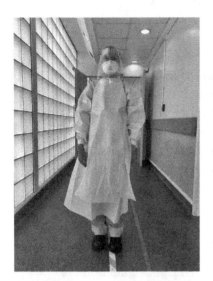
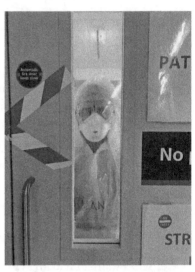
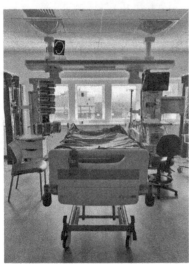
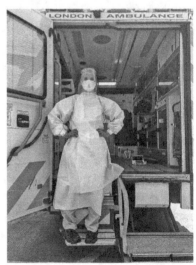

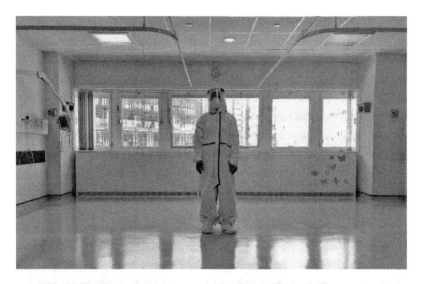

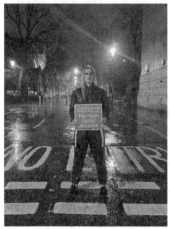

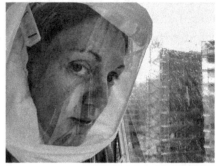

Photos by Hannah Grace Deller

I took my first photo of a colleague at work when I saw him staring out of a small window in the intensive care unit, bewildered and
afraid of what seemed an impending apocalypse. He was stuck behind
a door in the one-way system in the ICU unit, laden with rubbish bags
from the department that he had just cleared. I saw his face in the
window looking lost and bewildered. It reminded me of a character
from a movie I'd seen about a nuclear explosion. I knew I had to take
his picture and, of course, help him through the door. My photography
project had begun.

Photographs were my attempt to capture my colleagues' and my own experiences throughout the COVID-19 pandemic. I took photos whenever I felt it appropriate, as I instinctively knew I needed to document what was happening from the inside, to tell the stories. First, I had to make sure that my subjects were okay about being photographed. I also needed to ensure that the photos were ethical and respectful to all. I was extremely busy, and nothing ever really went to plan, but I managed to get my images when the moment was right, or around shift change times when people were changing in and out of PPE.

It was nice to connect with my colleagues when photographing them, and we'd talk about how they were feeling, if they were struggling, if they needed anything, and what had just happened on shift, especially if it was a tough day or night or there had been another death. They were scared. In their eyes I could see fear, tiredness, sadness—but also hope, anticipation, and even pride as they approached the unknown. The hardest part sometimes was just walking through the door.

I have found that even in the darkest times there are extraordinary emotions at work—in the holding of a hand in someone's last moments, in the intimacy you share with your patients when you're nursing them, and in that special moment you celebrate when your patient is discharged and sent home. It was life changing, and I'm grateful to have been involved in it.

I hope my photos will take you on your own reflective journey of the extraordinary life experience we have all shared throughout this pandemic. For me, making photographs has been very therapeutic. I would have never thought of merging my creativity with my nursing work. I always kept nursing separate, but this time I needed my photography more than ever to get me through the times I was experiencing. As I write this, the pandemic is not yet over, and there are rumblings of another wave, but my hope is that when this pandemic is finally over, we can come together, united and stronger, regardless of our differences.

I have seen some extremely sad and upsetting things that that have changed me forever. I have also experienced unbelievable connection, love, and kindness from all of the people I have met. Whether they were patients, families, artists, musicians, it did feel like we were in this together. I was determined to tell our story through photography, and the hope was always that one day I would look back and say, "Do you remember that time when COVID-19 hit the world and we all smashed it?"

Spring 2020: Hannah Grace Deller, Photographer (www.hgdart.com) and Nurse, Paediatric Matron, Children's Ward Became Adult COVID Unit and Adult ICU, London, United Kingdom

FINDING SANCTUARY
◆

Recovery after stressful times begins with safety—a space that can offer us shelter from the damaging elements, a sanctuary. During the Middle Ages, sanctuaries were asylums, places of protection for those in danger. They were sacred spaces that provided refuge and respite. To harm a person who sought shelter in the sanctuary was sacrilegious. In her book *Creating Sanctuary*, Sandra Bloom (2013) says that in order for healing to begin, we must start with a place of safety. Physical safety does not come empty-handed: sanctuaries also provide emotional and social safety.

The images you see on the preceding pages may remind you of the harrowing pictures of you and your colleagues working during the pandemic. As you well know, there is much more beneath the layers of paper, plastic, and fabric. Noted London photographer and nurse Hannah Grace Deller captured the powerful experiences of her colleagues throughout 2020. Photography became her salvation—making pictures of the people and the work she loves so dearly. One of Hannah's favorite poets is Kahlil Gibran; she finds great comfort in Gibran's verse. "On Joy and Sorrow" is the poem that speaks to her most. "It really met the moment of what nurses have been doing," she said. She paused, and simply asked, "Where do I put the sorrow?" Then she answered her own question, "I believe that doing my creative work, making photographs and talking about them, became something beautiful in the midst of such sadness."

SANCTUARY

◆

How do you know when you are safe? The presence of safety depends on four essential elements: a physically safe environment, psychological safety, social safety, and the ability to trust yourself and other people. The final element is behavioral safety, or knowing that you will be secure with the appropriate structures, limits, and expectations in place. Play, investigation, and learning can also be found in sanctuaries. Sanctuary isn't always found at home; a number of settings can lend themselves to sanctuary-like environments, places that offer an opportunity to develop attachments (Bloom, 2013).

We all need social support and the ability to control outcomes for healing. These are assured when we listen to each other. But talking about your fears and worries can be difficult, especially for children and adolescents. Finding the right words to describe our pain requires alternative approaches to healing. These strategies might include bibliotherapy, writing, photography, journaling, bodywork (which refers to massage and movement awareness), drama, guided imagery, dance, music, meditation, and yoga.

When we are confronted with stressful experiences, our lives can be transformed—positively, negatively, or both. Whether we are personally affected or witnesses to the experiences of others, such as families, friends, or colleagues, we need to take time to process these moments. In chapter 1, we introduced you to Rumi's "The Guest House" writing exercise, and an exercise on how to discover your well-being strategies. They are good places to start. Even during the most challenging of times, there is great potential for personal growth and learning. But we need to find the right tools—the ones that work the best for us.

At first, these strategies might not be obvious. This chapter will encourage you to take a new look at your own unique gifts and turn them into strategies that can heal and reduce stress. Some of these activities go beyond the traditional and often mentioned tools of meditation, yoga, and mindfulness. We want you to think creatively. Perhaps you'll write poetry, stories, or plays, or paint, photograph, and even make music.

You're probably saying to yourself, "I could never do these things, I don't have the talent." Our guess is that you have the passion, and that is exactly the inspiration and motivation you need. Take your time, explore the options, read, listen, look, and watch the work of others—until you are ready to try your hand at a new way of expressing yourself and telling your story. You'll find a list of resources that can help at the end of the book.

Let's start with a warm up-activity to help you find your sanctuary.

Writing about deep and traumatic matters is good for our physical health. Vivid writing stimulates our brain areas. Our pulse slows and our blood pressure lowers, our T-cells increase, and our immune system is boosted. By writing, we air what is on our minds and share it with the page. As soon as the words are written down, they don't have power over us.

> "Simply to line up words one after another upon a page is to create some order where it did not exist, to give a recognizable shape to the chaos of our lives."—Lee Smith, Dimestore: A Writer's Life

---

PUTTING IT INTO PRACTICE

Finding Sanctuary through Writing

Goal: To discover your inner sanctuary

Time and place: 15–20 minutes, a quiet space, maybe outdoors

What is sanctuary? Imagine an inner landscape where you can go at any time, a sanctuary that brings relief and a sense of calm.

▸ Sit comfortably, and feel your bottom as you sit on the chair. Place your feet on the floor in front of you. Lift your head toward the sky.
▸ When you think of a sanctuary that you know or would like to know, begin with a sensory experience:
  • What do you see? What can you touch? What do you hear? What do you smell? Can you taste anything, and what is it?

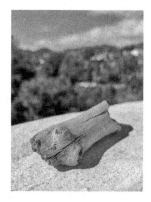

(continued)

▸ Let an image of a special place, your own healing place, come to you.

▸ When you see it and feel it, walk around in it. Take a good look from every perspective.

▸ Now pick up your card/notebook and begin to write. Allow as many senses as you can to be involved.

▸ Write for five minutes.

▸ Reread what you wrote, but do not do any editing.

▸ Keep the card or notes with you, either on your phone or in your pocket. Take it out when you need it most. Many times, you will remember a real place of sanctuary that brings you comfort and peace. Perhaps there is a shell, piece of driftwood, or small stone that you've found while visiting this sanctuary. Keep that physical reminder in your pocket. When you need to visit your sanctuary, hold that object and feel its surface, turning it over in your hand. It will help bring you to that place, that moment of peace and clarity.

This exercise was created with special thanks to author and writing coach Carol Henderson (http://carolhenderson.com).

WORDS

◆

Books and poems by nurse authors have filled library shelves for hundreds of years. Consider the voices of Walt Whitman and Louisa May Alcott, who were nurses during the Civil War. Below is Whitman's elegy to the wound-dresser on the battlefield.

> Bearing the bandages, water and sponge,
> Straight and swift to my wounded I go,
> Where they lie on the ground after the battle brought in,
> Where their priceless blood reddens the grass, the ground,
> Or to the rows of the hospital tent, or under the roof'd hospital,
> To the long rows of cots up and down each side I return,
> To each and all one after another I draw near, not one do I miss,
> An attendant follows holding a tray, he carries a refuse pail,
> Soon to be fill'd with clotted rags and blood, emptied, and fill'd again.

Other nurses spoke their truth in verse and narrative, including Mary Seacole, a nurse during the Crimean War; Vera Brittain, a British nurse and feminist during World War I; Margaret Sanger, American author and birth control activist; and *New York Times* author and columnist Theresa Brown.

Molly Case is a spoken-word artist, writer, and nurse who was born in South London. In April 2013, she performed her poem "Nursing the Nation" at the Royal College of Nursing, where she is the First Writer in Residence. Christie Watson, author of *The Language of Kindness: A Nurse's Story* (2018), also wrote *The Courage to Care: A Call for Compassion* (2020).

Such books can inspire and prompt us to write our own essays and stories. Expressive or reflective writing has a positive influence on how we adapt and cope. Researchers from the University of Parma (Tonarelli et al., 2017) found that writing can facilitate the clarification and solution of various problems, increase cognitive abilities, and promote social interactions. Putting words on paper allows us to describe our experiences, and express thoughts and emotions in distinct ways.

Writers have long translated the transformative experiences of their lives through their art. In her book *The Year of Magical Thinking*, Joan Didion wrote, "Grief turns out to be a place none of us know until we reach it." Reading the works of others encourages us to place their experiences in the context of our lives. The list of resources at the end of this book will offer a start for your explorations.

THE PRESCRIPTION OF FICTION
◆

Writer Dustin Grinnell perfectly captures the purpose of fiction and poetry in his three-part series on bibliotherapy with the four words introducing this section—the prescription of fiction. Great books stay with us long after we've turned the last page. We become immersed in the story and the characters, and don't want to leave them behind (Seifert, 2020). We know that books can heal, from the youngest children to the oldest among us, and we have found books to be restorative, food for our souls. The ancient Greeks believed in the spiritual power of books so completely that they designated libraries healing places of the soul. The word "bibliotherapy," from the Greek, means "book healing."

How can fiction heal us and give us strength to make changes in our personal and professional lives? We meet a narrator or protagonist who emerges as a friend, role model, storyteller, or even a reliable advisor. The story becomes an opportunity for self-revelation, problem-solving, and social support. There can be physical changes as well; reading stories activates neural representations of visual and motor experiences (Speer et al., 2009). And when we read together, it is easier to begin discussing and even debating the important issues. Readers may become inspired to write, paint, photograph or film their own experiences.

While teaching at Columbia University, Donna created a bibliotherapy program for young girls in elementary school. These "Growing Heroines" embraced every moment with their peers and the graduate students who facilitated their groups. They owned their books thanks to the generosity of publishers. They never lost them or forgot them. They wrote their own rules and were quick to point out any infractions. During one session, they read a passage from the Newbery Award–winning book *Dicey's Song*, which is the story of a courageous young girl who must deal with family tragedy and the challenges of growing up.

> "My granddaughter needs a bra," Gram said. Dicey looked away.
> She looked back at Gram, angry. She looked at the sales lady
> who was staring at her. She glared at her. This was a trick, a rotten
> trick. (Voigt, 1984, 89)

At that moment, one of the girls in Donna's group of third graders, spoke out with exasperation, "It really hurts to be a girl!" She followed those words with a plea to her peers, "Could we just talk today?" And they did.

Creative bibliotherapy uses imaginative literature—novels, short stories, poetry, plays, and biographies—to improve psychological well-being (Oatley, 2016). We are guided on a journey of self-discovery and consciousness raising. We gain new insights into our own life experiences. It is a unique forum for discussion and introduces us to new ideas. Fiction encourages a sense of shared humanity, and by allowing us to walk in another's shoes, we become more expert in understanding others. In short, we are allowed to lead many lives, not just one. Through fiction, our empathy and social understanding is enhanced.

Stories and fiction might even be as essential as reading academic articles and scientific texts (Dovey, 2015). Donna found that to be true when preparing nurses to understand the needs of sexual assault survivors and their roles as sexual assault nurse examiners. Before the five-day workshop began, participants were assigned two works of fiction: *Speak*, by Laurie Halse Anderson (2019), and *We Were the Mulvaneys*, by Joyce Carol Oates (2001). Anecdotal reports from participants suggested that they understood not only how sexual violence affects survivors, but also how their families are also changed. These works of fiction extended the individual experiences of the nurses and became topics of discussion in the class, raising consciousness and empathic engagement.

Researchers have used functional magnetic resonance imagery (fMRI) to measure brain activation while subjects are reading fiction. Neuroscientists are increasingly concluding that when we read a story and really understand it, we create a mental simulation of the events described by the story. This is the work of "mirror neurons," or brain cells that allow us to feel what others are experiencing as if it were happening to us (Keen, 2006).

The phrase that one becomes "lost in a book" has real significance. Fiction can take us from the endless stream of thoughts and worries in our minds. We can step outside of ourselves and our egos and escape (Grinnell, 2019). Reading fiction can take us away from the daily busyness and stresses of our lives. A study at the University of Sussex found that reading can reduce stress by up to 68%. It may even be a more effective stress reliever than other relaxation methods, such as listening to music or sipping a cup of tea (Lewis, 2009).

Choosing what to read is a personal choice, but recommendations from friends, book clubs, or reviews are a good start. The Resources section at the end of this book provides a list of websites and books that may be of interest to you.

HEALING NARRATIVES
◆

Researchers have explored the healing power of storytelling and writing. James Pennebaker became the first researcher to apply writing to the theoretical model of emotional regulation. Many other researchers, authors, and nurses have integrated expressive writing into educational and therapeutic programs and approaches.

Pennebaker (1993) found that writing about an upsetting event for as little as 15 minutes a day for four days can have a positive impact on your mental health. Pennebaker's writing prompts include:

Something that you are thinking or worrying about too much
Something that you are dreaming about
Something that you feel is affecting your life in an unhealthy way
Something that you have been avoiding for days, weeks, or years

THE SCIENCE OF EXPRESSIVE WRITING

Expressive writing engages the writer through the process of writing about stressful or significant life events. Journaling encourages the expression of emotions without the need to control, suppress, or avoid themes, thoughts, or feelings (Pennebaker, 1997; Pennebaker et al., 1997). Hypotheses explaining the effectiveness of expressive writing propose that the writing experience acts as means of emotional catharsis, exposure to the stressful event, and a way to cognitively process both emotions and thoughts (Baikie and Wilhelm, 2005). Studies confirm that cognitive processing plays an essential role in the expressive writing process, as the development of a clear narrative seems to help reorganize traumatic events into more psychologically adaptive, internal self-schemas (Pennebaker and Chung, 2012). Expressive writing provides relief by facilitating the transformation of traumatic events into clear and organized narratives (Smyth et al., 2001).

References

Baikie, K. A., & Wilhelm, K. (2005). Emotional and physical health benefits of expressive writing. *Advances in Psychiatric Treatment* 11: 338–46.

Pennebaker, J. W. (1997). Writing about emotional experiences as a therapeutic process. *Psychological Science* 8(3): 162–66.

Pennebaker, J. W., & Chung, C. K. (2012). Expressive writing and its links to mental and physical health. In: Friedman, H. S., ed. *Oxford Handbook of Health Psychology*. New York: Oxford University Press.

Pennebaker, J. W., Mayne, T. J., & Francis, M. E. (1997). Linguistic predictors of adaptive bereavement. *Journal of Personality and Social Psychology* 72(4): 863.

Smyth, J., True, N., & Souto, J. (2001). Effects of writing about traumatic experiences: the necessity for narrative structuring. *Journal of Social and Clinical Psychology* 20: 161–72.

Pennebaker created the Pandemic Project (http://www.exw.utpsyc .org/), which provides exercises, resources, and popular books on how to write your story. His main website at University of Texas at Austin offers more exercises and articles. (https://liberalarts.utexas.edu /psychology/faculty/pennebak#writing-health).

Louise DeSalvo, author of *Writing as a Way of Healing: How Telling Our Stories Transforms Our Lives*, also believes that stories can heal. Several studies have used DeSalvo's work with nurses (Tonarelli et al., 2017).

DeSalvo (2000) suggests these five writing characteristics to enable healing:

- Write in rich detail
- Connect feelings to event
- Balance positive and negative emotions, even if the piece describes difficulties
- Search for insight and reflection
- Write a full and comprehensible story

Finally, she recommends "going public" as the last and most crucial step in her model. She calls the sharing of personal written stories "the most important emotional, psychological, artistic, and political project of our time" (216).

While we all have the opportunity to create our own stories, personally and professionally, there are times when the actions of others shape how we view ourselves. Hilde Lindemann Nelson (2001) suggests we can transform our narrative, especially during those times that others decide what we can or can't do or know. During the COVID-19 pandemic, many nurses talked about how they couldn't accomplish what they needed to do for their patients—not enough staff, time, or personal protective equipment. These are the times we can feel helpless, exploited, or deprived of opportunities. Lindemann Nelson (2001) offers a unique tool to transform harmful stories: writing counterstories. As a first step, she urges us to communicate with each other and share our understanding of our stories. This cluster of histories, anecdotes, and other narrative fragments weave together a counterstory. They identify and shape who we are. And we can only do this in community with our colleagues.

In a report from the Hastings Center in the United States, the authors focused on fostering nurses' moral agency (Liaschenko and Peter, 2016). Emphasizing Lindemann Nelson's work on counterstories, they noted that only when health care organizations come together in community—with all levels of employees coming to the table—will they truly be moral communities, "because it is only when all who contribute to the ends of patient care are able to participate that a counterstory to the corporatism that sacrifices care to economic gain will be generated and voiced" (S20). If any time in nursing history calls for a collective sharing and creating of a counterstory, it is now.

THE HEALING POWER OF POETRY
◆

In her powerful thesis, "A Call to Create: Poetry as Healing and One Nurse's Self-Discovery," ICU nurse Kim Henry (2021) wrote, "I never knew I carried all these experiences inside until experiencing their release through the experience of regular expressive writing. Writing poetry to prompts has offered me to the work and privilege of giving shape to my memories. These writings have given voice and permission to express emotion; I have entrusted those traumatic memories into a safe space" (75). Her words confirm what researchers have found, that poetry has the power to heal (Carroll, 2005).

IN THEIR OWN WORDS

Nursing Shift
KIM HENRY

This worded work I lay before you,
solemnly taking your questions while listening
to defend. You must understand, in fact,
that throngs of my patients lived and thrived.

Coughed when they were asked.
Accepted suctioning when they didn't.
Asked for bedpans, when necessary,
and never pulled out a tube.

They mustered the strength,
to grasp bedrails at every two-hour turn.
Squeezed my hands tight and
wiggled their toes, all upon my command.

They didn't complain too much,
when made to sit up for hours.
Accepted my stern authoritarian command
to stand up straight and walk.

They breathed deeply, permitting
my cupped hands to percuss their
chests in search of phlegm, and lay
stoically silent during enemas' invasion.

They managed their pain, never
begging for more than their fair share.
They trusted, trying, adhering and
complying to hold hope in healing's journey.

Hear me: This work is not theirs.

Their names are now denoted
among the living. Memories erased,
they decline persistent attempts to prod me weekly,
now, even over forty-years past.

Rather, this worded work speaks of
those patients who fought valiantly and failed,
whose tortuous defeat haunts and returns to me again
and again. Their lives are the stories I tell my family.

Of those strong patients, we listen.

Kim reflected on this particular poem, "Why are my poems so filled with such graphic dark memories? My answers lie in trauma theory and how traumatic experiences are not processed inside the brain in the same manner as healthy experiences. Moreover, my answer speaks to the nurses' struggle with clinical objectivity and personal nursing experience. These contrasts remain impressed on my brain . . . This poem is my own answer to the 'Why' in my poetry's disclosures" (68).

Cortney Davis is not only a nurse practitioner but a renowned poet as well. In an interview from *Scrubs Magazine* (2012), she spoke eloquently about the power of poetry.

> Being a nurse helps me be a better poet. Because I am alert to the body's messages, I can allow my poems to be sensual, replete with sights and sounds and smells, with cries of suffering or songs of joy. Because, as a nurse, I am engaged in the very human activity of caring for others, I can pour that reality into poems, grounding what I do in the real world and, at the same time, allowing what I do to be creative and open to imagination.

Davis writes about the challenges of her patients and the profession, as well as about the fullness and weight of her own life—outside of hospital and clinic walls. Below are the powerful words she writes of her daughter's illness.

IN THEIR OWN WORDS

Radical Gratitude
CORTNEY DAVIS

Thanksgiving Day 2020

In the US, now more than 256,000 have died
of COVID-19. So far, my children,

my grandchildren, my husband, me—we are safe.
And all month I've been trying to practice

radical gratitude for this safety,
for the vaccines that may soon be ready,

for a newly elected not-yet-in-office president,
for the nurses who pierced my daughter's

veins, for the toxic red chemo that did
not help her, not even a little, for how

today's glossy, crimson cranberries
brought all this back and made me weep.

Most of all, I'm thankful for my daughter's
beautiful smile when we Face Timed last week,

for her strong voice when she told me
about the new hip pain, the elevated enzymes

that signal more bone damage, the mild
narcotic prescribed *just in case*,

for the phone number for Palliative Care,
although the doctor said, *you're not ready*

for hospice just yet. I'm thankful too that
once I studied poetry with Yehuda Amichai,

an Israeli poet, now long dead. In Jerusalem,
young soldiers going to war carried his poems

in their pockets. And I'm grateful
for the poems I'm writing, as if by writing

them I might stop my daughter's cancer,
trap its destruction in words,

like scorpions embedded in amber.
In class, I wrote down everything

Yehuda taught. *When words fail*, he said,
that's when poetry begins. And yet, he added,

in the midst of violent conflict, in times
of greatest suffering, even poems can't save us.

Reprinted with permission

Several nurses have shared their experiences with personal as well as professional loss in this book, and we have included an entire section on grief and loss in chapter 10, "Navigating the Challenges of the Health Care Landscape." It is a topic we do not talk about enough in nursing.

In 1984, Minerva: The Quarterly Report on Women and the Military published Diane Carlson Evans's poem "Our War." From 1968 to 1969, Evans served as a combat nurse in Vietnam in the burn unit of the 36th Evacuation Hospital in Vũng Tàu and at Pleiku in the 71st Evacuation Hospital. Upon her return home, she carried the psychological baggage of that year. "Our War" foreshadowed the journey that would become her destiny. As Evans (2020) painfully describes, "In 1984, I had come to Washington, D.C., for the dedication of the *Three Servicemen* sculpture [by Frederick Hart]. In his remarks, not once did President Ronald Reagan mention anything about women having served. Actually, about 10,000 women, more than eighty percent of them nurses, were stationed in Vietnam during the war" (20). Diane knew that she had to find her voice and help other women find theirs as well. She became an activist and champion for all women who served in Vietnam and founded the Vietnam Women's Foundation. In 1993, after 10 long years, the Vietnam Women's Memorial was dedicated as part of the Vietnam Veterans Memorial, near Maya Lin's Wall of names.

IN THEIR OWN WORDS

Our War
DIANE CARLSON EVANS

I don't go off to war, so they say,
I'm a woman.

Who then has worn my boots?
And whose memories are these,
of youth's suffering?

I'm a woman and I've tasted man's war.
Our war.
And he knows that I love in no greater way
than to share in his life or his death.

What are the rules?
Man or woman,
we are prey to suffer and survive together.

Please don't forget me.
I've been through war's hell and if only you will listen,
I've a story of those chosen to sacrifice for us all.

Reprinted with permission from Diane Carlson Evans,
Vietnam 1968–69, Chair and Founder, Vietnam Women's
Memorial Project, Inc.

In her work with nurses, Janel Sexton et al. (2009) found that expressive writing offered at least three therapeutic benefits when writing about difficult experiences. Writing offers an opportunity to uncover difficult emotions, making them more manageable or at least understandable. Putting pen to paper allows us to think about difficult or traumatic events in different ways; seeing the words in front of us causes us to reflect. Writing about difficult events helps us to regulate emotions in new ways, allowing us to cope more effectively.

Authors Anderson and Mac Curdy (2000), in *Writing and Healing: Toward an Informed Practice*, further describe how writing contributes to our emotional well-being. "By writing about traumatic experiences, we discover and rediscover them, move them out of the ephemeral flow and space of talk onto the more permanent surface of the page, where they can be considered, reconsidered, left, and taken up again. Through the dual possibilities of permanence and revision, the chief healing effect of writing is thus to recover and to exert a measure of control over that which we can never control—the past" (7).

Perhaps there is no greater purpose than putting our words on paper and then reading them—to ourselves and each other.

NARRATING THE STORIES OF OUR PATIENTS
◆

If writing appeals to you, and you'd like to explore different opportunities, look no further than narrative medicine and narrative nursing programs. Rita Charon first proposed narrative medicine in 2001; she is considered the architect of narrative medicine. Charon (2008) said that narrative medicine (or nursing) allows us to "recognize, absorb, interpret, and be moved by the stories of illness" (4). Some studies have concluded that narrative work enhances empathy in health care providers (Yang et al., 2018). For more on narrative medicine, see the programs and other resources listed at the end of this book.

IMAGES
◆

For centuries, artists have explored the emotions of anger, fear, and grief through their craft. While a painting, photograph, or sculpture cannot eradicate the turmoil left by such life-altering events, the arts can allow one to move beyond words and find other ways of expression. Nigerian visual and performance artist and writer Oroma Elewa is creating new spaces to exist emotionally: "I am my own muse, I am the subject I know best. The subject I want to know better" (Ukoha, 2019). Renowned painter Mary Cassatt lost her sister and two other siblings. She often painted images of women; mothers and children became a major subject of her work.

PHOTOGRAPHY
◆

The work of Hannah Grace Deller introduced this chapter about finding your sanctuary. Others who tell their stories with a camera (or mobile phone) include nurse Karen Cunningham (2020). Her photo essay "A City Nurse" chronicles how she photographed her friend and colleague, some 20 years younger, over the course of two shifts in a New York City intensive care unit. British photographer Kirsty Mitchell recalls how her world fell apart after her mother's death from a brain tumor. Photography became her "only escape" when she could no longer talk about how she felt. She produced pieces that "echoed the memories of her stories" (https://www.kirstymitchellphotography.com).

MAKING ART: DRAWING, PAINTING, AND CARTOONING
◆

In this new world of graphic novels, anime, and comic books, it seems only natural that a nurse would use comics to contemplate the complexities of illness and caregiving. MK Czerwiec, also known as the Comic Nurse, is an award-winning cartoonist and nurse. MK drew the panels that appear below, just for this book. In these illustrations, she makes the case for telling your story with pen and sketch pad. Take a look at her website Comic Nurse (https://www.comicnurse.com/) and the website she co-manages, Graphic Medicine, which is dedicated to the intersection of comics and health (https://www.graphicmedicine .org/). You might also enjoy MK's award-winning books *Menopause: A Comic Treatment* (2020) and *Taking Turns* (2017).

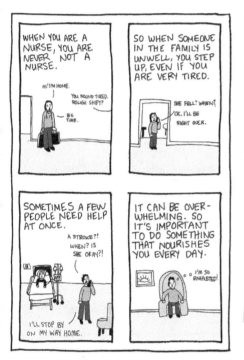
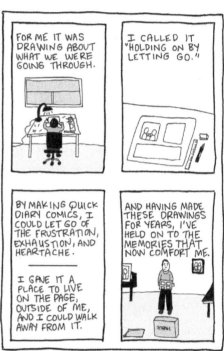

MK Czerwiec, RN, MA, www.comicnurse.com

Art therapy has been used extensively as a means of helping patients process their emotions and express their view of the world. Words are not necessary to fully express what is in our hearts.

Dr. Suzanne Drake, a nurse psychotherapist, encourages her patients to paint or draw their feelings. She suggests using the exercises on the website of artist and art therapist Youhjung, Thirsty for Art, to help connect to and own your emotions. On her website, Youhjung states, "Art accesses the deep-seated memories, images, and emotions within our mind and our body and allows us to release the ones that keep us stuck."

Unsticking Your Emotions

Goal: To visualize and re-create the shape, color, and texture of your emotions

Time and Place: 15–30 minutes, at home or outdoors, in a space where you can spread out your materials on a flat surface

If you wish, try one of the exercises from Youhjung's website (www.thirstyforart.com/blog/how-to-draw-feelings), and then follow Dr. Drake's instructions below.

- Begin with a few minutes of breathing and mindfulness.
- Bring your attention inward. What are you feeling? What is the emotion? Where do you feel it in your body?
- In your mind's eye, see if you can identify its size and shape.
- If it had a color, what color would it be? What kind of texture would it have? Hard, soft, squishy?
- Is it like a solid? Liquid? Gas? Gel?
- What about temperature? Is it hot, cold, room temperature?
- Just notice it without judgment. Let it be what it is.
- Stay with the feelings and images while you pick up the pencil or paintbrush.
- Simply put it on to paper as you experience it.
- Don't worry about what it looks like, just draw/paint what you feel.

Some programs, such as Literacy through Photography, blend photography, art, and writing. Although Literacy through Photography was originally developed for children by photographer Wendy Ewald, adults have also found that writing in combination with photography is a unique way to express healing and growth-promoting thoughts and emotions (Ewald and Lightfoot, 2001). The words and images produced facilitate healing and self-expression in response to experiences that have transformed our lives, in this case stress or traumatic work situations.

MUSIC TO OUR EARS

◆

No doubt you've heard the saying above; perhaps you've even used it yourself. This common idiom originates from nearly 200 years ago, and it means that we've heard something that's soothing, pleasing, or brings us happiness. Music, songs, instrumentals, and even lyrics have been found to be an effective way of reducing stress and enhancing well-being (de Witte et al, 2020). Listening to music decreases physiological arousal by lowering our heart rate, reducing cortisol levels, or decreasing heart rate and blood pressure, while affecting the psychobiological stress system (Thoma et al., 2013). Music may also affect our emotions, especially those related to worry or anxiety (Knight and Rickard, 2001). Music affects the structures in our brains and can influence the production of endorphins, the neurotransmitters that contribute to a sense of well-being, evoking feelings of pleasure and happiness. Music interventions for patients have been used with great success, whereby listening, making music, or singing are focused on specific patient needs. But what about the health care providers themselves? Can music serve caregivers as well as patients? The answer is yes.

Today, music is one of the hottest trends in wellness. According to the Global Wellness Summit, wellness music is a new trend that takes a number of forms (McGroarty, 2022). Streaming sites like Spotify offer a wide range of musical genres to suit your needs and interests, whether it is a playlist for workouts or one of their newest offerings, like the Ultimate Happy Playlist (see the Resources for the link). One of the most fascinating examples of the new wellness music trend is the rise of generative music apps and streaming services that create custom-made, always-adapting soundscapes that use algorithms and your own biofeedback to improve your well-being. As McGroarty (2022) describes, "You've got the healing music in you, and when combined with smart algorithms and AI, these custom sound frequencies can function like an always-there playlist you can turn to if you need to de-stress, focus or sleep."

Take a listen to the website My Noise (mynoise.net), and experiment with creating sounds and music that can calm and relax you. But how do you choose the music you need? We all have our preferences, and we may create playlists for any occasion. Tempo, instrumentals, and lyrics are important moderators. Meditative music is slow and correlates with a slower heart rate, resulting in greater relaxation (Knight and Rickard, 2001). Instrumental music that does not contain lyrics also has an effect. Several studies have found that lyrics can be more distracting and stimulating instead of calming (Hu and Downie, 2010), while others have discovered that lyrics can be comforting. Nurse Manager Anna Henderson, who works in palliative care at Vanderbilt University Medical Center, recounted, "It was all I could do to keep singing, but I did. But, you know, it's times like that, music and this job just go hand in hand."

Nurses have shared their voices and made music as so many others have. Consider the remarkable songs of Winona Judd or the folk-rock songwriter of the Lumineers, who sang of his father's death in "Long Way from Home."

Let's revisit the story of Hannah Deller's photographs. After her photographs were published in UK newspapers, musician Chris Difford of the band Squeeze brought together a collection of artists and songwriters to curate an album, called *Song Club*, to celebrate frontline nurses. All funds raised from the album are donated to the Royal College of Nursing COVID Support Foundation. The first single from the album is titled "Working on the Frontline," performed by actor and singer Jessie Buckley. The song is a powerful representation of life on the front line of the National Health Service and features Hannah Deller. Below are QR codes to access the music on YouTube and Amazon, respectively.

Hannah Grace Deller

Hannah Grace Deller

In Nashville, singer-songwriter and nurse Megan Palmer (2020) has incorporated music into her practice as well as her own wellness program. She joined Anna Henderson and several other colleagues who wrote songs and played for their patients during the coronavirus pandemic. Megan gave us permission to include the lyrics for one of her songs, "Kite." The song was written and recorded at home during the pandemic and released as a single. Take a listen on YouTube; the link is in the list of resources at the end of this book.

> I hold this string of hope
> To keep me grounded
> Praying for lightning not to strike again
> Rooting down, as I hold
> While it flails
> I sing a version of let's go fly a kite.

IN THEIR OWN WORDS

As I made my way to Anna's house outside Ashland City, Tennessee, I was so grateful to have a day off. Lately, life on 5 Round Wing, the Palliative Care Unit at Vanderbilt University Medical Center (VUMC), had been chaotic at best. I'd spent the last seven years there, while also growing my music/songwriting career. I'd always crafted nursing this way—relying on it as the gift that keeps on giving while also capitalizing on the flexibility of a nurse's schedule. But since COVID-19 became a household name, my music life had suddenly evaporated, and the hospital's needs were creeping up quickly. I had thrust myself into working more and more and had yet to realize my carefully curated career was at high risk for injury.

My friend Graham Weber from The House of Songs, a cowriting organization I had worked with in the past, called and asked what I thought about trying to write some songs with my coworkers. They offered to sponsor lunch for the sessions and see what happens. "Maybe something great could come out of it," he said. My immediate answer was, "Yes."

I needed this more than I wanted to admit. I was hungry for a task, or an assignment besides the two-dimensional livestreams I'd been doing from my home studio. It wasn't that I missed *performing*, but I was lacking *connection*.

Nursing creates many opportunities for empathetic interactions, especially in my unit, where I am frequently participating in end-of-life care, establishing a plan, and having conversations about what to expect. There is rarely time to process and integrate the intensity of the work. I was drawn to palliative/hospice care because I felt like I intuitively knew how to do it. I felt "called" to help people transition from this world. I had always leaned on music as a way to dissipate some of my stress after deeply connecting with people I'd most likely never see again after an intense time. Lately, I'd been experiencing some compassion fatigue and felt stress building in my system without a discharge plan.

My coworker Anna Marie Henderson is a ray of light. She is one of those people you are so happy to be on the unit with. Soon after she joined our team, I knew she was a natural-born healer. One day, I heard the most joyous sound coming from one of her rooms, and it was her gorgeous voice singing "Amazing Grace" with her patient. I knew I wanted to write with her.

She enthusiastically said yes and invited me out to her house on a day we both had off. She said she hadn't written many songs, but she loved to play gigs with her husband, Lenny. She had been performing since a young age and wanted to "help me out." The day before our session, I'd gotten a call from the Associated Press asking if they could sit in on our cowrite. To me, that was a strange question because it felt a little like inviting the media on a date, but I also understood nursing was currently under a microscope and the world was looking for a feel-good story. I didn't know if we could achieve anything great, and I didn't know how Anna would feel about it, but being the star that she is, she wholeheartedly agreed.

When I walked into her immaculately adorable home out in the country, I was at ease. We sat down to chat before the journalist from the Associated Press showed up. I brought my favorite sandwiches, and we each had a small glass of wine. She began by telling me about her 25 years of experience in hospice care, taking care of her parents, and also a special patient she'd cared for recently.

This woman was in room 5448, and she was very, very sick. She was alone. She asked me to stop for a minute, sit down, take a rest and hold her hand. I had a lot of things to do that day, but something in her voice told me that's what I had to do at that moment. I remember it was raining, and I could see the trees through the window and it looked like teardrops falling off the branch. She told me she could see in my eyes that I understood her, and then she relaxed and fell asleep. It was a simple thing, but it meant a lot to me that day to just *stop*.

I had chills hearing this story. The pause. The courage and compassion it takes to truly stop and be present with someone. What a gift. I jotted down some of her words because I wanted to take them with me as advice, but also maybe this is what we needed to write about. She went on.

"You know, I spent the time with her that day, and she died at the end of my shift. I came home and Lenny was there waiting for me, with dinner on the table. He could see I had a hard day, and I just fell apart in his arms. He held me while I cried and comforted me, and I'm so thankful that I have this wonderful man that I get to come home to after a day like that."

I said, "Anna. I'm crying. That is a beautiful story. Let's write that song."

There was a knock on the door. The Associated Press arrived with their cameras and bright lights. We set up, and "Stop for a Minute" wrote itself. We ignored the cameras and got to work, feeling the connection to the wellspring of emotion that invoked the muse to join us.

The song wasn't finished that day exactly, but its bones were formed. The AP wrote a great story that was picked up by many news outlets, and eventually we tied up some loose ends and took it to the studio. Along with Anna's song, I wrote more songs with Rebecca Hixson, Paul Raymond, Dara Downs, Suzie Brown Sax, and Emma Berkey that turned into an album called *Take Good Care*. As we created this body of work, it became clear to me that the work we do is important, but also caring for each other and ourselves is imperative to surviving as a nurse, especially in tumultuous times.

As I prepared to release the music in spring 2021, the pandemic was still raging on, and life on 5RW had gotten even more intense, as we cared for many COVID patients who did not survive. But now, I had a special connection with my writing partners, and we'd find ourselves quoting our lyrics to each other across the nurses station.

Rolling Stone featured "Stop for a Minute" in its publication, and local news channels shared our story as well. I felt a sense of healing through finding creative expression and began to feel a shift in myself as my two career paths suddenly seemed to have merged.

As all this was happening, I also faced another challenge with my own health. In 2016, I experienced breast cancer and went through treatment. In 2021, I unfortunately had a recurrence of the same cancer in my lymph nodes. It pained me to share the news and take a leave of absence from the job that I truly cared about. I felt a sense of guilt and frustration about it, but there was a bigger lesson to discover, and it looped me back to the wonderful songs we created. Surely they would not expire over time. They would go on to become even more meaningful and teach me more about the "calling to care" for myself, my fellow colleagues, and humanity in general.

April 29, 2021: Megan Palmer, BSN, RN, QTTP, Palliative Care/Hospice Nurse, Nashville, Tennessee, USA

Take a listen to what might be an anthem for collective support and action, "One Voice" by the Wailin' Jennys, as sung by the US Navy Band (to access the link to the song, see the Resources section), or the original version sung by the Wailin' Jennys (also in the Resources).

> This is the sound of one voice
> One spirit, one voice
> The sound of one who makes a choice
> This is the sound of one voice
>
> This is the sound of voices two
> The sound of me singing with you
> Helping each other to make it through
> This is the sound of voices two
>
> This is the sound of voices three
> Singing together in harmony
> Surrendering to the mystery
> This is the sound of voices three

This is the sound of all of us
Singing with love and the will to trust
Leave the rest…

Reprinted with permission from Ruth Moody (2004)

The music and lyrics of songs speak volumes about our profession and who we are. Songs have been used by nurses as a way to understand their world and how they can survive in it, or change it. "The Weight," originally written by Robertson (1968) and performed by The Band, was covered from a woman's perspective by female Canadian singing duo Dala. Just hearing the first line—"Pulled into Nazareth, was feelin' about half past dead"—evokes images of nurses pulling shift after shift of heartbreaking duties. Dala's rendition of the song, with its refrain about taking off and sharing a burdensome load, is powerful and meaningful to nurses; we believe that it not only proclaims the tremendous burden the nursing profession has carried over the past several years, but also heralds the collective support and action that nurses have taken. The song continues:

I just need some place where I can lay my head
"Hey, mister, can you tell me where a girl might find a bed?"
He just grinned and shook my hand, "No" was all he said

The song "Hero and the Sage," by Tara Beier (2016), could also be considered an anthem for the nursing profession. Tara gave us permission to include the lyrics, which paint a picture of an evolving world and how nurses can be the change.

Hero and The Sage
TARA BEIER

What's on your mind dear friend?
Just say what you want to say.
Why does power and grief still prevail today?
Living in a world of constant complexity,
What will it take,
For us to have peace?

Let's make a change,
Says the hero and the sage.

I just might contradict what I have to say.
We buy freedom in this modern age.
Divide the line between love and hate,
And make a choice,
On what side to take.

We must believe.
And we can make a change.
We must believe.
That we can make a change.

So, I ask,
Are you okay?
There will be,
Better days.
So, I have had to ask,
Are you okay?
There will be better days.

We must ask ourselves what we're here for.
God I wish, there's gotta be more.
So, close your eyes dear friend,
And dream a dream,
And find a place,
To make it what you mean.

We must believe,
That we make a change.
We must believe,
That we make a change.

Says the hero and the sage.
Says the hero and the sage.

As Beth Hudnall Stamm (1995) so eloquently points out, we have the essential need for wellness and caring in community: "It is important...as professionals, clinicians, and families, as we go about the work of healing—to build strong sustaining communities."

In addition to music, art, and writing, drama has found its way into and about nurses' lives. Consider the plays *That Kindness: Nurses in Their Own Words*, written by V (formerly Eve Ensler), or *The Line*, which takes viewers into the front line of the fight against COVID-19. Based on interviews with nurses and other health care providers, the words heard during the performance are real, but spoken by actors. Links to all of these performances and music are in the Resources section.

FINDING YOUR FLOW STATE
•

As humans, we are drawn to optimal experiences where we are fully immersed in the moment, at the task at hand. When this happens, it is called "flow." Psychologist Mihaly Csikszentmihalyi, who was the first to describe flow, calls it "an almost automatic, effortless, yet highly focused state of consciousness" (Csikszentmihalyi et al., 2018). It is in this flow state that individuals feel fully alive, competent, and creative, which leads to improved well-being overall. We hope that you will find your flow state and create.

Closing out this chapter is Gail Pfeifer, who found art in her hands.

IN THEIR OWN HANDS

> *"Paying close attention to the simpler steps and enjoying
> the process, while keeping the end goal in mind, makes all the
> difference—in good pottery and in good nursing care."*

I learned how to throw on the potter's wheel when I was about eight months pregnant with our second child. I took lessons to have something of my own, on Saturdays, while my husband spent time with our 3-year-old son. I wasn't sure at the time whether to go back to clinical nursing, to resume studying for a postgraduate degree, or to continue staying home with two small children. Pottery helped me decide. That may sound odd, as the connection between throwing clay on a wheel and a nursing career isn't something most nurses—or potters—would think of. And neither did I at the time.

Making functional and beautiful wheel-thrown pots depends on the materials used, the skills of the potter, and the vagaries of glazing and firing. While the finished pot may appear to be a simple, functional form, precise steps are involved in wheel throwing. The first, centering the clay, is the most important. Each subsequent step in the throwing process builds on this first step, and each subsequent step must be well done, too. The potter's hand position and mindfulness affect centering and the steps that follow—if the clay is off-center for any reason, the potter has less control over the final shape, function, and quality of the pot.

Not that any handmade pot can match the perfection of the machine made. But perhaps therein lies the beauty of creation. In fact, well-accomplished Japanese potters of the Zen tradition value the beauty of transience and imperfection, and they will sometimes alter a pot that looks too perfect by giving it a tap. Although the form is altered by that tap, the function of the pot remains.

All nurses are familiar with the term "patient-centered care," which is taught in nursing schools and colleges but often disregarded in clinical practice. In many ways, it is the same essential first step as centering the clay. Throwing a good pot is not much different from good nursing care, where the materials are different but the outcome is dependent on how well centering is done. The materials in nursing care are the disease process in this particular patient, the skills of the nurse, and the vagaries of the health care system in which all these things operate and which may sometimes be opposing forces. A nurse who is mindful of the importance of excellence in performing simple tasks will have more, if hardly absolute, control over quality care. If a nurse is assigned too many patients to care for, it's almost impossible for him or her to keep the patient as the center of care. Throwing clay on the wheel and nursing are both, at times, messy processes, and while they may appear at first to comprise simple tasks, those tasks—done well and carefully—make all the difference in final outcomes.

Both careers have the potential to reach out and touch another person. If you've ever been a patient, especially a hospitalized patient, you understand how important a good nurse can be. He or she speaks past the disease you are being treated for and reaches you, the whole person with a unique family, a home, a job, and sometimes none of these. If you've ever purchased a handmade piece of art, it's likely that it also spoke to you in some way, to who you are and to what is important to you.

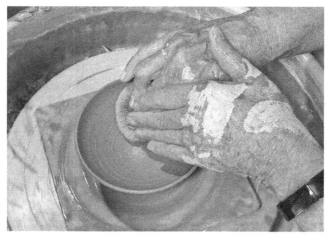

Gail Pfeifer

I did decide to stay home to raise our kids full-time. When our youngest started school, I continued to want something for myself, but free time stayed elusive. The centering required of wheel-throwing helped me center not only the pots I created but also myself. Yet I had less time for it. And I didn't want to return to clinical practice, where I felt I would use up too much of myself and have nothing left for my family. I felt I would be knocked off center. So, I began to write, something I always loved to do and could do at home when the kids were in school.

I wrote for free, about motherhood in a little publication called *Welcome Home*. I wrote—and got paid for writing—about pottery. Then one day I said to myself, "Why not try writing for nursing magazines and newspapers. You know nursing even better than you know pottery."

I landed some assignments for *Nursing Spectrum*, a nursing newspaper, then for journals like the *American Journal of Nursing*, *Critical Care Nursing*, and others. As our children approached their teenage years, I applied for a part-time job with a medical communications company, which ultimately led to full-time jobs as the executive editor for several medical journals and projects. I negotiated working at home before it was popular and went into the office on my husband's days off. It was a perfect fit.

Now that the kids are grown and living their own lives and my husband has retired, I've moved back to freelance writing and to focusing once again on making pottery. And I'm still a nurse, advising family and friends within my scope of knowledge when they ask medical questions. I've come full circle, and I'm centered on what I love to do.

Although science is important in both pottery and nursing, neither wheel throwing nor nursing can be reduced to plain science or performed perfectly. The clay, the patient, and your life affect every step. Yet both have the potential to become forms of art. And both can provide a feeling of accomplishment like nothing else. Paying close attention to the simpler steps and enjoying the process, while keeping the end goal in mind, makes all the difference—in good pottery and in good nursing care. And, for me, in a centered, if imperfect, life.

Summer, 2020: Gail Pfeifer, MA, RN, Medical Writer, Editor, Consultant, and Potter, Stone Harbor, New Jersey, United States

What does art in your own hands mean to you? Consider why you take on creative endeavors such as writing, creating art, or making music. If you are intrinsically motivated, meaning you do so for the enjoyment of the activity rather than desired outcomes, you are more likely to achieve flow states that can improve your craft and well-being over time.

Read, look, and listen to nurses who are authors, poets, writers, artists, and filmmakers in the Resources section of this book. Better yet, create your own art, music, and writing.

REFERENCES
Anderson, C. M., & Mac Curdy, M. M. (2000). *Writing and Healing: Toward an Informed Practice. Refiguring English Studies.* Urbana, IL: National Council of Teachers of English.
Anderson, L. H. (2019). *Speak,* 20th ann. ed. New York: Farrar, Straus and Giroux.
Associated Press. (2020). Nashville nurses sing to comfort patients in midst of pandemic. *New York Post,* June 11, 2020. https://nypost.com/2020/06/11/nurses-musical-voices-give-comfort-in-midst-of-pandemic/
Beier, T. (2016). "Hero and the Sage." On *Hero and the Sage.* Los Angeles, CA: Red Raven Records.
Bloom, S. L. (2013). *Creating Sanctuary: Toward the Evolution of Sane Societies.* New York: Routledge.
Carroll, R. (2005). Finding the words to say it: the healing power of poetry. *Evidence-Based Complementary and Alternative Medicine* 2(2): 161–72.
Charon, R. (2008). *Narrative Medicine: Honoring the Stories of Illness.* Oxford: Oxford University Press.

Csikszentmihalyi, M., Montijo, M. N., & Mouton, A. R. (2018). Flow theory: optimizing elite performance in the creative realm. In Pfeiffer, S. I., Shaunessy-Dedrick, E., & Foley-Nicpon, M., eds. APA Handbook of Giftedness and Talent. Washington, DC: American Psychological Association, 215–29.
Cunningham, K. (2020). "A city nurse." New Yorker, May 4, 2020. https://www.newyorker.com/magazine/2020/05/04/a-city-nurse
Czerwiec, MK. (2017). Taking Turns: Stories from HIV/AIDS Care, vol. 8. University Park: Pennsylvania State University Press.
Czerwiec, MK, ed. (2020). Menopause: A Comic Treatment, vol. 19. University Park: Pennsylvania State University Press.
Davis, C. (2012). A portrait of the nurse as a poet. Scrubs Magazine, April 26, 2012. https://scrubsmag.com/a-portrait-of-the-nurse-as-a-poet/2/
Davis, C. (2021). Daughter. West Hartford, CT: Grayson Books.
DeSalvo, L. A. (2000). Writing as a Way of Healing: How Telling Our Stories Transforms Our Lives. Boston: Beacon Press.
de Witte, M., Spruit, A., van Hooren, S., Moonen, X., & Stams, G. J. (2020). Effects of music interventions on stress-related outcomes: a systematic review and two meta-analyses. Health Psychology Review 14(2): 294–324.
Didion, J. (2005). The Year of Magical Thinking. New York: Alfred A. Knopf. Quote from pg. 188.
Dovey, C. (2015). Can reading make you happier? New Yorker, June 9, 2015.
Evans, D. C. (1984). Nurse. Minerva 2(3): 22.
Evans, D. C. (2020). Healing Wounds: A Vietnam War Combat Nurse's 10-Year Fight to Win Women a Place of Honor in Washington, D.C. Brentwood, TN: Permuted Press.
Ewald, W., & Lightfoot, A. (2001). I Wanna Take Me a Picture: Teaching Photography and Writing to Children. Boston: Beacon Press.
Grinnell, D. (2019) The anatomy of bibliotherapy: how fiction heals, part I. Hektoen International: A Journal of Medical Humanities 11(3).
Henry, K. C. (2021). A call to create: poetry as healing and one nurse's self discovery. English Theses 6: https://repository.belmont.edu/english_theses/6
Hu, X., & Downie, J. S. (2010). When lyrics outperform audio for music mood classification: a feature analysis. Presented at the 11th International Society for Music Information Retrieval Conference, ISMIR 2010, Utrecht, Netherlands, August 9–13.
Keen, S. (2006). A theory of narrative empathy. Narrative 14(3): 207–36.
Knight, W. E., & Rickard, N. S. (2001). Relaxing music prevents stress-induced increases in subjective anxiety, systolic blood pressure, and heart rate in healthy males and females. Journal of Music Therapy 38(4): 254–72.
Lewis, D. (2009). How Reading Can Reduce Stress. Sussex, UK: Galaxy Stress Research, Mindlab International, Sussex University.
Liaschenko, J., & Peter, E. (2016). Fostering nurses' moral agency and moral identity: the importance of moral community. Hastings Center Report 46: S18–S21.
Lindemann Nelson, H. (2001). Damaged Identities, Narrative Repair. Ithaca, NY: Cornell University Press.

McGroarty, B. (2022) Wellness music. Global Wellness Summit. Accessed August 2, 2022. https://www.globalwellnesssummit.com/2020-global -wellness-trends/wellness-music/

Moody, R. (2004). "One Voice." Recorded by The Wailin' Jennys. On 40 Days. St. Paul, MN: Red House Records.

Oates, J. C. (2001). We Were the Mulvaneys. London: Penguin.

Oatley, K. (2016). Fiction: simulation of social worlds. Trends in Cognitive Sciences 20(8): 618–28.

Palmer, M. (2020). "Kite." Nashvillle, TN: M. Palmer.

Pennebaker, J. W. (1993). Putting stress into words: health, linguistic, and thera- peutic implications. Behaviour Research and Therapy 31(6): 539–48.

Robertson, J. R. (1968). "The Weight." Recorded by The Band. On Music from the Big Pink Vinyl. Los Angeles, CA: Capitol Records.

Seifert, C. (2020). The case for reading fiction. Harvard Business Review, March 6, 2020. https://hbr.org/2020/03/the-case-for-reading-fiction

Sexton, J. D., Pennebaker, J. W., Holzmueller, C. G., Wu, A. W., Berenholtz, S. M., Swoboda, S. M., Pronovost, P. J., & Sexton, J. B. (2009). Care for the care- giver: benefits of expressive writing for nurses in the United States. Prog- ress in Palliative Care 17(6): 307–12.

Smith, L. (2016). Dimestore: A Writer's Life. Chapel Hill, NC: Algonquin Books.

Speer, N. K., Reynolds, J. R., Swallow, K. M., & Zacks, J. M. (2009). Reading stories activates neural representations of visual and motor experiences. Psychological Science 20(8): 989–99.

Stamm, B. H. (1995). Secondary Traumatic Stress: Self-Care Issues for Clinicians, Researchers and Educators. Derwood, MD: Sidran Press.

Thoma, M. V., La Marca, R., Brönnimann, R., Finkel, L., Ehlert, U., & Nater, U. M. (2013). The effect of music on the human stress response. PLoS One 8(8): e70156. https://doi.org/10.1371/journal.pone.0070156

Tonarelli, A., Cosentino, C., Artioli, D., Borciani, S., Camurri, E., Colombo, B., & Artioli, G. (2017). Expressive writing: a tool to help health workers. Research project on the benefits of expressive writing. Acta Bio Medica: Atenei Parmensis 88(Suppl. 5): 13.

Ukoha, E. (2019). Then and now—a conversation with Oroma Elewa. Medium, July 1, 2019. https://nilegirl.medium.com/then-now-3114840f352e

Voigt, C. (1984). Dicey's Song. Greenwich, CT: Fawcett.

Watson, C. (2018). The Language of Kindness: A Nurse's Story. New York: Random House.

Watson, C. (2020). The Courage to Care: A Call for Compassion. New York: Random House.

Whitman, W. (1898). The Wound Dresser: A Series of Letters Written from the Hospitals in Washington during the War of the Rebellion. Boston: Small, Maynard.

Yang, N., Xiao, H., Cao, Y., Li, S., Yan, H., & Wang, Y. (2018). Does narrative medi- cine education improve nursing students' empathic abilities and academic achievement? A randomised controlled trial. Journal of International Medical Research 46(8): 3306–17.

CHAPTER 9

•

Seeking Empowerment
through Advocacy and Activism

*"It was scary at first, but while deepening my knowledge,
I started gaining confidence, a little bit of courage, and
a new sense of determination. I reasoned that because
the climate crisis was mostly a human-made problem, it
meant that humans could also provide the solution.
I started to feel more powerful."*

Until I became a mum, I always thought of myself as a "tough" one. After Alessandro was born, in 2017, everything started to seem scary:
"How am I supposed to take care of my son, to protect him?"
This new level of vulnerability went exponential when Marta, my daughter, came along in 2019. My fear became panic, and my worries deteriorated into anxiety and postpartum depression. That was when I started to hear more about climate change, and everything became even worse:
"How am I supposed to protect my children while the entire world is literally burning?"
For a few months I felt desperate. Going to sleep became a routine of panic attacks and endless nightmares of my kids living in a world without clean water or breathable air. Then, one day, I realised I had to do something, because I could not handle the idea of my kids looking at me in 30 years' time and asking me why I hadn't done anything about it.

So, I did what I do best: I went online and studied everything I could find on climate change and the impact that it has on human health. It was scary at first, but while deepening my knowledge, I started gaining confidence, a little bit of courage, and a new sense of determination. I reasoned that because the climate crisis was mostly a human-made problem, it meant that humans could also provide the solution. I started to feel more powerful.

I decided to take some actions in both my personal and professional life. My partner and I began our personal journey toward sustainability with small steps; we changed the way we ate, we shopped, or we moved. In 2020, I went back to work with the determination to bring my motivation into my workplace. As I am an anaesthetic nurse, I spend 10 hours a day in an operating theatre. The environmental impact of my job is massive: energy and water supplies, plastic and clinical waste, anaesthetic gases. All of these contribute to greenhouse gas emissions and the climate change crisis.

On my first day back, when I went to talk to my managers about bringing sustainable initiatives into the operating theatre, I was told that I could take care of the bins in the tea room and improve the recycling waste, if I wanted. I was so disappointed. How could they not understand how important this is? How could they not see? But then I realised that change is scary, it is hard work, and it is usually a slow process that comes with a lot of resistance. I had to start small, with little steps, and be patient.

A month later, Ireland was hit by COVID-19, and as with the rest of the world, nothing else mattered. I had to wait until February 2021 to finally have the chance to start my first project, and gain my space and trust from my colleagues as "the green person."

The first few months were not easy, but I feel like an all-new journey has begun at this point in my life. I don't really know where this journey into sustainability is going to bring me. I realise that I am not going to change the world by myself. But knowing that I am trying my best to address the climate change issue and give my children the possibility for a better future has definitely changed my world.

2019 to February 2021: Federica Pirro, BSc, MA, RN,
Anaesthetic Nurse, Operating Theater, Dublin, Ireland

The pages of this chapter are filled with examples of how nurses are speaking out, taking action, and becoming part of the solution—on many issues, whether related to climate change, professional practice, racism, or a concern that is deeply personal. You might be thinking that you don't have time to engage in these activities, but remember, you advocate every day—for your patients, their families, communities, and yourselves. Take a look at social media, where the hashtags #NurseTwitter, #NursesVoice, and #NursesAreNotOk are trending, and you will see nurses speaking out and taking action on staffing ratios, unsafe practices, racial injustice, and other hot-button issues facing nurses, health care, and the world today.

You may ask how advocacy or activism contributes to your well-being. Living a purposeful life is among the six core dimensions of Carol Ryff's model of well-being (Ryff, 2014). Purposeful life engagement includes life goals and a sense of directedness, meaning-making, and beliefs that give our lives purpose. Those who score high on purpose in life accrue numerous health benefits: living longer, less dysregulation of physiological systems, fewer negative disease outcomes, and practicing more preventive health behaviors (Ryff et al., 2016). The benefits continue as we age. Formal volunteering, where one contributes time and talent to an organization, has been shown to be protective in dealing with the negative effects of later life role changes (Greenfield and Marks, 2004). Volunteering is closely associated with empowerment. As a result of our volunteer actions as advocates or activists, we build our purpose and passion, transforming us.

Nurses have been activists for centuries. You have probably read about pioneers such as Clara Barton and Florence Nightingale in your educational programs, but there are many more— British-Jamaican nurse and entrepreneur Mary Jane Seacole; suffragette Lavinia Dock; Grace Neill, a nurse and social reformer who crusaded for nurse registration laws in New Zealand; Jessie Sleet Scales, born in Ontario, Canada, who hosted the last stop on the Underground Railroad and became a pioneer in public health nursing; and Canadian nurse Moyra Allen, credited with developing standards for nursing programs around the world. What can we learn from activists and their commitment to make change? First, let's look at how the intertwined concepts of advocacy, activism, and social justice apply to the nursing profession.

CREATING SOCIAL AND PROFESSIONAL CHANGE:
THREE CORE IDEAS
•

Peggy Chinn (2018) defines activism as "taking informed, deliberate actions to bring nursing values into the public sphere in ways that challenge the status quo that threatens human health and well-being" (99). The architect of the nurse activist website NurseManifest (https://nurse manifest.com/), Chinn argues that the voice of the nurse should be heard in these discussions, as it is unique, significant, and powerful.

Advocacy, according to the American Nurses Association (ANA), is an essential element of the nursing mission to advocate for individuals, families, communities, and populations (ANA, 2010). Grace (2001) emphasizes that through "professional advocacy," nurses can address the needs of both the individual patient and society specifically through political action, collaborating with other disciplines, and conducting research that fulfills nursing's goals. Nurses also need to advocate for themselves and their profession, individually and collectively.

It is the collective professional responsibility of nurses to address systems and structures that are unjust (ANA, 2015). Grace and Willis (2012) argue that social injustices occur "when all persons are not treated with equal moral concern...their lives are significant and meaningful just because they are human beings" (199). Social justice is critical for our work.

LESSONS FROM HISTORY
•

During the early years of the AIDS epidemic, the mainstream media brought attention to the work of activists who raised awareness and played a key role in securing governmental funds for research (Brodie et al., 2004). For people living with HIV/AIDS, there was shame and social alienation, especially for those coping with mental health disorders. Our conversations with HIV/AIDS nurses at the beginning of the 2020 pandemic confirmed the research on nurses' experiences with HIV/AIDS patients decades ago (Sherman and Ouellette, 1999). Nurses caring for patients with HIV/AIDS and nurses caring for COVID patients had nearly identical reactions—fear of contracting

HIV, helplessness, problems getting up-to-date information, grief, and inadequate referral resources, as well as concerns over discriminatory treatment of client groups (Olivier and Dykeman, 2003).

HIV/AIDS activists were clear about how their movement could succeed (Burns, 2010). They knew that they had to be represented and driven by "user activists," specifically, people who were living with HIV and mental illness. A group of activists and survivors healed and became stronger as a result of their collective actions, developing a sense of agency, empowerment, and personal growth (Rabkin et al., 2018).

Although the activists themselves were subjected to the trauma and grief of losing friends and colleagues from AIDS, they persisted in their efforts. Facing a relentless disease that was cloaked in shame and public ignorance, they joined together in solidarity.

The success story of the South African Treatment Action Campaign (TAC) bears mentioning. Founded in 1998 and spearheaded by a group of people with HIV, they were no longer willing to be passive victims of an unjust system. TAC is now one of the world's most effective AIDS groups, providing prevention and treatment to vulnerable populations. With 182 branches in Africa, they have reshaped their focus in light of the current public health crisis with the Resilient Advocacy in the Time of a Pandemic Project.

Today, nurses are also dealing with shame and stigma. Not from a misunderstood disease such as HIV/AIDS, but from an array of coronavirus myths and misinformation open to public opinion and fodder for ongoing debate. Nurses readily express their reluctance to seek mental health care or admit they need help for fear of embarrassment that they may not be "strong enough" to do their jobs. Other nurses tell us about being targeted and threatened for doing their jobs—wearing scrubs, caring for COVID patients, promoting the need for vaccinations and mask-wearing, or even sending sick students home from school for quarantine and testing. And they are victims of racist harassment and discrimination as well. The COVID-19 pandemic has brought many issues to the surface, but the reality is that nurses have been facing some version of these issues their entire careers. Now, as a light is cast on the deep-rooted issues in nursing, we must ask ourselves: How can nurses advocate for each other?

Advocacy and activism relate to your well-being. As so many studies have confirmed, advocacy and activism are *intimately* connected to our personal and collective sense of well-being.

Caution: The following story may be distressing to some readers, as it includes descriptions of sexual assault and violence. This is a reminder to take care of yourself. Please see the Resources section at the end of the book for more information.

IN THEIR OWN WORDS

> *"I used to wonder why I had to endure this horrific trauma,*
> *but I have come to realize that 1994 did not happen to me*
> *because of what I had done; it happened because of*
> *everything I would do."*

I met Ron at a dinner party in 1989. He called me the next day and asked me out on a date. We saw each other often after that and were married in August 1990.

Fast forward to June 1994. Ron went out to get the morning paper. The telephone rang. It was a woman, and she asked to speak to him. I said, "He's not home right now. This is his wife. Can I take a message?" The woman on the other end gasped, "Oh my God. I have to talk to you." We talked on the phone for more than two hours. She told me that she had been seeing my husband for several years and that they had a son together.

I wrote down her every word; I was going to confront Ron about everything. I told him about the phone call and repeated each and every detail. He was furious, and we argued for hours. I don't remember if he denied anything; I just remember his rage. Finally, around 8:30 that evening, I decided to stop arguing. I felt a change in Ron. I could see him getting angrier and angrier. I had a strange feeling in the pit of my stomach. I was sure that if the argument continued, he would hit me.

Barely an hour later, we began to argue again. He said, "I ought to punch you in the face and break your jaw." Instantly I told him, "If you put your hands on me, I will call the police." Ron reached into the nightstand on his side of the bed. When he turned around and looked at me, he had a knife in his hand. He placed the knife just under my chin and began to scream at me, "Who did you say you were going to call?" He said those words over and over. I refused to answer him but never took my eyes off the knife. I remember thinking to myself, "Just be quiet, and he will calm down." Eventually he did calm down, and as he turned away from me to put the knife back in the drawer, I eased off the bed and ran out of the bedroom.

I ran in my t-shirt and underwear. My feet were bare. I ran out the door. I didn't stop running until I was two blocks from the police station. When the police checked the house, Ron wasn't there. Neither was the knife. The police completed their report and told me that I needed to go to court in the morning to get an order of protection.

At court the next day, I told my story to the judge, a woman. Halfway through, she stopped me and said, "I've heard enough." She gave me a temporary order of protection. The police would meet me at my home at 3 pm to remove Ron from the premises.

When I woke up on the morning of July 9, 1994, and opened my bedroom door, Ron was standing there. He was wearing only a pair of boxer shorts. In his hands were ropes and that same knife! He punched me in the middle of my chest, and I fell backward onto the bed. He got on top of me and pinned me down. He grabbed a scarf and stuffed it into my mouth. I remember thinking, "I'm going to die." He tied my wrists to the headboard. He tied my ankles to the footboard. He raped me.

I called 911 as soon as Ron left the bedroom. I whispered the details of what had just happened into the phone. I heard Ron running out of the apartment. Within minutes, the police came, and I was taken to the hospital to have a rape kit done.

A physician entered my cubicle in the emergency room. He walked over to the counter, opened the evidence collection kit, and started to read the directions. I had been an ER nurse long enough to know that if evidence is not collected properly, it might not be used in court. I had to show this doctor how to do my own rape kit. In that instant, I knew I was no longer the victim—I became the nurse in charge! Ron was eventually arrested, pled guilty, and served seven years in prison.

Several years after the rape, my county started a program to train nurses to perform forensic exams. I attended the training and became the coordinator of one of our state's first Sexual Assault Nurse Examiner Programs. For the past 23 years, I have been board certified to perform forensic examinations on adults, adolescents, and children; now more than 3,000 forensic exams. I am committed to improving the care of sexual assault patients in the hospital. As a technical advisor, I've traveled across the United States as well as to Kenya, Jordan, and Columbia to train nurses and physicians to perform forensic exams. I have provided expert witness testimony in court and spoken publicly about my own experiences as a marital rape survivor. Speaking out helped me heal.

I am an advocate for women, men, and children who are victims of rape or sexual abuse. I believe that rape feeds on a conspiracy of silence, and that those who can, must speak for the thousands who cannot.

1994 was the worst year of my life.

I used to wonder why I had to endure this horrible betrayal, this unspeakable trauma, but I have come to realize that 1994 did not happen to me because of what I had done; it happened to me because of everything I would do. I turned a mess into a message.

July 9, 1994: Karen Carroll, RN, SANE-A, SANE-P,
Westchester County, New York, United States

Karen's story is powerful, personal, and pivotal to her life's work. Her story underscores decades of outrage against sexual assault and harassment—an outrage that has made its way into headlines and our way of life in television, films, best-selling books, and social media campaigns. Writers and activists refer to any one of these events as pivotal, a watershed moment, or a turning point where, finally, the way sexual assault survivors are treated in society will be different. Survivors will be believed, injustices corrected, legislation signed, and prevention efforts will take hold in new and powerful ways. Yet, somehow, like a wave receding from the shoreline, these moments tend to disappear from the public discourse. Until the next time.

As Karen's story so clearly illustrates, nurses are not only experts at empowering their patients, they also call attention to societal injustices and ongoing health inequities. By helping to shape the conversation around sexual assault and the role of nurses, lasting change in the prevention of sexual assault and harassment becomes possible.

As mentioned above, lessons from history can inform the journeys of both advocates and activists. In 2006, Tarana Burke, seeking to bring attention to violence that confronts women and girls of color, created the grassroots campaign "Me Too" as a way to unify survivors (Ohlheiser, 2017). Burke was a civil rights activist and a sexual assault survivor herself. This remarkable movement may have been the first time survivors felt heard and supported by others.

Kate McNair, a women's health nurse practitioner, is one of those empowering voices. In the midst of the #MeToo movement, she tweeted about her newly published *Huffington Post* article, "I've Seen the Effect #MeToo Has Had on Sexual Assault Survivors." In the post, she shared how some of her patients disclosed they had the courage to come forward based on the testimony of other women on social media. McNair (2018) emphasized that while the movement helped women and men come forward, there has not been enough attention on the role of sexual assault nurse examiners (SANE). She underscored the need for systemic change and addressing inequities in post-assault care: more funding and access, ending the backlog of evidence collection kits, and education. Kate and Donna wrote and researched extensively about activism and nursing; some of the words in this text were the result of our collaboration.

According to annual Gallup polls in the United States, nurses have consistently outranked 15 other disciplines as the most trusted professionals, a result of unflinching commitment to professional standards and ethics (Brenan, 2017; Saad, 2020). Nurses also make up the largest segment of the health care profession, with almost 22 million nurses and 2 million midwives across the globe. Nurses have always had the potential to move mountains; after all, the profession's history is securely rooted in social and political activism (Puglionesi, 2020). But these are difficult times that require a renewed call to action. With every coronavirus pandemic surge across the globe, a rising chorus of voices—your voices—have increasingly demonstrated this collective power.

Researchers (Davoodvand et al., 2016) have identified numerous opportunities in nursing for the expansion of patient advocacy roles. Nurses are not only the first advocates for patients but also the link between the patient and the health care system. During the early days of a public health crisis, nurses are often the only health care provider consistently at the bedside of a patient, who may be fearful or otherwise alone. In many cases, they are the only advocates for patients and their patients' families during these pivotal moments.

As nurses, you've advocated for your patients individually, but since early 2020, your roles are no longer limited to providing physical care and emotional support behind the doors of a patient's room. You are speaking up for your patients, for changes in the health care system, and for each other.

RAISING YOUR VOICES
◆

The pandemic has shone a light on the glaring issues in patient care and in the nursing profession. Nurses are well equipped to see public health problems through both a holistic and ethical lens owing to their unique perspective, history, and foundation. The goals and responsibilities of the nursing profession include advocacy, research, education, and participation in shaping health policy (International Council of Nurses, 2012). The ANA (2017) even describes how ethics, human rights, and nursing combined to act as a "formidable instrument" to confront and address social justice issues that intersect with health (Willis et al., 2014).

Numerous authors have described the many ways that nurses can and should try to take action (Gelinas, 2018; Salvage and Stilwell, 2018). Among these tangible strategies are organizing and starting grassroots efforts, speaking to federal and state representatives, connecting with stakeholders, serving on boards and/or committees, voting, participating in peaceful marches, and writing op-eds and letters to the editor. Nurses must tell their own stories. The public, government leaders, and the profession itself need to hear these powerful messages.

In terms of research, nurse scholars can develop the practice; identify social injustices; conduct research while being thoughtful of the methodology used; and disseminate that scientific evidence via academic journals, lectures, and presentations. In education, courses and nursing curricula can address social justice, policy, and avenues to activism (Florell, 2021).

Professional nurses should become knowledgeable about issues in the profession as well as any recent legal changes or reforms. This information can be disseminated via blogs, social media platforms, and among colleagues. If you find misleading information about the profession, your practice, or role in print or electronic media, write letters to the editor—it is crucial to clarify, reinterpret, reiterate, and emphasize. Advocacy and activism can also address positive changes in the profession itself: improved salaries, better working conditions, and appropriate resource allocation. We have seen hundreds of articles that chronicle the extreme working conditions of nurses during the pandemic, from nurses feeling forced to take on double shifts because of a lack of staffing to hospitals refusing to implement hazard pay. As dismal as these stories sound, we have to remember that there are regional and global differences, and this type of treatment is not commonplace everywhere and should not be accepted as the "norm." We need to find the nuggets of gold—the success stories—and promote them to the rest of the world.

Working conditions and salaries have been at the forefront of nurses' concerns and have stoked the ire of nurses who have spent the past two years of their lives, maybe longer, in the most difficult working conditions. The National Health Service in the United Kingdom has had an ongoing battle over nurses' salaries and benefits. In the spring of 2021, The Independent reported that the government suggested a 1% pay raise, but nurses protested and argued that 1% really wasn't a raise at all. They were already struggling to pay their bills and make ends meet. Interestingly, the author of the article pointed out that at the beginning of the pandemic in the winter of 2020, the public clapped for their health care workers every evening as the shifts changed. They were the heroes of the hour—for about 10 weeks. Then the fanfare and appreciation ended. Author Abi Jackson (2021) added, "Nurses are not just heroes of the hour—they're heroes full-stop; day in, day out, pre-pandemic and (hopefully) long after it."

Similar concerns were felt worldwide (Ford, 2021). Underpaid nurses in Wales were asking for a 12.5% salary increase (Smith, 2021); health care workers in Poland were protesting low wages and poor working conditions (Nowak and Weiss, 2021). But in a bizarre twist, the headline of a 2021 Motley Fool article read, "Travel Nurses Are Suddenly

Making Wall Street Caliber Money." Billing rates for travel nurses soared, increasing 40% over a 12-month period, with emergency room specialists seeing a 60% hike, and some weekly salaries grew as high as $8,000. In times of need or desperation, hospitals hire travel nurses to work alongside their staff nurses at vastly different salaries. Loyal staff nurses who have been with their hospital systems for years and decades tell us that it is just another "slap in the face." Hospital administrations are using stop-gap measures to meet demands of their patient population, but that may not solve long-term problems.

INNOVATION

♦

As nurses, you have always identified the most ingenious solutions. Your extraordinary problem-solving skill set can address issues with communications, patient care, programmatic innovations, and more. In early 2021, a group of staff nurses were frustrated with the daily information dump of the newest pandemic policies and procedural changes. Returning to work after one day off meant scrolling through pages of emails to find relevant information related to safety and patient care. At one New Jersey hospital, nurses took matters into their own hands and created an easy information-sharing system. They formed a small committee for this project and posted each update and the latest research on a large bulletin board to keep everyone informed. Nurses arrived at work and were able to quickly check the newest information, then immediately care for their patients. It was not only innovative but also time- and likely life-saving. When asked if the rest of the hospital adopted their information-sharing system, they looked puzzled and didn't know. Their action in creating this solution supported the needs of the nurses on their floor, but neither they nor their administrators had considered how this could be implemented on a larger scale, improving the nursing care at a hospital-wide level.

No doubt there have been many great ideas for resolving professional or patient care issues. Consider what's happened in your own work life. How did you share information about any of your projects? What was the response from colleagues and administrators?

Cultivating Great Ideas

Goal: To identify one solution to a problem or innovative strategy you've devised at work

Time and place: 10–15 minutes; write in a journal to keep at home or at work.

Use the prompts below to help you reflect on past strategies and nurture new ideas.

Describe the solution you devised. Remember to include time, place, situation, and outcomes.

Did colleagues join you in the planning and execution? Who?

Did you share the information? If you did, how?

Consider starting a great ideas notebook.

As nurse activist Paula Kagan (2013) points out in a powerful editorial, "Innovation means taking a profoundly critical look at where we are and how things are done and taking the risk to abandon habits of thought and action toward true change and accomplishment that betters human health and quality of life" (270). As with advocacy and activism, nursing innovation is a global phenomenon.

IN THEIR OWN WORDS

Sometimes, a small act of "helping" turns into a life-transforming experience.

I have been working with a chest surgery team in New Delhi, India since 2017, learning its nuances with great interest and contributing in my own small way. In December 2020, the team relocated to a new hospital, beginning a new chapter in my life. I moved up the ladder and was made leader of the nurses' team (3 specialist nurses and 40 general nurses), which pushed me out of my comfort zone with new challenges and responsibilities. These were COVID times, when the world had virtually come to a standstill, but nurses and doctors were working like angels to help the society, often at huge personal cost.

The head of our department, a man wedded to quality care, dreamt of making ours the best chest surgical unit in the country. Despite his efforts, however, there was a lacuna in the quality and continuity of clinical care due to COVID. There was a void of thoracic surgeons; they are a rare breed in India.

It was July 2, 2021, and I had just returned to the duty room after the morning rounds with a cup of tea in my hand. The room dimly lit, the window glass fogged from the rain outside. There I was, staring into the vacuum outside, drowned in thoughts on how to help the unit. Suddenly, there was lightning and a thought flashed in my mind.

What if three of us (specialist thoracic nurses) start doing longer shifts—a day, that night, and the next day, ending at 5 pm. The next nurse would start her shift at 9 am, so during any day, from 9 to 5, there will be two specialized thoracic surgery nurses, one from the previous day and one for that day, giving the much-needed continuity of care. We will be the workhorses; consultants will provide the cover.

I shared the idea with my two colleagues, who looked at me with shock and asked, "Are you out of your mind?" But I wanted to try it out and persuaded my two colleagues to take it to the head of the department. Surprisingly, he was toying with such an idea himself and accepted the proposal on a trial basis.

The experiment started on July 5, 2021, and I was assigned the inaugural duty. A chest surgery nurse doing a 32-hour shift, just like a resident—on one hand, the idea was filling me with pride, but at the same time, an unknown fear of responsibilities, decision-making, and a lot of uncertainty was tormenting me. I had no clue how the experiment would unfold or where it would take us, but I was determined to give it a fair try and make it succeed to help the unit.

I did the first duty, with the consultant taking an exhaustive round and available by phone for helpful tips. The day passed without incident, as did the first night and next morning, when I was joined at 9 am by my colleague for next day shift, and I passed on all patient details to her. We took a detailed round with the consultant. Suddenly, we all noticed that we were in better control of everything on the ward, and there was a continuity of care. My first 32-hour shift passed uneventfully. Before leaving at 5 am, I met the head of the department. I could see relief writ large on his face. He smiled at me and quipped, "Neha, you just created history!"

I had tears of joy rolling down my face. I left for home, exhausted but exhilarated.

As I returned after a day off, for second duty, the signs were clear that the experiment had paid off. The next few weeks were historic and changed our lives as we witnessed a thrilling cycle of positivity. The consultants would reach out to us and share useful information and tips for hours. Their input improved our output, which encouraged them to invest even more time in us. We were invited to unit meetings and learned how to work up new cases in the outpatient department, read X-rays, insert and remove chest tubes, scrub in operating room cases, and a lot more.

The positivity did not end there. We were invited to accompany the consultants for the academic program in various cities and asked to be part of the presentation. I was ecstatic when introduced to senior doctors as a vital member of the team. I was appointed the national clinical coordinator for a program our department conducts on safe insertion of chest tubes. I've also been asked about being sent abroad for more exposure.

The past few months have been a dream phase of my life, with new status and a new horizon. Little did I realize that a small but bold step by me would sow the seeds for the first-of-its-kind nurse-thoracic surgeon cadre in India.

I dream of a day where nurses will become the voices of the medical profession!

December 2020: Neha Tiwari, RN, Chest Surgery Nurse Coordinator,
Institute of Chest Surgery and Lung Care Foundation,
Medanta–The Medicity, Gurugram, India

ADVOCACY AND ACTIVISM ARE
GOOD FOR YOUR HEALTH
◆

There is a kindling point where empathy, innovation, passion, and commitment come together and drive us to act outside of our usual practice settings—hospitals, classrooms, or the community. As you read in the story above, nurses who are involved and take action contribute to their profession and to the world around them. Even in the most desperate situations such as community disasters, contributing time and taking a leadership role can have benefits, especially for the mental health and unity of the community (Bowe et al., 2021). Yet there is an even greater benefit—one that is personal and will build your reserve of resilience.

Advocacy and activism (Vestergen et al., 2017) can generate many psychological benefits: strengthened relationships, better work-life balance, building self-identity, empowerment, sustained commitment, enhanced self-esteem, general well-being, greater self-confidence, and organizing knowledge. Hernández et al. (2007) even describe activism as a potential antidote to vicarious trauma, building transformative skills and resilience. For example, researchers have found that writing about one's stressful or traumatic experiences can be the first step in activism—it additionally has the potential to improve coping strategies, clarify and solve problems, and facilitate social interactions (Pennebaker, 1997; Jacobson and Jeffries, 2018).

THE SCIENCE OF ADVOCACY AND ACTIVISM

The psychological benefits of advocacy and activism, and their contribution to well-being, have been confirmed in a number of studies. A June 2020 UK survey (Bowe et al., 2022) showed that coordinated community, such as resident group associations that provide practical and emotional support to vulnerable residents, predicted the psychological bonding of community members. Building a sense of community identification and unity by reaching out to the most vulnerable and isolated during the pandemic predicted increased well-being and reduced depression and anxiety.

Two online surveys of college students and a national sample of activists demonstrated that well-being was higher in participants who self-identified as activists (Klar and Kasser, 2009). Even those who engaged in brief activist behavior reported significantly higher levels of subjective vitality than the subjects who engaged in the nonactivist behavior. Using the Ryff Scales of Psychological Well-Being, the activism group was positively associated with life satisfaction, and positive affect.

In a large study based on data from the sixth round of the European Social Survey of 54,673 respondents aged 15 and older, Šarkutė (2017) confirmed that political activism is closely tied to higher levels of subjective well-being. Activism was positively correlated with a global self-evaluation of well-being, emotional well-being, vitality, community well-being, and supportive relationships. But the strongest positive correlations were found between political activism, community well-being, and supportive relationships.

Another study looked at 10 years of research focusing on the relationship between activism and well-being during adolescence (Testa and Cavallini, 2021). The researchers found that activism during adolescence enhances various types of well-being, personally and collectively. The group effect has considerable importance, empowering adolescents to build up their awareness, work collaboratively on issues of mutual concern, and expand their social connections, all leading to improved psychological well-being.

These adolescent behaviors can help to establish a lifelong commitment to advocacy and activism as well as collaborative practices, ultimately promoting a sense of well-being that has a ripple effect in all that they do.

References
Bowe, M., Wakefield, J. R., Kellezi, B., Stevenson, C., McNamara, N., Jones, B. A., Sumich, A. & Heym, N. (2022). The mental health benefits of community helping during crisis: coordinated helping, community identification and sense of unity during the COVID-19 pandemic. *Journal of Community and Applied Social Psychology* 32(3): 521–35.

Klar, M., & Kasser, T. (2009). Some benefits of being an activist: measuring activism and its role in psychological well-being. *Political Psychology* 30(5): 755–77.

Šarkutė, L. (2017). Does political activism induce subjective wellbeing? Evidence from ESS data. *International Journal of Psychology* 2017: 21.

Testa, D., & Cavallini, F. (2021). How activism correlates with well-being in adolescence: a systematic review. *Journal of Clinical and Developmental Psychology* 3(3).

Labor activists, nurses, and domestic workers make up the core of the labor movement in the Philippines. They have transformed their labor of care into a "feminist politics of care" (Sales, 2021). During the pandemic, Filipina nurses were increasingly visible as they appealed for government and employer accountability. When National Nurses United (NNU) heard about a new virus from colleagues in Asia, Zenei Triunfo-Cortez, the first Filipina president of NNU, the largest organization of nurses in the United States, immediately sent letters of concern to the World Health Organization and the Centers for Disease Control and Prevention. During Nurses Week, NNU held a vigil at the White House for nurses who died from COVID-19. In August, nurse activists demanded Congress pass the HEROES Act as one step toward "reenvision[ing] a world based on nurses' values of caring, compassion, and community" (NNU, 2020).

IN THEIR OWN WORDS

I was at home in New York on the morning of January 12, 2010, when I heard a report on NPR about an earthquake in Haiti. It was horrific. I thought about the people of that small island, barely 800 miles from shores of the United States. Haitians are our neighbors, already dealing with poverty, stagnant development, and inadequate government services, and on that day in 2010, they were suddenly living with devastation. Several hours later, I heard another report that struck deep inside of me. While the president of the country was driving around surveying the damage, he heard cries for help coming from what had been a school of nursing. I am a nursing professor, and that hit me in the gut.

I was determined to do something about it.

At our next faculty meeting, I talked about the tragedy and arranged a forum to discuss what we could do for the devastated nursing school in Port au Prince. The appeal resonated. One attendee, Joanna (an adult nurse practitioner), asked me if I knew Carmelle Bellefleur, a nursing professor, Haitian, and member of our alumni association. I did not, but we soon became fast friends. Joanna called Carmelle, who immediately boarded a train and was with us within an hour. Ultimately, four of us flew to Haiti to evaluate the nursing school in person and to understand what was possible. We stayed in the earthquake-damaged home of Carmelle's cousin. The family slept outside in a tent provided by UNICEF. They were too afraid of aftershocks to sleep inside.

Our investigation was based on face-to-face visits with public and private educators, government members, and providers. It was as complete as the circumstances would allow. We saw the devastation caused by the quake as we moved around the city, looking for facilities and for people who cared enough to help. We found unfortunate lapses in nursing education, nursing practice, and in health care delivery in general. It was so unsettling—the difference between knowing the existence of these issues from afar and feeling it directly, hearing it, seeing it. The events in Haiti that week were an assault on our senses and sensibilities: the destroyed city, the population living in filth, sewage running along the road, so many homeless. The most dramatic sight was of a dead baby in a crib in the courtyard of a hospital we visited, there for the entire world to see, including a terrified four-year-old boy.

Our team returned to Haiti frequently. We held a two-day conference in New York City for any nurse in the United States or Canada who was interested in helping in Haiti. The consensus of that meeting was that Haiti needed better nursing education if health care was to improve. As difficult as that sounded, we knew that the best medium- to long-term answer lay in training nurses, and training them in Haiti. After a series of meetings in Haiti and New York, our group founded a nurse practitioner program in one of the private nursing schools, which had only an undergraduate program. There was no graduate nurse education in Haiti at all; ours was the first. Three of us were nurse practitioners and nursing school graduate faculty, and we taught the program ourselves, based on the curricula developed at our home institutions. To effect change, you need infrastructure and organization, so we formed a nonprofit called Promoting Health in Haiti. We funded the organization ourselves. We have subsequently raised money, gained funding, and expanded our faculty; the start-up grew.

We have graduated 34 nurse practitioners with masters degrees, and we are still going strong, with well-educated primary care providers making a difference in health care outcomes and in the experience and education of their peers. By providing solid graduate nursing education in Haiti, the brain drain phenomenon is avoided. These men and women are living and working in their Haitian communities. The program has moved to Haiti State University, into the public domain, where we always wanted it to be.

I feel a sense of accomplishment in creating this paradigm shift, creating a new class of providers for Haiti, but I feel the work is incomplete;

there is still so, so much more to do. I know that health care in Haiti remains primitive. Access, quality, outcomes all need to improve. Our nurse practitioners are working hard, but we need more of them. The Haitian political process needs to evolve to effectively support primary care and to demonstrate that government cares about the health of ordinary people. That job we will have to leave to others.

January 12, 2010: Carol Roye, EdD, RN, CPNP, FAAN, Pediatric Nurse Practitioner, Westchester, New York, United States

YOUR COLLECTIVE VOICES
◆

As you can see from Carol Roye's experience in Haiti, it took the collective action of US nurses and nurses from Haiti to achieve their goals. The benefits of collective action have been well established (Foster, 2014). There are at least three important outcomes of communal effort: people are inspired by joining with others, they have greater confidence in the movement, and they have greater confidence in themselves and each other (Drury et al., 2015). Participants are self-assured and empowered, and as a result, their personal lives are changed for the better (Foster, 2014). Activists lead more fulfilled lives compared to non-activists (Klar and Kasser, 2009). While individual actions can have positive effects, the power of the group may carry more weight. According to Drury et al. (2015), "as an individual you can complain about injustice, but as a group you can change it" (23). Engaging and connecting with family members, friends, colleagues, or even posting on social media can lead to a greater sense of well-being by participating in a shared community.

While the job of an activist may seem overwhelming, we must be clear that one does not solve these issues alone. Collaboration with colleagues and those from other professions, in and outside of health care, is an important takeaway. Everyone can and should be a part of the conversation and deserves a seat at the table.

HEALTH CARE IS A HUMAN RIGHT
◆

IN THEIR OWN WORDS

So, it's 2005, and I'm in the second semester of my freshman year here at Michigan. The course was an honors seminar in health policy and its influences on health disparities.

Up until the moment I bought the *Policy and Politics in Nursing and Health Care* textbook, I didn't realize I could combine the two things that I felt the most passionate about—policy and nursing—into a career. I can tell you honestly: that class set me on my path to Congress. I knew I wanted to be a health care provider since I was a kid. I'd tell anyone who asked that I was going to be a pediatric cardiologist when I grew up. This was, of course, before I could spell pediatric cardiologist and way before I took organic chemistry.

Let's fast forward to 2017. I was 30 and wrapping up my abso-lute dream job at the Department of Health and Human Services. I had been appointed by President Obama to help guide the federal response to the Ebola epidemic, the Flint water crisis, and other public health emergencies. The incoming administration had made it clear that their intention was to overturn the Affordable Care Act and *take health care away* from millions of Americans. That's *not* why I became a nurse.

While the debate over the future of the Affordable Care Act was raging in Congress, [my congressional representative] pledged that he would not repeal health care coverage for people with preexisting conditions. I took him at his word. So, two weeks later, when that now *former* congressman voted for a version of ACA repeal that jeopardized the health care coverage for 300,000 people in my community—people with diabetes or depression or a heart condition like me—I made a decision. I was running for Congress.

One of the first things we learn in nursing school is our code of ethics. We're duty-bound to advocate for our patients' rights. We are guided by compassion, clinical excellence, and a commitment to health care as a human right. So when my community's health care was threatened, I felt a responsibility as a nurse to step up. That's not to say I wasn't scared. I was terrified.

But our professors didn't only teach us clinical excellence. They taught us to be the next generation of nurse leaders. I had my friend Sarah, who stepped up as my campaign manager. We built a website, constructed a policy platform, and we shot a campaign video.

In November 2018, against all odds, my first race for public office ended in a five-point victory. At 32, I became the youngest Black woman to serve in Congress.

Listen, I know that my story is unique. But remember this: You have been prepared for leadership too. I'm not saying you have to run for Congress. Nurses can be leaders in a clinic, a university, a C-suite, a public health board ... the opportunities are endless. What matters is that you share your expertise. Because listen: our communities need our leadership. Our voices and our expertise are critical, *especially* right now.

Just like I was, you have been prepared to be a leader. And you already have *everything* you need to make an impact.

So remember this: Those things that make you different make your leadership all the more powerful and all the more necessary. As nurses, we must recognize the power of our voices. As citizens, we must do the same. It's my responsibility to remind you that without active engage-ment, American democracy will falter. Our democracy is too precious, too essential, to let it slip away. And because this school nurtured my passion for policy, I want to encourage you to explore your own. Most everything you'll do as a nurse, from the treatments you administer, to how long a patient can stay in your unit, to how much you're getting paid, to the kind of PPE you have access to, involves political decision-making. As nurses, we can more effectively advocate for ourselves, our patients and our communities when we understand how policy decisions shape the care we deliver.

We must *dare* to provide health care for all.

Today, I'm asking you to recognize that as a political statement. To make good on that promise, we need nurses to be involved as *agenda setters, barrier breakers, decision makers*. At this moment in history, your leadership is critical. I know how challenging these past two years have been. And I want to recognize your resolve in the face of unprec-edented challenges. The majority of your clinical experience occurred during a once-in-a-century pandemic. Many of you have grappled with the challenges and inequities of our health care system before your career has even begun. At times, you may have felt your commitment and courage pushed to the limits. And now, you are uniquely prepared to drive transformational change in your communities.

I decided to mount my unlikely campaign for Congress because I felt that people of conscience needed to stand up for our shared values. I believe that is even more true today, and that this moment specifically requires nurse leadership. Stepping into leadership has a ripple effect: you show others what's possible, you inspire them to tap into their own strength.

That's the power you hold, and the responsibility you carry.

April 30, 2022: Congresswoman Lauren Underwood, 14th Congressional District, Illinois. University of Michigan School of Nursing Commencement, Ann Arbor, Michigan, United States

In the spring of 2022 when Congresswoman Lauren Underwood, RN (IL-14), gave that powerful commencement address at the University of Michigan School of Nursing, her words were met with cheers and applause. Her message was strong, but her story does not have to be unique. In fact, her words were a clarion call to nurses to get involved and take action—now more than ever.

Nurses have always appealed to their professional organizations for the protection of the interests of their members, and to advocate for their patients and the communities they serve. Issues such as standards of practice, workplace safety, patient privacy, and nurse-to-patient ratios are only a few of the issues facing the profession today. "In its core, advocacy seeks to ensure that the needs, rights, and wishes of vulnerable individuals are heard and safeguarded" (Davies, 2021).

COVID-19 tested the capacity of many nursing organizations as they struggled to address the profession's new and urgent demands—inadequate PPE, long hours, short staffing, and unsafe conditions. This was a crisis of epic proportions.

Provision 9.4 of the American Nurses Association (ANA) Code of Ethics (2015) states, "Professional nursing organizations must actively engage in the political process, particularly in addressing legislative and regulatory concerns that most affect—positively and negatively—the public health and the profession of nursing."

Erin Hartnett, a nurse practitioner in New York City, wants professional associations such as the ANA "to honor these declarations by using their platform to advocate and engage politically" (Chamlou, 2022). Hartnett emphasizes that "healthcare really depends on what laws get passed. So, if nurses don't know or understand the whole political arena … then they can't advocate." Her words speak volumes about an ever-widening chasm that prevents professional nurses from accomplishing their mission. Nurses do not focus solely on patients who are acutely ill—they promote health for the whole population, no matter where they may be.

To fill this chasm, Hartnett invited a group of colleagues to join a new grassroots organization, Nurses for America. The group supports nurses, democracy, and the policies that align with the values and positions held by the nursing profession. In addition, they have a keen interest in voter rights, health equity, reproductive rights, gun control, and candidates who support these policies. Their website (https://nurses foramerica.net/) is filled with position statements, letters to the editor, and candidate positions. They also publish a monthly newsletter to inform readers how to be involved.

Catherine Dodd, a longtime nurse activist from the San Francisco Bay area and member of Nurses for America (NFA), spoke with passion and commitment about the intersection of nursing, policy, and political action when she said, "I maintain my license and use my nursing education and experience each day that I analyze and advocate for legislation." She poses two important questions for all nurses to consider if they are to engage in a political organization: "Is our organization's mission to educate nurses about legislation? Or, is it about educating nurses about how policy/legislation and politics are inextricably linked?" (pers. comm., August 12, 2022).

Another member of NFA, Eileen Gordon, a pediatric nurse practitioner from Ohio and awardee of the Ohio Nurse Practitioner of the Year, is passionate about nurses being the change makers we need: "To make change, nurses, including new nurses, must be engaged in politics, both local and national. The future of our patients and our profession depends on it." She points out that the American Medical Association and other health professional groups have labeled voting a "health determinant," and urges nurses and nursing students to volunteer to sign up voters with Vote-ER, a nonpartisan effort by nurses and doctors using a QR code to direct people to register to vote (pers. comm., August 24, 2022). Those who vote have a better chance in determining their health as regulated by elected officials.

Elected officials determine the outcome of vital health legislation that, when positive, can regulate out-of-control prescription prices. When negative, it can keep lifesaving drugs like insulin out of reach for those who need it to stay alive. The threatened ending of Social Security and Medicare, leading to poorer health outcomes for our patients, is also in the hands of elected officials. Even the makeup of the US Supreme Court is subject to the political desires of elected officials. When the Supreme Court overturned a long-standing law respecting the right of our patients to bodily autonomy, it was in conflict with our code of ethics as nurses.

In addition to voting, nurses can write letters to editors on timely topics and engage in virtual and in-person activities to promote candidates to political office who stand for nurses, reducing gun violence, reproductive freedom, and the protection of all people, especially patients. New nurses can support local nurses who run for political office and will represent the needs of our patients, and not corporations.

Nurses cannot afford to sit on the sidelines.

FINAL THOUGHTS
•

The intent of this chapter is to spark thought and conversation, and to empower you and your colleagues. All nurses must engage at the complex intersection of social justice and health activism—it is the essence of what it means to be a nurse. While focusing on the most vulnerable populations—our patients—we must also address the problems that require changing the tears in the cultural fabric of our society and government.

Since early 2017, there has been a surge of activism, especially among women—they have taken to the streets to protect their rights in ways not seen since the women's suffrage movement and the civil rights era (Zernike, 2018). Young people are even starting their own movements, sowing hope for the future, demanding governments take action in fighting climate change, and promoting legislation for gun laws that could prevent school shootings (Mazzei, 2019). Resources are plentiful, with new organizations launching each year aiming to be the solution they have been seeking. Movements not only achieve political and policy change but are also the "engines of cultural change" (Berridge, 2007).

Nurses have the potential to wield immense power and will be inspired to find their own voices—not only to support those who did or will require your care in the future, but also to educate the public and advocate for policy and professional change.

All nurses must take action for both their patients and each other.

We cannot afford to be silent any longer.

It's time.

REFERENCES

ANA. American Nurses Association. (2010). *Nursing's Social Policy Statement: The Essence of the Profession.* Silver Spring, MD: ANA.

ANA. American Nurses Association. (2015). *Code of Ethics for Nurses with Interpretive Statements.* Silver Spring, MD: ANA.

ANA. American Nurses Association. (2017). *Ethics and Human Rights Statement.* Silver Spring, MD: ANA.

Berridge, V. (2007). Public health activism: Lessons from history? BMJ 335(7633): 1310–12.

Bowe, M., Wakefield, J. R., Kellezi, B., Stevenson, C., McNamara, N., Jones, B. A., Sumich, A., & Heym, N. (2021). The mental health benefits of community helping during crisis: coordinated helping, community identification and sense of unity during the COVID-19 pandemic. *Journal of Community and Applied Social Psychology* 32(3): 521–35.

Brenan, M. (2017). Nurses keep healthy lead as most honest, ethical profession. *Gallup News*, December 26, 2017. https://news.gallup.com/poll/224639/nurses-keep-healthy-lead-honest-ethical-profession.aspx?version=print

Brodie, M., Hamel, E., Brady, L. A., Kates, J., & Altman, D. E. (2004). AIDS at 21: media coverage of the HIV epidemic 1981–2002. *The Nation* 49: 68.

Burns, J. K. (2010). Mental health advocacy—lessons from HIV activism. SAMJ *South African Medical Journal* 100(10): 654. http://www.samj.org.za/index.php/samj/article/view/4427/2965

Chamlou, N. (2022). Nursing association under fire after "abandoning nurses" in time of need. *Nurse Journal*, August 12, 2022. https://nursejournal.org/articles/nursing-organizations-under-fire-after-abandoning-nurses/

Chinn, P. L. (2018). From the editor: the time for nursing activism. *Advances in Nursing Science* 41(2): 99.

Davies, N. (2021). Advocating for patients. *Independent Nurse*, August 27, 2021. https://www.independentnurse.co.uk/professional-article/advocating -for-patients/239940/

Davoodvand, S., Abbaszadeh, A., & Ahmadi, F. (2016). Patient advocacy from the clinical nurse' viewpoint: a qualitative study. *Journal of Medical Ethics and History of Medicine* 9: 5.

Drury, J., Evripidou, A., & van Zomeren, M. (2015). Empowerment: the inter-section of identity and power in collective action. In: Sindic, D., Barreto, M., & Costa-Lopes, R., eds. *Power and Identity*. New York: Psychology Press, 94–116.

Florell, M. C. (2021). Concept analysis of nursing activism. *Nursing Forum* 56 (1): 134–40.

Ford, M. (2021). Budget "worrying sign" that nurses will receive low pay rise, says RCN. *Nursing Times*, March 3, 2021. https://www.nursingtimes.net /news/policies-and-guidance/budget-worrying-sign-that-nurses-will -receive-low-pay-rise-says-rcn-03-03-2021/

Foster, M. D. (2014). The relationship between collective action and well-being and its moderators: pervasiveness of discrimination and dimensions of action. *Sex Roles* 70 (5–6): 165–82.

Gelinas, L. (2018). What #metoo means for nurses. *American Nurse Today* 13 (2): 4.

Grace, P. J. (2001). Professional advocacy: widening the scope of accountability. *Nursing Philosophy* 2 (2): 151–62.

Grace, P. J., & Willis, D. G. (2012). Nursing responsibilities and social justice: an analysis in support of disciplinary goals. *Nursing Outlook* 60: 198–207.

Greenfield, E. A., & Marks, N. F. (2004). Formal volunteering as a protective factor for older adults' psychological well-being. *Journal of Gerontology Series B: Psychological Sciences and Social Sciences* 59 (5): S258–S264. https://doi.org /10.1093/geronb/59.5.s258

Hernández, P., Gangsei, D., & Engstrom, D. (2007). Vicarious resilience: a new concept in work with those who survive trauma. *Family Process* 46 (2): 229–41.

International Council of Nurses. (2012). *The ICN Code of Ethics for Nurses*. Geneva: International Council of Nurses.

Jackson, A. (2021). Opinion: after the year we've had, can we not value our nurses enough to pay them better? *The Independent*, June 17, 2021. https:// www.independent.co.uk/life-style/opinion-boris-johnson-royal-college -of-nursing-nhs-england-b1867687.html

Jacobson, J., & Jeffries, P. (2018). Nursing, trauma, and reflective writing. *NAM Perspectives*, June 25, 2018. https://nam.edu/nursing-trauma-and-reflective -writing/

Kagan, P. N. (2013). Innovation in nursing: only radical change will do. *Advances in Nursing Practice* 36 (4): 268–70.

Klar, M., & Kasser, T. (2009). Some benefits of being an activist: measuring activism and its role in psychological well-being. *Political Psychology* 30 (5): 755–77.

Mazzei, P. (2019). Parkland students bask in Pulitzer mention: "They took us seriously." *New York Times*, April 16, 2019. https://www.nytimes.com/2019/04/16/us/pulitzer-parkland-stoneman-douglas-eagle-eye.html?search ResultPosition=2

McNair, K. (2018). I've seen the effect #MeToo has had on sexual assault survivors. *Huffington Post*, June 28, 2018. https://www.huffingtonpost.com/entry /opinion-mcnair-me-too-sexual-assault-survivors_s_5b242e22e4b0783 ae1294d4e

Motley Fool. (2021). Travel nurses are suddenly making Wall Street caliber money. August 31, 2021. https://www.fool.com/investing/2021/08/31/travel-nurses -are-suddenly-making-wall-street-cali/

NNU. National Nurses United. (2020). Thousands of nurses hold national day of action Aug. 5 to save lives during COVID-19 and beyond. Press release, August 3, 2020. https://www.nationalnursesunited.org/press/national -day-action-aug-5

Nowak, M., & Weiss, C. (2021). Mass protests against untenable conditions in the Polish health care system. World Socialist Web Site, September 14, 2021. https://www.wsws.org/en/articles/2021/09/15/pola-s15.html

Ohlheiser, A. (2017). The woman behind "Me Too" knew the power of the phrase when she created it—10 years ago. *Washington Post*, October 19, 2017. https://www.washingtonpost.com/news/the-intersect/wp/2017/10/19 /the-woman-behind-me-too-knew-the-power-of-the-phrase-when-she -created-it-10-years-ago/

Olivier, C., & Dykeman, M. (2003). Challenges to HIV service provision: the commonalities for nurses and social workers. *AIDS Care* 15(5): 649–63.

Pennebaker, J. W. (1997). Writing about emotional experiences as a therapeutic process. *Psychological Science* 8(3), 162–66.

Puglionesi, A. (2020). Nurses have a history of activism in the U.S., championing suffrage and health care access. *Teen Vogue*, July 14, 2020. https://www .teenvogue.com/story/history-activist-nurses-united-states

Rabkin, J. G., McElhiney, M. C., Harrington, M., & Horn, T. (2018). Trauma and growth: impact of AIDS activism. *AIDS Research and Treatment* 2018: 1–11.

Ryff, C. D. (2014). Psychological well-being revisited: advances in the science and practice of eudaimonia. *Psychotherapy and Psychosomatics* 83(1): 10–28. https://doi.org/10.1159/000353263

Ryff, C. D., Heller, A. S., Schaefer, S. M., van Reekum, C., & Davidson, R. J. (2016). Purposeful engagement, healthy aging, and the brain. *Current Behavioral Neuroscience Reports* 3(4): 318–27. https://doi.org/10.1007/s40473-016-0096-z

Saad, L. (2020). U.S. ethics ratings rise for medical workers and teachers. *Gallup*, December 22, 2020. https://news.gallup.com/poll/328136/ethics-ratings -rise-medical-workers-teachers.aspx

Sales, J. (2021). Activism as essential work: Filipino healthcare workers and human rights in the Philippines. *Diplomatic History* 45(3): 595–603.

Salvage, J., & Stilwell, B. (2018). Breaking the silence: a new story of nursing. *Journal of Clinical Nursing* 27(7–8): 1301–3.

Sherman, D. W., & Ouellette, S. C. (1999). Moving beyond fear: lessons learned through a longitudinal review of the literature regarding health care providers and the care of people with HIV/AIDS. *Nursing Clinics of North America* 34(1): 1–48.

Smith, M. (2021). Severely underpaid nurses in Wales calling for a 12.5% pay rise. Wales Online, April 2, 2021. https://www.walesonline.co.uk/news/health/severely-underpaid-nurses-wales-calling-20310575

Vestergren, S., Drury, J., & Chiriac, E. H. (2017). The biographical consequences of protest and activism: a systematic review and a new typology. *Social Movement Studies* 16(2): 203–21.

Willis, D. G., Perry, D. J., Lacoursiere-Zucchero, T., & Grace, P. (2014). Facilitating humanization: liberating the profession of nursing from institutional confinement on behalf of social justice. In: *Philosophies and Practices of Emancipatory Nursing: Social Justice as Praxis.* London: Taylor & Francis, 251–65.

Zernike, K. (2018). The year of the woman's activism: marches, phone banks, postcards, more. *New York Times*, November 3, 2018. https://www.nytimes.com/2018/11/03/us/politics/women-activism-midterms.html

CHAPTER 10

•

Navigating the Challenges
of the Health Care Landscape

"I get the feeling that I won't be able to handle things. It's draining,
it's exhausting. I think I need to decide what I'm going to do,
what I'm going do with the rest of my life. Maybe I'll go
back to school. I don't know ..."

IN THEIR OWN WORDS
_____

It was a really, really difficult weekend for me. I worked Friday, Saturday, and Sunday.

I had a 78-year-old patient; I knew she wasn't going to make it. Her daughter accused the staff of everything; it was all our fault. Although I have a good team on my unit, there are some people who leave everything for the next shift to do. It falls on me. I never have a chance to go back to baseline when I'm working. On difficult weekends, I run to my friend in the car on the way home. It's good to just have her listen, thank goodness.

But some nights it's just too much. I have to escape—I turn on reality TV, *Grey's Anatomy*, and *New Amsterdam*. Then I realize I'm not really escaping, so I turn on MTV reality shows. I keep a list of my symptoms; I'm worried about burnout. I am always tired, bone tired. I feel so fatigued. I try to leave my patients at work, but I can't get them out of my mind. I can't get work out of my head.

In the beginning, I worked overtime, but I stopped that. I'm so frustrated with management. I bottle up what I see. There's a lot of death. I push it down, turn it off. Seeing so much, so fast, there is no time to process things. You take care of one patient who is dying, then the patient dies, you have to clean the patient, the bed gets scrubbed, and then the next patient comes in. There is no time to process. I put everything on the back burner.

When we're short staffed, everyone agrees it's a problem, but nothing is done. Sometimes administration tries to check in with us. Making rounds, asking to make sure we're doing okay. Sometimes we get an email saying how much they support us. But they don't come on the weekends when I'm working. Some people don't help at all. Then I get the feeling that I won't be able to handle things. It's draining, it's exhausting. I need to decide what I'm going to do, what I'm going to do with the rest of my life. Maybe I'll go back to school. I don't know...

March 2020: Anonymous, Pulmonary Intensive
Care Unit, Western/Mid-Atlantic United States

BURNOUT
◆

"I don't know what I'm going to do." These are such powerful words. What is burnout, and what does it have to do with you? The syndrome of burnout has a long history. Almost 50 years ago, California poverty lawyers used the word to describe the process of their gradual exhaustion, cynicism, and loss of commitment to their work with the underserved. Christina Maslach is one of the pioneering researchers on job burnout and coauthor of the *Maslach Burnout Inventory*. Her work is the basis for the 2019 decision by the World Health Organization (WHO) to include burnout as an occupational phenomenon, with health consequences (www.who.int/news). The eleventh revision of the *International Classification of Diseases* describes burnout as a state of depletion that results in physical, emotional, and mental exhaustion. It is the inability to cope with our work environment owing to the ongoing demands and stresses of our daily work lives. Traumatologist Charles Figley (2015) contrasts burnout to secondary traumatic stress and describes it as a gradual process that leads to a state of extreme dissatisfaction with one's work, characterized by excessive distancing from patients, impaired competence, low energy, and increased irritability. The WHO calls burnout an "occupational phenomenon."

Maslach et al. (2001) visualized burnout as a triad of behaviors:

- Overwhelming exhaustion and fatigue, feeling worn out and depleted.
- Cynicism, an indifferent or negative attitude, or extremely detached reactions to people in the work setting—patients, colleagues, administrators.
- Diminished personal accomplishment, a self-evaluated feeling of incompetence, lack of accomplishment, and decreased productivity at work.

It is important to remember that a crisis in one's relationship with work in general is not necessarily a crisis in one's relationship with people at work (Maslach et al., 2001). Jenkins and Baird (2002) are clear that burnout is a defensive response to prolonged work exposure. This is particularly true for nursing. Nurses engage in demanding work and interact with people all day long. Inadequate support intensifies the psychological strain.

Want to find out where you stand on the burnout scale? A burnout self-test appears on the MindTools website (2022). Using a Likert scale format for 15 questions, you can respond to statements such as, "I feel run down and drained of physical or emotional energy," "I am harder and less sympathetic with people than perhaps they deserve," and "I feel that organizational politics or bureaucracy frustrate my ability to do a good job." While the self-assessment tool does ask about perceived workload, it does not factor in the intensity of your work. The *Maslach Burnout Inventory* is available for purchase on the Mind Garden website. You might consider suggesting that your hospital administration or nursing organization order copies of the *Maslach Burnout Inventory*.

Challenging clinical settings put health care workers at high risk for negative mental health outcomes, including burnout syndrome. Studies such as that by Magnavita et al. (2021) confirm that during the previous Severe Acute Respiratory Syndrome (SARS) and Middle East Respiratory Syndrome (MERS) epidemics, about one-third of health care workers reported symptoms of burnout. This is similar to the rates for those exposed to chronic occupational stress during non-epidemic periods.

Nurses are not alone. You may be living with or know someone who is struggling with burnout as well. According to a survey of more than

1,000 workers in the United States, conducted by the Business Insider website (2021), 61% of respondents were currently "at least somewhat burned out." The job-posting website Indeed published a report in March 2021 confirming that the majority of respondents said their burnout had worsened during the pandemic; 52% overall said they were currently burned out.

In her 2021 book *Can't Even: How Millennials Became the Burnout Generation*, journalist Anne Petersen looks at the infrastructure of the workplace. She compares burnout to a bridge falling in disrepair. If the bridge collapses, do we keep driving around it, or do we repair it? Petersen reminds her readers that we need to fix the bridge.

What is the cure for burnout? Perhaps we should start with prevention first. Bakker et al. (2008) have introduced the concept of work engagement: a positive, fulfilling, emotional state of work-related well-being. People who are engaged identify strongly with their work. They are energetic, dedicated, and engrossed. The positive experience of engagement is predicted by the presence of work resources. These individuals are autonomous, and they receive coaching and feedback from supervisors and mentors. They also possess the personal resources of optimism, self-efficacy, and self-esteem. You may recognize these qualities as characteristics of resilience. We'll talk more about that in chapter 11.

> "Burnout is . . . the sum total of hundreds and thousands
> of tiny betrayals of purpose, each one so minute that it
> hardly attracts notice."—GUNDERMAN (2014)

In an article about burnout that went viral, Kim (2021) points out that thinking of burnout as a form of betrayal is eye-opening. Suddenly, burnout is not your problem alone, and you don't have to fight it by yourself. And you can't heal from burnout by yourself. As Kim so clearly points out, burnout is "a relationship in conflict." The relationship? You and your employer. It's time to reframe the problem of burnout and ask yourself how the relationship can be repaired.

In spring of 2022, Vivek Murthy, Surgeon General of the United States, issued *Addressing Health Worker Burnout: The U.S. Surgeon General's Advisory on Building a Thriving Health Workforce*. In this sweeping, action-oriented report, Murthy stresses that burnout is not an individual mental health diagnosis; rather, it is "a distinct workplace phenomenon that primarily calls for a prioritization of systems-oriented, organizational-level solutions." While most risk factors for burnout existed well before the pandemic, the report emphasized that women, people of color, and those who work in rural and tribal communities are at greater risk for burnout.

The advisory details a multipronged, whole-of-society approach that addresses the burnout crisis in health care. The goals include protecting the health and safety of all health care providers, ensuring that mental health care is accessible and available without punitive policies, reducing administrative burdens, transforming organizational cultures to give precedence to employee well-being, recognizing social connections as a core value in health care, and investing in public health and an expanded health care workforce through research and education. Preventing or treating burnout does not fall to an individual nurse, although individual support may be required. It is a system-wide problem and can only be solved as such.

PUTTING IT INTO PRACTICE

A Journaling Self-Assessment

Goal: To identify emotions, thoughts or behaviors associated with burnout or empathic distress

Time and place: 15 minutes each day, a quiet space, after work

Is it burnout or something else? Use the following prompts to write and think about your experiences, and to help answer this question. Use pen and paper or your phone to track your thoughts. Choosing to write has advantages—a notebook that soothes or inspires, a favorite pen. Keep your writing instruments next to your bed; if you wake up in the middle of the night, jot down your thoughts. A pen that lights will guide your way across the page without the overstimulation of a lamp or phone screen. Note patterns and frequency, along with what alleviates your reactions or symptoms.

Describe your reactions or symptoms.
    What?
    When?
    Where?
    How often?
What relieves those reactions or symptoms?

What or who are your triggers? How often do you experience them?
    At work?
    At home?
    Arriving at work?
    Leaving work?

Name one resource (person, place, information, or strategy) that alleviates your stress at work.
    When and how did you use this resource?
    What was the result?

Think about your personal and professional history to the present day.
    What do *you think* contributes to your vulnerability to burnout?
    Age?
    Gender?
    Education?
    Type of job?
    Time at your job?
    Other factors?

Now ask a colleague the same question, and share your thoughts.

Prevention Strategies

Goal: To identify burnout prevention strategies that are helpful and easy to use

Time and place: 10–15 minutes each day, in a quiet space. Allow for more time if discussing with a peer or support person.

Name at least one strategy for each category. Review your answers from the previous practice as a guide to discover your strategies.

- Physiological
  - Movement, exercise
  - Sleep
  - Eating well
- Social
  - Who supports me?
  - Who are my resources?
  - What did I do to take action?
    - Who did I talk to?
    - Have I identified the problem and the solution?
    - Did I write down my concerns and memorialize them?
- Professional
  - Who supports me?
  - What and who are my resources?
  - What did I do to take action?
    - Who did I talk to?
    - Have I identified the problem and the solution?
    - Did I write down my concerns and memorialize them?

Sometimes it helps to visualize how we hold on to worry, stress, and negative emotions.

Try the activity below, then share it with a friend or colleague. If you have children, they can try it too, maybe at bath time. They might even think about SpongeBob SquarePants!

PUTTING IT INTO PRACTICE

The Weight of the Sponge

Goal: To visualize how you hold on to stress, worry, or negative emotions

Time and place: 10–15 minutes, in a place where you have access to water, a bowl, sink, bathtub, or pool

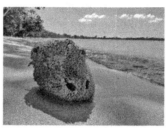

Visualize a free-form natural sea sponge, not the rectangular pink or blue ones from the grocery store. If you can, hold one in your hand. Look at its color and texture, the holes and crevices hiding in plain sight. Squeeze it, feel how light it is. Place the sponge in a bowl of water or a small sink. Watch it float.

By Michele Calabretta on Unsplash

Now, submerge the sponge under water. Hold it until the sponge becomes heavier and sinks to the bottom of the bowl or sink.

As you submerge the sponge, think about the things you carry, things that trouble or worry you. Maybe you are worried about a friend or a patient. When we completely take on other people's sufferings as our own, every pore of our being takes on those burdens. We become heavier. In time, their distress becomes our own personal distress; we feel threatened and overwhelmed. We are sinking to the bottom of the bowl. We put ourselves at risk for burnout. Try to be receptive to other people's feelings without absorbing those emotions as your own.

Pull the sponge out of the water and gently squeeze it, releasing the water trapped inside.

As the water cascades into the bowl, imagine those worries, concerns, and troubles leaving you, just as the water leaves the sponge. You don't have to hold on to it, and it is no longer so heavy that it sinks.

VICARIOUS TRAUMA AND
SECONDARY TRAUMATIC STRESS
◆

Caring for patients who are critically ill can put nurses at risk for vicarious trauma or secondary traumatic stress (Newell and MacNeil, 2010). While these concepts are similar, there are differences in how they affect health care professionals.

- Vicarious trauma results from ongoing direct practice with patients who are injured, critically ill, or traumatized; it affects the way you think about the world and your work (Pearlman and Mac Ian, 1995).
- Secondary traumatic stress occurs as a result of knowing about a traumatizing event experienced by a significant other (or colleague) and helping or wanting to help this suffering person. Secondary traumatic stress causes symptoms that are similar to those seen in posttraumatic stress disorder (PTSD) (Figley, 2015).

Li et al. (2020) conducted a study in China during the first wave of the COVID-19 pandemic that found that vicarious traumatization scores for frontline nurses were significantly lower than those of nonfrontline nurses. The researchers pointed out that vicarious traumatization scores of the general public were significantly higher than those of the frontline nurses. The severity of vicarious traumatization in nonfrontline nurses was significantly higher than that of frontline nurses who were in close contact with COVID-19 patients. In addition, married, divorced, or widowed nurses had higher vicarious trauma scores than that of unmarried nurses. The researchers hypothesized that vicarious traumatization arises from an empathic response to their acutely ill patients. However, non-frontline nurses not only felt sympathy for patients with COVID-19, but were worried, anxious, and felt helpless for their frontline colleagues.

IN THEIR OWN WORDS

> *"What kept me going, despite the devastation and incompre-*
> *hensible conditions, was the resilience, strength, gratitude,*
> *hope, and spiritual grace of the people of Haiti. It was evident*
> *with each patient encounter, and again each evening when*
> *the haunting sound of 30,000 voices from the tent city below*
> *would join together in prayer and song."*

Of all the accomplishments in my nursing career, I am most proud of the opportunity to be a part of a federal medical team that responds to disasters. It has allowed me to serve my country in a way I never dreamed possible, but it has also been the most difficult. Working in a disaster situation challenges the physical and mental stamina of both responders and victims. Sleep easily rejuvenates the body. It's the emotional impact that can take its toll.

Disaster medicine wasn't a career goal. In fact, I knew nothing about it until Hurricane Katrina occurred. There was a desperate call for medical help, so I volunteered but wasn't deployed until Hurricane Rita struck Louisiana three weeks later. A disaster medical team was on-site in Lake Charles, Louisiana, and I joined them, working 12- to 16-hour shifts. Many patients were evacuees from fishing towns along the coast that were decimated from storm surge. Some were searching for family members who had refused to leave. As each story became more heartbreaking, I recognized how much of a toll the experience was taking on my own mental health. Journaling each night after my shift helped a great deal to memorialize the experience and process the sadness I was feeling for my patients. I also began to look for at least one positive aspect of each patient encounter and focus on it. It was amazing how suddenly the resilience and strength of these individuals was so apparent and so contagious.

There have been several deployments since that time, but the most memorable was the 2010 earthquake in Haiti. By that time, I had joined a federal disaster medical team. I never questioned whether I could handle the physical and emotional demands of Haiti that lay ahead. It just didn't cross my mind.

Nothing could have prepared us. We arrived at Port au Prince airport to extreme heat and the putrid smell of burning garbage, tires, and human remains. Running water and electricity were nonexistent, and toilets were cardboard boxes lined with plastic. Under military guard, we were transported in the back of dump trucks to our assignment. The team commander warned of horrific damage, intense odors, and bodies lying in piles along the road. That was the moment when I recognized the importance of "filtering out" those sights too difficult to handle emotionally. It became a tool used frequently in the next three weeks—learning not to look at the horrors present, and to focus on the job to be done.

At our base of operations, sleeping was a communal arrangement on the ground. Baby wipes became the mainstay for cleanliness, and toilet paper was a coveted commodity. We washed clothes in plastic tubs with toilet plungers and took turns giving each other haircuts when the oppressive heat demanded a shorter style. Vanity was no longer a part of anyone's repertoire.

Medical operations were two tents set on the top of a massive hill. At the bottom of the hill was a tent camp of 30,000 earthquake victims. Each day, young Haitian men from the camp would climb the hill and volunteer as translators, or carry patients back and forth. Their stamina and determination to help were inspiring. It was here that disaster triage became the core of our day-to-day operations. Decisions had to be made as to who was most likely to survive and therefore warrant care, and who was "expectant" to die and therefore go untreated. These concepts contradicted everything we believed in as medical professionals. Our training was to save lives, not choose who would live or die. Disaster medicine necessitates making tough decisions so that the most good can be done for the greatest number of people. Since health care in Haiti is virtually nonexistent, and living conditions are a breeding ground for disease and malnutrition on the best of days, to provide a level of care that could not be supported afterward meant the individual would most likely succumb regardless of our actions. But many others with a greater potential to survive could be treated effectively. It was fundamental mass casualty field triage and agonizingly painful. Many of us would sit at night and talk through the decisions made, knowing that our choices of care would have been much different in our country. We cried and supported each other, and the conversations became a nightly therapeutic ritual.

Treatment required an enormous amount of ingenuity and demonstrated the practice and art of nursing and medicine at its finest. Wet nurses were found to breastfeed orphaned babies since formula didn't exist, and medical records were pieces of paper taped to a patient's chest. Incubators for newborns were made with cardboard boxes and heat blankets. For all the difficult decisions that were made, we celebrated this creativity. These challenges became our greatest gift when they were successful, and kept our spirits high.

We did the best we could in an extremely difficult situation, and I truly believe we gave sound medical care that made a significant difference in the lives of many Haitian people. I know that they definitely touched my life in more ways than I have yet to understand. What kept me going, despite the devastation and incomprehensible conditions, was the resilience, strength, gratitude, hope, and spiritual grace of the people of Haiti. It was evident with each patient encounter, and again each evening when the haunting sound of 30,000 voices from the tent city below would join together in prayer and song.

Each mission since my first deployment has helped me understand the trauma of disasters for both responders and victims. What I have seen in common with each is the strength of the human spirit if we allow ourselves to process our experiences in whatever way works best. Journaling was the means I chose during Hurricane Rita, and it helped, but I found what worked best for me was to share my feelings with fellow teammates who validated I wasn't alone with my emotions.

But truth be told, it has always been the patients I've cared for during these missions that gave me the ability to cope with whatever was happening. I had been sent to help them as victims of a disaster, and yet it was they who gave me strength and resilience. I call it the therapeutic human spirit.

August 2005 and January 2010: Donna Barry, DNP, APN, FN-CSA,
Nurse Practitioner, Beaufort, South Carolina, United States

RISKS AND PREVENTION
◆

How can you prevent the consequences of trauma in your personal and work lives? And how do you know if you are at risk for vicarious trauma or secondary traumatic stress? Before we offer some suggestions and strategies, let's take a look at the science.

THE SCIENCE OF TRAUMA

Researchers have studied the impact of trauma work on mental health professionals, disaster workers, and health care providers. Some studies found that certain experiences can put professionals at risk (Kanno and Giddings, 2016). These circumstances stemmed from personal histories as well as work experiences. A prior history of a traumatic experience, especially as a young child, can make professionals more vulnerable, but it can also make them more aware and sensitive to how current work circumstances will affect them. Education and training, including mastery of content focused on trauma theory and interventions, provide protection for health care professionals. Supervision and the opportunity to talk through difficult work situations is key to protecting your own mental health. External supervision and support, both formal and informal, allow professionals to recognize that their experiences and reactions to difficult work are common among others in their profession. Researchers confirm, however, that informal support, such as peer support groups, was identified as the strongest predictor of prevention of traumatic stress (Bonach and Heckert, 2012).

Studies have found that vacation time helps workers reflect positively about work, improves mastery of knowledge, and induces relaxation (Fritz and Sonnentag, 2006). When employees return to work, their sense of well-being and performance-related outcomes improve. Tucker et al. (2008) found that exercise and activities that relied on lower mental effort were associated with better-rated sleep, as well as improved recuperation and diminished fatigue the next day.

Portuguese researchers found that well-being promotion and trauma-informed strategies reduced nurses' symptoms during the COVID-19 pandemic. They looked at physical and relaxation activities, recreation, diet, and water intake, as well as maintenance of social supports that facilitated shared emotions.

Risk factors do not only sit within individuals, however. There are organizational risk factors as well—work settings, administrative constraints, inadequate supervision, lack of resources, and insufficient support from colleagues and administrators (Dunkley and Whelan, 2006).

Repairing the damage done to a profession and its members must be a priority that requires a multidimensional approach. There is global acknowledgment that the stressors and psychological needs of health care providers must be addressed, not only from the perspective of individuals but also from an organizational position (Søvold et al., 2021).

References
Bonach, K., & Heckert, A. (2012). Predictors of secondary traumatic stress among children's advocacy center forensic interviewers. *Journal of Child Sexual Abuse* 21(3): 295–314.

Dunkley, J., & Whelan, T. A. (2006). Vicarious traumatisation: current status and future directions. *British Journal of Guidance and Counselling* 34(1): 107–16.

Fritz, C., & Sonnentag, S. (2006). Recovery, well-being, and performance-related outcomes: the role of workload and vacation experiences. *Journal of Applied Psychology* 91(4): 936–45.

Kanno, H., & Giddings, M. M. (2016). Hidden trauma victims: understanding and preventing traumatic stress in mental health professionals. *Social Work in Mental Health* 15(3): 331–53. https://doi.org/10.1080/15332985.2016.1220442

Søvold, L. E., Naslund, J. A., Kousoulis, A. A., Saxena, S., Qoronfleh, M. W., Grobler, C., & Münter, L. (2021). Prioritizing the mental health and well-being of health-care workers: an urgent global public health priority. *Frontiers in Public Health* 9: 679397.

Tucker, P., Dahlgren, A., Akerstedt, T., & Waterhouse, J. (2008). The impact of free-time activities on sleep, recovery and well-being. *Applied Ergonomics* 39(5): 653–62.

PUTTING IT INTO PRACTICE

Ways You Can Protect Against the Effects of Trauma, Vicarious Trauma, and Secondary Traumatic Stress

Goal: To evaluate the impact of your work on your personal and professional lives

Time and place: This is an ongoing practice. Take time each day to reflect on these questions and prompts.

- Personal approaches
  - Life and work balance
    - How do you balance the intensity of your work?

(continued)

- What activities or events take you "away" from your job?
- When was the last time you engaged in those activities?
- Relaxation
  - What do you do to relax?
  - How often?
  - How do you know you are relaxed? (Describe your thoughts, emotions, behaviors.)

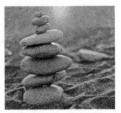
By Nadin Mario on Unsplash

- Humor
  - When was the last time you had a good laugh?
  - What was the occasion?
  - At work?
- ▸ Professional considerations
  - Balance
    - Think about balancing your practice: Do you rotate to different work settings or stay on the same unit, with the same patients all the time?
    - If you could take a break from your current responsibilities and work in a different location, where would it be?

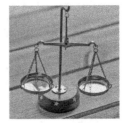
By Elena Mozhvilo on Unsplash

  - Boundaries
    - When have you drawn the line and said "no"? "No" to overtime, "no" to extra shifts, "no" additional patients?
    - How do you process intrusive or traumatic images?
    - How did the process feel to you, both in the moment and then later on?
    - Do you need more boundary practice?
  - Getting support: formal and informal
    - Who do you go to for support?
    - Formal: How did you find the group? Consider investigating Schwartz Rounds in your hospital, university, or online (see https://www.theschwartzcenter.org/programs /schwartz-rounds/ and https://njnew.org/programs /virtual-schwartz-rounds/).

- Informal: Do you go to a café or bar after work? Send texts or make phone calls?
- Plans for coping
  - What are your plans for coping strategies?
  - Do you have them handy?
  - Consider keeping a daily diary to monitor intrusive images or memories.
  - Consider carrying a ProQol Pocket Card (see chapter 1 and the Resources section at the end of this book).
- Ongoing learning: external training, education, trauma-informed approach
  - When and what was the last course you attended?
  - Was it work-related or you-related?
  - How did you hear about it, and who did you tell about it?
- Evaluate healing
  - How are you doing now compared to six months or a year ago?
  - What are your goals for the next six months?
  - Who shares your goals? A friend, colleague, family member?
- Skill development
  - What new skills have you learned?
  - Do you like them, and do they work for you?

COMPASSION, EMPATHY, AND EMPATHIC DISTRESS FATIGUE

•

By now, the stories are all too familiar. Ferguson. London. Sandy Hook. New Orleans. Ukraine. New York. Oslo. Paris. Haiti. Pakistan. Wuhan.

It seems that tragedy befalls humanity in ever increasing numbers and with ever increasing regularity. Whether such tragedies are caused by forces of nature, human conflict, or a catastrophic public health emergency, everyone is a potential witness to the resulting social, physical, and emotional devastation. Nurses are not immune or isolated from any of these events. In fact, they are often called to action by hospitals, communities, and disaster response teams. Technology and social media extend the reach of disease, injury, and loss, changing the world we live in. Somehow, people and communities, wounded and dazed, come together in a spirit of selfless collaboration to help, to heal, and to learn from tragedy and its aftermath. More than anyone else, nurses know that empathy and compassion are the essential components of this human response to another's need.

How does empathy affect your professional life, the nursing profession, and your family or community? The concept of empathy is not new, but it has evolved since experimental psychologist E. B. Titchener coined the term in 1909. "Empathy" was first translated from the German *Einfühlung*, "to feel one's way into," by way of the Greek *empatheia*, "in" (*en*) "suffering or passion" (*pathos*) (Titchener, 1909). Plainly stated, empathy is the ability to share the emotions of another or anticipate how an individual is likely to feel in a particular situation (Eisenberg, 2002). It is not emotional mirroring, nor is it sympathy. Sympathy is feeling the emotion *for* the other person rather than feeling the emotion *as* the other feels it (Eisenberg et al., 2010). Empathy is being attuned and responsive to the emotional states of others. Cognitive empathy is one's ability to *understand* the emotional experience of the other person, while affective empathy is *feeling* the other's emotional response (Shamay-Tsoory, 2009).

Compassion

While empathic individuals are often compassionate, compassion is not the same as empathy. The word "compassion" means to "suffer together." It is the feeling that surfaces when one witnesses another person's distress *and* has a strong desire to help relieve the other person's suffering (Goetz et al., 2010; Goetz and Simon-Thomas, 2017). The empathetic person can take the perspective of another person and feel their emotions, deeply and with understanding, but may not necessarily have the desire or take action to relieve their distress.

Compassion arises when we witness another person's suffering. We are motivated to help them, to relieve their pain. As nurses, you will recognize that moment—the emotions and subjective feeling of warmth, empathic concern, and a real sense of understanding the other's perspective and intentions. Not only do you have the desire to help, but you also act on that desire.

THE SCIENCE OF COMPASSION

Helping and caregiving have the potential to positively transform our lives, leaving us with a sense of satisfaction. There is a sense of fulfillment for making a commitment and satisfying an obligation. Cohen et al. (2002) found that the very act of helping and associated companionship contribute to a feeling of gratification.

The neuroscience of compassion and empathy provides powerful evidence that caring is good for us. Empathy and compassion are processed along two distinct neural pathways: a socio-affective (empathy) pathway and a socio-cognitive (compassion) pathway. Scientists report that compassionate behaviors activate the pleasure circuits in the brain (Wu and Hong, 2022). In other words, there is an intrinsic reward to compassion, one that could help outweigh any negative reactions or risks to the caregiving professional.

Compassion is linked to reward and affiliation processing within the brain, stimulating oxytocin and vasopressin receptors that promote positive emotions toward those who are suffering (Gilbert, 2019). Compassion activates networks that provide a protective action from stress. Researchers have found that during situations that evoke compassion, the heart rate decelerates (Kirby et al., 2017). Compassion training lowers stress hormones and strengthens the immune response, enhancing resilience and minimizing stress (Klimecki et al., 2013).

References
Cohen, C. A., Colantonio, A., & Vernich, L. (2002). Positive aspects of caregiving: rounding out the caregiver experience. *International Journal of Geriatric Psychiatry* 17(2): 184–88.
Gilbert, P. (2019). Explorations into the nature and function of compassion. *Current Opinion in Psychology* 28: 108–14.
Kirby, J. N., Doty, J. R., Petrocchi, N., & Gilbert, P. (2017). The current and future role of heart rate variability for assessing and training compassion. *Frontiers in Public Health* 5: 40.
Klimecki, O. M., Leiberg, S., Lamm, C., & Singer, T. (2013). Functional neural plasticity and associated changes in positive affect after compassion training. *Cerebral Cortex* 23(7): 1552–61.
Wu, Y. E., & Hong, W. (2022). Neural basis of prosocial behavior. *Trends in Neurosciences* S0166-2236(22)00126-6.

Nurses have described to us the appeal of bedside nursing, finding satisfaction and a sense of accomplishment, and "knowing they are in the right place." Even when they take new positions in education or administration, some continue bedside care through per diem work.

Empathy

Author and psychologist Carl Rogers (1975) believed that empathy was the cornerstone of the human relationship. He described empathy as a dynamic process, not a state of being: "To be with another in this [empathetic] way means that for the time being you lay aside the views and values you hold for yourself in order to enter another's world without prejudice ... In such situations deep understanding is, I believe, the most precious gift one can give to another." Empathy is the cornerstone of nursing practice as well, not only at the bedside but in the classroom and the community.

Empathy is essential for understanding others' emotions, but when we excessively take on the emotions and suffering of others as our own, we are at risk for negative emotions and distress.

Empathic Distress Fatigue

We've all heard or even used the term "compassion fatigue" when referring to the negative effects of providing nursing care, especially during highly charged, intense emotional circumstances. We're prompted to ask the question: How does it differ from burnout or vicarious trauma? Neuroscientists have contributed groundbreaking research to better understand how empathy and compassion can affect your practice and your life.

How can nurses protect themselves from distress while still remaining empathic and compassionate? How can you respond to your own suffering while still taking action to alleviate or prevent it from overwhelming you? We urge you to revisit chapter 1, which addresses self-compassion specifically.

Learning about compassion can enhance your well-being and your practice, leading to a greater understanding of your own need for self-compassion and receiving compassion from others. The trajectory of the COVID-19 pandemic clearly illustrates this need. In early 2020, health care providers were lauded and honored for their courageous work. They

THE SCIENCE OF EMPATHY

There are three steps necessary for a healthy empathic response (Hofmeyer et al., 2017). First, we take the perspective of another person, imagining what it is like to be in their situation (Valk et al., 2017). The second step is one of self-awareness and recognition of self-other boundaries. We distinguish ourselves and our mental state as separate from the suffering person (Ekman and Krasner, 2017). Finally, we are able to regulate our own emotions (Thompson et al., 2019). Although we witness the affective state of the other person, we will not experience the same emotions.

Singer and Klimecki (2014) studied how the brain processes empathic experiences by activating neural networks similar to those that process first-person experiences. When we feel empathy for someone who is distressed, our brain shows activation of neural circuits similar to those of the suffering person.

References

Ekman, E., & Krasner, M. (2017). Empathy in medicine: neuroscience, education and challenges. *Medical Teacher* 39(2):164–73.

Hofmeyer, A., Toffoli L., Vernon R., Taylor, R., Klopper, H. C., Coetzee, S. K., & Fontaine, D. (2017). Teaching compassionate care to nursing students in a digital learning and teaching environment. *Collegian* 25(3): http://dx.doi.org /10.1016/j.colegn.2017.08.001

Singer, T., & Klimecki, O. M. (2014). Empathy and compassion. *Current Biology* 24(18): R875–R878.

Thompson, N. M., Uusberg, A., Gross, J. J., & Chakrabarti, B. (2019). Empathy and emotion regulation: an integrative account. In: Srinivasan, N., ed. *Progress in Brain Research*. New York: Elsevier, 273–304.

Valk, S. L., Bernhardt, B. C., Trautwein, F. M., Böckler, A., Kanske, P., Guizard, N., Louis Collins, D., & Singer, T. (2017). Structural plasticity of the social brain: differential change after socio-affective and cognitive mental training. *Science Advances* 3(10): e1700489.

cared for the sickest of the sick and comforted families and each other. Throughout the rollercoaster of surges and politicization of COVID treatment and prevention strategies and vaccinations, nurses, long the most trusted professionals in the United States, became the target of anger and rage. They were ignored or pushed away at the bedside and in hospital administrative offices. Their voices rang hollow in the face of angry, dying patients who didn't believe they had COVID or bitterly demanded medications that were not approved for COVID treatment. They spoke out, using social media as their megaphone. Few listened. Nurses began to think about making life- and career-changing decisions. Feeling unsupported by administrators and overshadowed by traveling nurses who were able to make their own schedules and received hefty salaries, nurses saw compassion dry up around them, yet they were expected to exude compassion for their patients. Physically and emotionally exhausted, underappreciated and questioning their chosen field, they resigned or changed practice settings. Some nurses reported that administrators didn't even ask why they were leaving or persuade them to stay. As one nurse reported to us, the lack of respect from administration only confirmed they were making the right choice.

THE SCIENCE OF COMPASSION FATIGUE

Relying on recent studies in neuroscience, German pioneers in the field of empathy research (Klimecki and Singer, 2012) and now nurse researchers (Hofmeyer et al., 2020) confirm that compassion does not cause fatigue. As you've read in the section above, it has the opposite effect—a positive emotional state that can enhance our sense of well-being.

These researchers suggest replacing the term "compassion fatigue" with "empathic distress fatigue," which is defined as "a strong aversive and self-oriented response to the suffering of others, accompanied by the desire to withdraw from a situation in order to protect oneself from excessive negative feelings" (Singer and Klimecki, 2014, R875).

Studies using functional magnetic resonance imagery (fMRI) (Klimecki and Singer, 2012; Singer, 2015) show that empathic distress fatigue is triggered when the "self-other" distinction is blurred, when the clinician experiences a patient's distress as their own. Emotional regulation skills maintain clear "self-other" boundaries. We adopt another's pain and negative emotions, leading to an intense neurological response and overwhelming pain and distress. There is an urgent need to withdraw from the presence of suffering people to protect ourselves. That separation results in personal distress as well as poor role performance.

References

Hofmeyer, A., Kennedy, K., & Taylor, R. (2020). Contesting the term "compassion fatigue": integrating findings from social neuroscience and self-care research. *Collegian* 27(2): 232–37.

Klimecki, O. M., & Singer, T. (2012). Empathic distress fatigue rather than compassion fatigue? Integrating findings from empathy research in psychology and social neuroscience. In: Oakley, B., Knafo, A., Madhavan, G., & Wilson, D. S., eds. *Pathological Altruism*. New York: Oxford University Press, 368–83.

Singer, T. (2015). Empathy is not compassion: showing evidence for differences in their neuronal and experiential signatures as well as their plasticity. Paper presented at the International Convention for Psychological Science (ICPS), Amsterdam, March 12–14, 2015.

Singer, T., & Klimecki, O. M. (2014). Empathy and compassion. *Current Biology* 24(18): R875–R878.

While we are just beginning to understand the complexities and contributing factors that have driven nurses away from the profession, a powerful essay, "Nurses Have Finally Learned What They're Worth," gives us pause (Hilgers, 2022). The author of this thoroughly researched article pulls in the historical elements of the business of health care as background, and layers on top of it the deadly and devastating impact of the pandemic—the burnout, empathic distress, the loss of dignity, and the evaporation of compassion—for patients, for colleagues, for staff, and for oneself. It's not only about the money; it is also about value and being valued.

Nurses have told us since the beginning of 2020 that their ideas to solve problems at the bedside and in the boardroom are not always shared with colleagues or brought to the larger organization. But we've also heard from nurses in hospitals with nurse practice councils. These councils take an active role in shaping nursing roles and practices, and their voices are heard. They are valued and respected. They make a difference.

Compassionate leadership in health care cultures seems to have gone missing. Or at the very least, it is invisible to nurses. Nurses cannot and should not take on prevention or alleviation of empathic distress fatigue as their problem alone. It belongs to the system.

You and your organization may want to consider compassion education programs. These programs include burnout prevention skills, mindfulness, self-compassion, and loving-kindness meditation. The intent of the sessions is not to reduce or remove negative emotions, but to increase activation of areas in the brain associated with love, affiliation, positive emotions, hope, and reward as a protective factor to prevent empathic distress (Mills et al., 2018).

There are a number of compassion training programs around the world. The Compassion Cultivation Training (CCT) was developed by the Center for Compassion and Altruism Research and Education (CCARE) at Stanford University by Thupten Jinpa, a Tibetan Buddhist scholar, former monk, and academic (Jazaieri et al., 2013). In collaboration with contemplative scholars, psychologists, and scientists, the program is now located at the Sanford Institute for Empathy and Compassion at the University of California, San Diego, and adapted for health care professionals (https://www.compassioninstitute.com/healthcare). The goal of CCT is to provide a structured and systematic way of cultivating daily-life skills needed to strengthen qualities of compassion, empathy, and kindness to oneself and others. The institute has trainers in 23 countries and offers a free care package for health care providers (https://www.compassioninstitute.com/healthcare/carepackage).

LOSS AND GRIEF
◆

IN THEIR OWN WORDS

April 12, 2020. Easter Sunday.

One of the hardest days of my life. And a day that I will never forget.

Work continued to be overwhelming, more health care workers getting sick, less staff available, frequent huddles, policies changing by the minute, cohorting positive COVID patients together, beds filling up, more patients being intubated, doctors deciding who to intubate first.

More patients dying. Fear of the unknown. The stress continued.

It was so heartbreaking and made me so sad to see our patients die alone.

My 87-year-old patient was actively dying. My heart was telling me to call her daughter. I had to let her know that her mom was not doing well. The call was really hard. Her daughter cried loudly over the phone, as she wanted to see her mother and say goodbye. It was destroying me inside.

I asked if she wanted to FaceTime. "Yes, please, anything you can do for me to see my Mama, I will appreciate it from the bottom of my heart." I set up the video call, held the phone in front of my patient, and watched as she spoke to her mother for 10 minutes.

She told her mother how much she loved her. How sorry she was for what she was going through, and how she wished that she could just be with her to hold her hand.

And then she said, "Goodbye, Mama."

She cried loudly as my patient took her last breath.

I will remember this moment forever.

God brought me into this world to help people. I love being a nurse, and I always will. In the beginning of the pandemic, we tried to limit our exposure as much as possible because we still didn't know enough about the virus, but while I held the phone for my patient, my fears were set aside. I was next to my patient and didn't even realize the time. I just wanted my patient to spend her last minutes "Not alone," and for her daughter to say her final goodbyes.

My patient's daughter called me a week later to thank me. She said, "Because of you, I was able to say goodbye to my mother, and for that, I will never forget you." Several months later, she called me again. This time she wanted to meet me. We met in September, and she told me that a weight had been lifted off her shoulders. She wanted to hold my hand and give me a hug so badly, but due to COVID regulations, she couldn't.

I'm grateful that I was able to be there for my patient's daughter during such a difficult time. I'm grateful that my patient was not alone when she took her last breath.

I wouldn't be able to do what I do without the support and help of my colleagues. We have such an amazing team. It was important for us to talk to each other, to lift our voices, to solve our problems, and to have that positive energy to heal our wounds during the COVID crisis.

That Sunday afternoon, after my patient died, I told my colleagues we needed to take a minute and pray. We walked to a quiet place and made a circle, held hands, and prayed together—to give us strength, to keep us safe and strong. We prayed for our patients. We prayed for the families. And we prayed for this nightmare to be over soon.

I'm thankful that we were able to pause for a minute during a horrible day, to put our heads down, take a breath and pray. Our unit secretary happened to take a picture of us and posted it on social media.

An artist from New York saw our photo and created a beautiful painting from it.

He submitted his work to the Rockefeller Center Flag Project, and it was selected for display. Our flag was displayed in August 2020, and again in March 2021, when we were invited to Rockefeller Center to tell our story. The staff was amazing and were honored to meet us. Our day was like a dream.

They lowered our flag from the flagpole; we were able to see and hold it in our hands.

We thought about that Easter Sunday almost a year before. Then we took pictures with the Rockefeller staff. It was an amazing day. We're astounded at how the community came together to show us love and support through our toughest times, and the recognition we received, even one year later.

And for that we are so grateful.

Claudia Nogueira, RN-BC, Neuroscience/Spine Unit,
Freehold, New Jersey, United States

Since the beginning of 2020, death, grief, pandemic statistics, and images of grieving nurses and families have dominated the airwaves and occupied more space in our heads and hearts than we ever thought possible. As you read in the story above, nurses are frequently the go-between, the soothing messenger between patients and their families in the final moments of life.

Many nurses have also told us about the other, not so calm or soothing times with families. When those last conversations are wracked with remorse, anger, or pleas for dying relatives to hang on, not give up, and come home, how do you process those moments when you bear the grief of another? How do you respond when a family makes accusations that you somehow caused their loved one's death? How do you hold your own grief, of a mother or close friend, while supporting a family?

> "No one ever told me that grief felt so like fear. I am not afraid, but the sensation is like being afraid. The same fluttering in the stomach, the same restlessness, the yawning. I keep on swallowing ... There is a sort of invisible blanket between the world and me. I find it hard to take in what anyone says. Or perhaps, hard to want to take it in."—C. S. Lewis, A Grief Observed

The words of C. S. Lewis capture the feelings that so often accompany grief. There is a sense of losing one's mind, of being alone, and the belief that no one else can understand or even appreciate this personal and devastating experience. Few things in life are as painful as the sudden, tragic death of a special person in our lives. There is no opportunity to say goodbye. Traumatic losses can be untimely or violent, or surrounded by countless other deaths.

Researchers such as Verdery et al. (2020) have heightened concerns about the loss of life attributed to the pandemic. As we write this, worldwide mortality rates from COVID-19 continue to soar. The deaths of family members, especially for children and grandchildren of the deceased, correspond to particularly adverse emotional outcomes. In addition to the risk of poor mental health associated with grief and bereavement, there is also the impact on economic resources. The authors estimate that, on average, under diverse epidemiological circumstances, every death from COVID-19 will leave approximately nine bereaved in the United States. The number of people at risk for losing a grandparent, parent, sibling, spouse, or child for each COVID-19 death is likely underestimated. Nurses are not only exposed to these bereaved family members, but they may also be grieving their own losses, if not from the pandemic then from earlier times in their lives.

One year after the research above was published, two new studies were released with updated information on the plight of children left behind as a result of the pandemic. A team of international researchers (Hillis et al., 2021a, b) developed estimates of pandemic-related orphanhood and caregiver deaths using mortality and fertility data to model estimates and rates of COVID-19-associated deaths in 21 countries. From March 1, 2020, to April 30, 2021, they estimated 1,134,000 children experienced the death of primary caregivers, including at least one parent or custodial grandparent, and 1,562,000 children experienced the death of at least one primary or secondary caregiver. Between two and five times more children lost fathers than mothers.

A similar study focused on US caregiver deaths between April 1, 2020, and June 30, 2021. Those findings suggest that more than 140,000 children under age 18 in the United States lost a parent, custodial grandparent, or grandparent caregiver from COVID-19-associated orphanhood or death of a grandparent caregiver. These caregivers provided the child's home and basic needs, love, security, and daily care.

The implications of these studies warn of another pandemic, one that centers on the mental health of children and families. Needs of bereaved children and their families will tax the mental health system across the globe. In January 2022, a letter was sent to the White House from the COVID Collaborative, making the case for the mental health of bereaved children. As of November 2021, roughly 1 in 450 children in the United States have lost at least one caregiver to COVID. Arizona, Mississippi, New Mexico, and Texas had the highest rates of caregiver loss.

Schools and school nurses have been and will continue to be key players in this new and urgent mental health crisis. The Northeastern University School Health Academy (NEUSHA) has committed ongoing education to school nurses in regard to their ever-changing and more demanding roles as lead public health providers in communities. Identifying children in need of mental health services will be their next challenge. The current research on child bereavement does not even take into account the far-reaching impact of these deaths on the lives of people in the larger community. Neighbors, teachers, coworkers, and classmates are also among the number of people affected. Nurses in all practice settings must address these issues in their patients, patients' families, and communities.

Grief has a way of reappearing, often when we least expect it, and certainly when we are not prepared. Talking about death with family, friends, and colleagues is challenging. But we know it helps and allows us to share the burden. We remember the people who were with us, stood by us, and propped us up when we didn't think we could stand anymore.

Listen to the words of a nurse who was leaving for a new position. At a small goodbye gathering, her colleagues expressed their gratitude for her kindness. "Stacy came up to me with tears in her eyes. We went through those first months of COVID together. Then Stacy told me that I was there for her first death, and I was so helpful. I asked her what I did, since I couldn't remember—there were so many patients who died on our unit. Stacy recalled how I sat with her after her patient died. She was crying and didn't know what to do. I did what I could do best. I comforted her. She thought for a moment and added, 'I guess we have a bond etched in tears.'"

THREE CAUTIONARY TALES
♦

Conversations surrounding death and grief prompt thoughtful and sometimes uncomfortable questions. If you are grieving or talking to those who have experienced a loss, there are several caveats that will serve you well. First, recognize that there are some myths that surround death and grief in our society, such as the need to define stages or markers to gauge our recovery, searching for closure, and erasing painful images.

Stages Are Not the Markers of Grief and Healing
"Phases" or "stages" of grieving suggest there is a prescribed, optimum way to work through grief, and that you can only move in a straight line, forward or backward. This is not true; grief is a journey that begins with loss and takes many twists and turns. There is no one starting point, nor is there a final end point. "Resolving" is another word frequently used to address the grieving process. Resolution implies that you can find a solution. Grief is shaped by multiple factors: earlier experiences; attachment to significant others; the nature of death and surrounding circumstances; age; and support of family, friends, and colleagues. The process is much more circular, like a feedback loop.

Beware of Closure
"Closure" is a word often used to define an event or occurrence that leads to "the act of closing or condition of being closed." This word

surfaced in media reports after Timothy McVeigh's sentencing and execution in response to the Oklahoma City bombing that killed 168 people and injured 680 others in 1995. Journalists wrote that the victim's families' "search for closure" would come to an end with McVeigh's death. Can a physical event really end the painful grieving process? It is human nature to search for a way to end our pain. The identification of one signature event that pronounces "no more suffering" may be wishful thinking. Grieving is one of the greatest human challenges. Consider replacing "closure" with the more appropriate concept of "integration." The real work of integrating a loss into the tapestry of our lives is just beginning. We will always grieve, although not with the same intensity or pain.

Don't Erase Death

Be cautious of others who may be eager to erase our history. Some communities and cultures want us to feel better, to not feel pain or to be sad. By editing sights and sounds that might remind us of the death, we mistakenly think people will feel better. But there is a danger in hiding or removing reminders of those we have lost, no matter how long ago. It feels as though the people and places never existed; as a result, we deny our own history.

Grieving includes strong feelings of yearning or longing for a loved one. It is an attempt to fill the empty space in our hearts and minds. With traumatic loss, this yearning often leads to reminders or painful images of the traumatic event, such as a traumatic hospitalization. Thinking of this loved one is then accompanied by agonizing images and thoughts, further complicating the grieving process. Grief is often described as a generalized pain or heaviness in the chest, feeling depressed and hopeless about the future, and a sense that things that were once important do not seem to matter anymore. We cry easily, lose interest in eating, or experience physical discomfort.

Many nurses are parents who had concerns about their children during the pandemic. Their children, in return, had just as many concerns about them, and the dangerous nature of caring for COVID patients. One young boy asked his mother every day before she left for work, "Are you going to be okay? Are you going to die?"

The impact of the pandemic has had far-reaching consequences for all bereaved families. The Cambridge University Hospitals National Health Service Foundation Trust followed national guidelines to restrict visiting, but there were unavoidable aftereffects. The personal belongings of deceased patients began to accumulate in clinical areas. In a paper describing their work, Debbie Critoph and Stephanie Smith (2020), two nurse clinical communication skills tutors, were redeployed by the trust for end-of-life care and to address this sensitive issue. Mourning was a lonely journey for these families—regardless of cause of death—and the absence of rituals normally seen after a death, such as visits from family and friends and face-to-face meetings with hospital teams, were no longer available. The authors created a new service to reunite bereaved relatives with their loved ones' personal effects. In their own words, the authors described their experience as both heartwarming and heartbreaking.

Nurses do grieve for their patients. Endacott (2019) found that the quality of the patient's death, their suffering, and loss of dignity have been significantly associated with emotional distress in nurses. Caring for dying patients prompts us to consider our own mortality. Nurses fulfill many roles: confidante, educator, advocate, cultural liaison, and translator, at times attempting to mitigate conflict. You can also feel vicarious grief for mourning family members. The very sharing of another's sorrow serves as a reminder of our own losses and thus reactivates any of our own earlier grieving. It is not unfinished grief, as all grief is unfinished to some extent; perhaps "revisited grief" is a better term. The images we see on mainstream and social media, particularly the televised media, serve as a catalyst for vicarious grieving (Sullender, 2010).

Pausing for a moment of reflection after a patient's death allows us to reconnect as caregivers. It rejoins patients, family members, and providers with the essence of health care: humanity. Jon Bartels created The Pause when he was inspired by the actions of a hospital chaplain who requested the health care team stop and pray after an unsuccessful resuscitation. Bartels (2014) noted, "During one of our intense resuscitations, I had noted that when we were done, we kind of just walked away from the situation … I realized that we had lost a ritual of honoring."

The Pause poses minimal risk (Cunningham et al., 2019) and has considerable benefits, including increased perceived team cohesion, a moment for reflection, and a way to honor a deceased patient. It also allows nurses to feel more present to meet the needs of the next patient they care for during a shift. See the script for The Pause as suggested by Jon Bartels below; you can modify it to suit your needs.

PUTTING IT INTO PRACTICE

The Pause

Goal: To pause for a moment of reflection after the death of a patient

Time and place: Barely a minute or two. Try it at work with your colleagues.

"Could we stop and honor this patient who was alive prior to coming in here, who was loved by others, who loved others, who had a life—and also take the moment to honor all the efforts we put into caring for the patient? I ask that we hold the space, to honor this patient in your own way and in silence."

Saying these words and pausing in silence for one minute allows staff to own the practice and honor a patient's last rite of passage.

GRIEVING WITH YOUR PEERS
♦

Dr. Robert Neimeyer (2012) offers sound advice on grieving with your peers. First, embrace the power of presence. Words are not always needed. You don't have to fix anything or take away your friend's pain. You don't need to find answers, or solve problems, or do anything. Learning to be fully in the moment with a friend or colleague takes some thought, reflection, and perhaps some changes in ourselves. Clinicians Miller and Cutshall (2001) remind us that we may need to explore our individuality, humanness, and prejudices, as well as our brokenness.

Kathryn Mannix, author of *Listen: How to Find the Words for Tender Conversations* (2021), says there are no difficult or challenging conversations, only conversations that require a more delicate approach. She calls them "tender conversations." And the word "conversation" is important, as this exchange between peers is not about giving advice or imposing your views but rather offering respectful empathic engagement among peers.

Provide a safe and healing setting by creating a stable relational container, a space that can be fluid, not restraining, for a retelling of the story of a patient's death. Listen to the narratives of the death to more fully take in the unspoken meaning of one's grief. This does not mean the "details" but the story. The goal is to integrate the loss into the larger narrative of your lives and your practice. Remember that self-compassion and being in touch with one's emotions will help to capture the full spectrum of human responses.

TOOLS FOR HEALING

◆

What is grief, and how do you process it? What does it look like? Conversations surrounding death and grief prompt thoughtful and sometimes poignant questions. Turn them into tender conversations. Grieving is not one emotion but a constellation of many emotions. Our grief is universal but also unique, as we all have different life experiences and cultural backgrounds. Think about comforting yourself and those around you. Grieve and take in the world around you through the five senses.

Here are some suggestions:

- Be with people: friends, family, and colleagues, at work, school, and in your community.
- Find familiar ground, a space that can be in your own home, perhaps in your room. A private place of solitude, comfort.
- Seek out people and places important to you, giving you a sense of familiarity and comfort.
- Value quiet moments and times of solitude.
- Live in your body. Seek out contact with others—shake someone's hand, give them a hug, get a massage, dance, take a warm bath, pet your dog or cat.
- Enjoy comfort food. Do not deprive yourself of the things you love.
- Pay attention to your physical reactions in the aftermath of loss. Know when you are irritable or sad. Let other people know what you are experiencing.

- Take care of your body. See your primary care provider or dentist. Get a haircut, massage, or a manicure/pedicure.
- Be patient and conscious of your healing. What felt good when you were younger may feel good now. Reread a favorite book or story.
- Do something to order your universe. Clean and organize a desk or closet, redo an address book, take on a project, craft, or home-owner project. Paint, plant, clean.
- Be mindful of triggers: monitor the television, social media, and news you consume.
- Follow your spiritual path: meditate, pray, walk in natural settings.
- Exercise your body. Sweat. Move for at least one hour; walk, swim, bike, dance, or run.
- Sleep with as much regularity as you can, not too little and not too much.
- Give yourself permission to make mistakes, and acknowledge them when you do.
- Recognize your emotions every day, positive and negative.
- Let someone do you a favor. Ask for and accept help from others.
- Eat healthfully, and take clinically approved vitamins and/or supplements to fill any gaps in your nutrition.
- Read and write every day. Keep a journal and a book by your bedside.
- Keep a gratitude diary.

Now for the hard part: sharing and expressing words of sympathy.

THE ART OF EXPRESSING CONDOLENCES

•

When someone close to you dies, you want to reach out to others who are also grieving—family, other colleagues, and friends. But remember that you are grieving as well. Many nurses have lost peers and associates during the pandemic; some of you have lost family members. You are desperate to say the right thing, to find meaningful words. Perhaps we are much more aware of condolences, given our current climate of violence, death, and sorrow. The customary words "my thoughts and prayers are with you" seem overused and hollow. Have they become meaningless, and do they actually help share the burden of bereavement?

The following suggestions and tips provide guidance on how you can express your sympathy, support, and friendship or affection to a family member or friend who has lost an important person in their lives. Bear in mind that there are unique cultural and regional expressions important to families. Be sensitive to those differences when writing.

A condolence message or note should have at least these three elements:

- Your own feelings regarding the death of the person
- What the (deceased) person meant to you and how you knew them
- How you can support the recipient of your message

In Your Own Hand

Commit to words of sympathy with paper and pen. As Bruce Feiler (2016) noted in the *New York Times*, the rules of expressing sympathy have been swept into the wave of our contemporary digital communications. It may seem easier to embellish our words with not one or two emojis, but a string of icons that are supposed to reflect what we are feeling. Why not just express those emotions in words and on paper? Families often reread condolences weeks and months later, finding comfort and support. If you wish, send an email immediately and follow up with a handwritten note. A handwritten card or letter allows a more personal connection than a card with preprinted words. If you do want to use a sympathy card, be sure there is minimal text inside. Your words will be far more important to the person reading the card.

How to Begin a Condolence Note or Letter

It's okay to acknowledge that words do not come easily to you, but be sure to avoid focusing on yourself. Do not make the note about you or how you reacted upon hearing the news.

- Instead of: "I cried for hours after I heard the news about your father."

- Try something like this: "Many times, I have sat down to write, but no words have come, or words were wholly inadequate to express even a part of what I am feeling."

On the occasion of President John F. Kennedy's assassination, Prime Minister Indira Gandhi wrote an eloquent letter to Jacqueline Kennedy. Gandhi spoke of how she could not find the words to adequately express her sorrow. The words above are hers.

When should you send your note? It's never too late. Take your time. It might help you feel better if you send a note immediately, but sending a note or a follow-up letter after a few weeks will be greatly appreciated.

Tell a Story

Share a warm and inspiring memory of the person who has died. Telling a story about the deceased allows the family to see their important person through the eyes of others. Describe that moment in rich and warm detail.

- Instead of: "I remember him well."
- Try something like this: "Your dad always made me laugh. I remember the time he took us to Cub Scouts for the Pinewood Derby, and we got a flat tire along the way. You and I were freaking out, so worried we would miss the start. Your dad changed the tire so fast, I couldn't believe it. He was laughing and made us laugh, too."

Use words as they are meant to be used. Do use the words death and died. Avoid euphemisms, unless there are accepted cultural or regional preferences. "Loss" and "passing" are not only vague and ambiguous but can also be forms of denial or confusion, especially for children.

- Instead of: "I am so sorry to hear about the passing of your father."
- Try something like this: "I am so sorry to hear about the death of your father."

Avoid clichés. The standard "He's in a better place," "God wanted him in heaven," or "Everything happens for a reason" can offend. In fact, any sentence that begins with "at least" or "if only" should be eliminated from your note. There is no comfort to be gained when those words are used in a condolence note.

Involve Your Children

Don't delegate condolence writing to adults only; if your children knew the person who died, then they can and should write a short note as well. This is an ideal time for a family to sit together and write the note, finding words that may not be perfect but authentic.

- Instead of: "My children are thinking of you and your family."
- Try something like this: "Please find enclosed a few words (pictures) from my children, (name them). We talked about (name of the deceased) today, and they wanted to let you know that they are thinking about all of you."

Add Inspiration from Literature and Poetry

If you are having trouble coming up with your own words of sympathy and support, use those of poets and authors. Collect quotations, phrases, lyrics, and poetry that speak to the essence of grief and friendship. Sometimes the words of others resonate and make clear what we are feeling inside. Embed these eloquent words in your note, perhaps beginning with your own words and ending with a quotation.

Preface the quotation with a brief introduction of what it means to you: "Anne Lamott is one of my favorite authors. She speaks with eloquence and candor about the most painful moments of life and how we can heal and recover."

Here are a few favorites:

"What we have once enjoyed we can never lose. All that we love deeply becomes a part of us."—Helen Keller

"Friendship is unnecessary, like philosophy, like art ... It has no survival value; rather it is one of those things which give value to survival."—C. S. Lewis, *The Four Loves*

"The friend who can be silent with us in a moment of despair or confusion, who can stay with us in an hour of grief and bereavement, who can tolerate not knowing ... not healing, not curing ... that is a friend who cares."—Henri Nouwen

"Only grieving can heal grief; the passage of time will lessen the acuteness, but time alone, without the direct experience of grief, will not heal it."—Anne Lamott

And for those of you with children, some of the most inspiring and comforting quotes come from the pages of children's literature. Mr. Rogers provides sensitive words for some of life's most difficult moments:

"When I was a boy and I would see scary things in the news, my mother would say to me, 'Look for the helpers. You will always find people who are helping.'"—Fred Rogers

"In times of stress, the best thing we can do for each other is to listen with our ears and our hearts and to be assured that our questions are just as important as our answers."—Fred Rogers, *The World According to Mister Rogers: Important Things to Remember*

Other children's authors have captured the essence of friendship and support:

"There is nothing sweeter in this sad world than the sound of someone you love calling your name."—*The Tale of Despereaux*, by Kate DiCamillo

"Promise me you'll always remember: You're braver than you believe, and stronger than you seem, and smarter than you think."—Christopher Robin to Pooh, *Winnie the Pooh*, by A. A. Milne

Giving the Gift of Your Time

Finally, give your grieving colleague, family member, or friend the gift of your time. Don't ask them to let you know what they need; it is impossible for them to identify their needs through the fog of grief. They don't know what they need until they come face-to-face with it. Anticipate their need for help, and frequently check in with them.

• Instead of: "Let me know if there is anything I can do."
• Try something this: "I want to help you in any way I can. I'll get lunch tomorrow."

You are reaching out to those for whom you care a great deal.

We are sorry that so many of you have endured death and grief in your practices and in your personal lives. Certainly, nurses confronted death long before the pandemic. Coronavirus magnified and intensified these difficult moments.

Take good care. Remember, you are not alone.

MORAL DISTRESS

•

The coronavirus pandemic has forced the greater health care community to recognize what many nurses already knew: moral distress not only affects quality of care but also has consequences for a professional's quality of life. A negative impact on quality of life can increase vulnerability, causing self-doubt, and ultimately lead to questioning our commitment to the nursing profession.

What is moral distress? You've felt it and observed it in your colleagues. You may have also heard the terms "moral injury," "moral outrage," "moral apathy," and "moral residue." Let's examine this concept and how it pertains to the nursing profession.

Originally defined by philosopher Andrew Jameton in 1984, moral distress arises when nurses know the right thing to do, but organizational or structural constraints make it nearly impossible for them to pursue the right course of action. In the aftermath, nurses are left with painful and distressing emotions along with psychological disequilibrium. The intimate nature of the nurse–patient relationship contributes to the prevalence of moral distress; another human being is depending on you for safety, healing, and survival. When you cannot provide the best possible care, there can be a sense of guilt and betrayal. Confronted with institutional obstacles, failures, and conflicts, it is not unusual for nurses to react with heightened emotions of anger, frustration, and anxiety. Later on, after those initial acute emotions dissipate, reactive distress or moral residue lingers. There is no clean slate for starting over; you carry the remnants of the last event, waiting for it to happen again.

The American Association of Critical-Care Nurses (2006) points out that moral distress is a complex, challenging problem with damaging repercussions, which are often minimized or even ignored by administrators in health care settings. An element of burnout, moral distress is also a threat to nurse retention. When you are not able to fulfill your nursing obligations because of continuing value conflicts, ineffective and fractured communication, poor teamwork, organizational oversights, or staffing policies that do not address current needs, then you are at risk for moral distress.

What are the psychological and physical consequences of moral distress? How do you react when you are prevented from caring for your patients in the way you believe is appropriate and based on best practices? Moral distress is not a recent development. Long before the pandemic, we have heard nurses talk about their frustration, anger, psychological and physical exhaustion, helplessness, distress, and depressive moods (Wiegand and Funk, 2012). Studies such as that by Hanna (2004) have confirmed the physical consequences of moral distress— sleeplessness, migraines, and gastrointestinal symptoms.

Researchers investigating major causes of moral distress in nurses caring for COVID-19 patients found themes of uncertainty and lack of knowledge; being overwhelmed by the depth and breadth of the illness; fear of exposure to the virus; constraints on their ability to provide care; tensions and miscommunications among professionals; and the impact of scarce resources (Silverman et al., 2021).

MORAL DISTRESS AND SYSTEMIC INJUSTICE

•

Moral distress is a consequence of systemic injustice, racism, and gender inequality. These injustices permeate every part of our society, including the nursing profession, educational institutions, and hospital administrations. When nurses' knowledge is dismissed, undermined, or ignored, especially among Black, Indigenous, Hispanic, and other nurses of color, nurses are left with anger, frustration, and shame.

You've probably heard people describe the impact of the pandemic with the well-worn phrases "COVID-19 doesn't discriminate" or "We're all in the same boat." But nothing could be further from the truth. Since the earliest days of the first wave of infections and deaths, discriminatory attitudes, structures, and policies have only intensified preexisting

racial disparities, and COVID-19 has affected persons of color at disproportionate rates.

As overwhelming as it is to contemplate the damage to human life
resulting from the 2020–21 pandemic, it is equally overwhelming to
fathom the existence of dual pandemics—COVID-19 and racism. At
a recent panel presentation on the mental health of nurses at Rutgers
University in New Jersey, researcher and professor Charlotte Thomas-
Hawkins described these two concurrent pandemics and the many
nurses of color who have experienced them. Not only are patients of
color most severely affected by COVID-19, so too are their nurses of
color. In addition, nurses may feel especially vulnerable to contracting
the virus and bringing it home to their families. Thomas-Hawkins et al.
(2022) noted that the second pandemic—racism occurring in and outside of the workplace—emerged with heightened global attention after
the murder of George Floyd.

Along with her research team, Thomas-Hawkins surveyed 800
hospital-based nurses, of all races, living throughout New Jersey. Overall, nurses reported a high level of emotional distress, with three out
of every four nurses admitting they were burned out. In addition, 57%
reported anxiety, and nearly half had severe levels of distress. Most
notably, nurses of color reported higher levels of emotional distress,
higher levels of worry about COVID-19, and more negative racial
climates in their workplace. They also experienced a higher number
of racial microaggressions, with Black nurses reporting the highest
number of microaggressions and the most negative racial climates.
In summary, Thomas-Hawkins confirmed that workplace racism is a
reality for hospital-based nurses, especially for nurses of color, as is the
psychological impact of racism they experience.

In September 2020, the nursing activist website Nursemanifest: A
Call to Conscience and Action launched a new initiative called "Overdue Reckoning on Racism in Nursing." Their goal is to open and explore
conversations that focus on coming to terms with racism in nursing.
This reckoning is long overdue and acknowledges the reality of racism,
especially in health care and specifically in nursing. The founders emphasize that it also begins a process of healing and change. Ongoing
events include a series of webinars, blog posts, email lists, a comprehensive reading list, and important resources. Discussions bring the voices

of BILNOCs (Black, Indigenous, Latinx, and other Nurses of Color) to the foreground. Two monthly discussions are held, one for nurses of color to explore avenues for antiracism actions. The second meeting, facilitated by nurses of color and open to all nurses, focuses on different topics related to antiracism activism in nursing.

> and when we speak we are afraid
> our words will not be heard
> nor welcomed
> but when we are silent
> we are still afraid
> So it is better to speak
> remembering
> we were never meant to survive
>
> —Audre Lorde, *The Black Unicorn: Poems*

Moral injury, initially identified in the military population (Litz et al., 2009), refers to unprecedented traumatic events where a soldier perpetrates, fails to protect, or bears witness to events that break the rules of their moral code and values. Many of these events relate to death and traumatic injury, especially if a soldier couldn't save his buddy's life. Recently, researchers have theorized that health care providers, especially during the early days of the pandemic, are in precisely the same situation as soldiers (Williamson et al., 2020). Moral distress and moral injury may appear to be similar, since both are under the umbrella term of moral suffering. Moral injury primarily refers to death-related or violent events. Moral distress refers to moral dilemmas experienced by health care providers in their day-to-day practice—such as disagreement on treatment protocols, inadequate staffing, or not enough protective equipment.

Researchers suggest that the loss of a patient's life (especially at a young age), unsupportive administrators, exposure to traumatic events, and minimal or lack of social support can put nurses and other members of the health care team at risk for moral injury (Williamson et al., 2020). Even so, not everyone exposed to these traumatic events develops moral injury. Awareness, social support, and collective resilience strategies are key to both preventing and recovering from this common condition.

Zen Buddhist teacher Roshi Joan Halifax (2018) defines moral apathy as a denial, lack of caring, or willful ignorance that makes it possible for us to ignore situations that cause harm to others. Moral apathy is the act of ignoring the suffering of others, especially those we are serving. It can arise in response to burnout, losing the capacity to care. Moral apathy is not freedom from moral feelings.

Moral distress can also drive us to take action. Cynda Rushton, who has written extensively about moral distress and critical care nurses and the impact of the pandemic (Rushton et al., 2021), describes moral outrage as anger, frustration, or disgust in response to a real or perceived violation of a moral principle. Nurses are justified and seek accountability (Carse and Rushton, 2017, 2018). Look no further than social media to see evidence of moral outrage in the political arena and among our colleagues.

Rushton (2013) asserts that moral outrage may be an antidote to moral distress. Principled moral outrage is grounded in reflection, knowledge, and compassion; it is not an emotional, unplanned action. In other words, cooler heads prevail. Rushton (2013) identified the necessary tools and strategies for fostering principled moral outrage. Her approach incorporates a series of steps that range from greater awareness of mind and body to exploration of alternatives and to making organizational change. See Rushton (2013) for an eloquent discussion of the specific strategies she recommends.

Nursing educators and their students are not immune to moral suffering. In fact, they may be at greater risk because they are coping with multiple organizational and environmental settings—administrative decisions and positions at the highest university/college level as well as those decisions made at the individual professional school. Clinical agency requirements and expectations may place additional demands and further complicate personal decision-making. In addition, faculty and students may have different perspectives regarding support and expectations of each other.

Graduate students may be at increased risk of moral suffering if they work full or part time in a clinical setting in addition to carrying a course load. Family commitments can push individuals to the breaking point, resulting in burnout or empathic distress fatigue. Moral distress can negatively affect patient care, causing nurses to avoid certain clinical situations and ultimately leave the profession.

IN THEIR OWN WORDS

Things are really bad. I can't even wrap my head around what I am seeing... the sheer number of patients, and they are so sick. I can't bear to say this, but I've had to lower my expectations. We have no resources. I can't get my work done. Management is doing the best they can, but it's not enough.

When I come to work, I hit the ground running. But my relief nurse shows up late, again. When it is time to go, it is TIME to go! Where is my relief? I want to go home.

I have an assignment of seven patients; others have two or three patients. What is that about? When a family member calls, I talk to them. I tell them to call me back. Some nurses don't talk to family because they "don't have time." They seem not to have the capacity to care.

Last Monday, I lost it with my nurse manager, and I didn't even care what I said. I just couldn't hold it in anymore. I exploded and ranted. I've never been so upset. I am embarrassed and ashamed. I shouldn't have been so angry and emotional. I was right about my concerns, but not right about how I expressed them to my nurse manager.

Luckily, I got a chance to clear the air. I apologized for the way I spoke to her, but not about my concerns. Lesson learned.

April 2020: Anonymous, Graduate Nursing
Student, New England, United States

As you can see from this story, moral outrage drove this nurse's emotional outburst, but it also prompted greater reflection and acknowledgment. A lesson was learned, although painful, and set the stage for more lessons to come.

We have seen and heard many nurses talking about the issues that precipitate moral distress and compromise patient care. In some cases, organizations and hospitals are striking back with penalties and removing professionals from their positions. But those voices have to be heard. We have to have realistic hope that these constructive protests and creative ideas will be taken seriously.

Moral distress is not a personal, moral, or character defect. Think about moral distress as an opportunity to reflect, raise your voice, take action, and address the challenges inherent in nursing practice and in all settings. In the direst, most morally harmful situations, there is opportunity for growth, for building moral resilience. Nurses draw upon their inner resources, allowing them to work under the most difficult conditions, but not without reflection and acknowledgment that they are facing an ethical challenge. Studies confirm that moral resilience is associated with lower burnout rates (Antonsdottir et al., 2021). Identifying potential interventions at all points in clinical practice, even in the face of increasing morally distressing circumstances, allows nurses to see that change is possible.

REFERENCES

Burnout and Vicarious Trauma
Bakker, A. B., Schaufeli, W. B., Leiter, M. P., & Taris, T. W. (2008). Work engagement: an emerging concept in occupational health psychology. *Work and Stress* 22(3):187–200.
Business Insider. (2021). The Great American Burnout Is Just Getting Started. Business Insider, June 2021. https://www.businessinsider.com/the-us -workforce-is-feeling-more-burned-out-than-ever-2021-6
Figley, C. R., ed. (2015). *Compassion Fatigue: Coping with Secondary Traumatic Stress Disorder in Those Who Treat the Traumatized*. London: Routledge.
Gunderman, R. (2014). For the young doctor about to burn out. *The Atlantic*, February 25, 2014. https://www.theatlantic.com/health/archive/2014/02 /for-the-young-doctor-about-to-burnout/284005/
Jenkins, S., & Baird, S. (2002). Secondary traumatic stress and vicarious trauma: a validational study. *Journal of Traumatic Stress* 15: 423–32.
Kim, W. (2021). Is that all there is? Why burnout is a broken promise burnout. *Refinery* 29, September 29, 2021. https://www.refinery29.com/en-gb /burnout-great-resignation
Li, Z., Ge, J., Yang, M., Feng, J., Qiao, M., Jiang, R., & Yang, C. (2020). Vicarious traumatization in the general public, members, and non-members of medical teams aiding in COVID-19 control. *Brain, Behavior, and Immunity* 88: 916–19.
Magnavita, N., Chirico, F., Garbarino, S., Bragazzi, N. L., Santacroce, E., & Zaffina, S. (2021). SARS/MERS/SARS-CoV-2 outbreaks and burnout syndrome among healthcare workers: an umbrella systematic review. *International Journal of Environmental Research and Public Health* 18(8): 4361.

Maslach, C., Jackson, S. E., & Leiter, M. P. (1997). *Maslach Burnout Inventory.* Menlo Park, CA: Mind Garden. https://www.mindgarden.com/312-mbi -general-survey

Maslach, C., Schaufeli, W. B., & Leiter, M. P. (2001). Job burnout. *Annual Review of Psychology* 52(1): 397–422.

Murthy, V. (2022). *Addressing Health Worker Burnout: The U.S. Surgeon General's Advisory on Building a Thriving Health Workforce.* Washington, DC: US Department of Health and Human Services Office of the US Surgeon General. https:// www.hhs.gov/sites/default/files/health-worker-wellbeing-advisory.pdf

MindTools. Burnout self-test. Accessed August 5, 2022. https://www.mind tools.com/pages/article/newTCS_08.htm

Newell, J. M., & MacNeil, G. A. (2010). Professional burnout, vicarious trauma, secondary traumatic stress, and compassion fatigue. *Best Practices in Mental Health* 6(2): 57–68.

Pearlman, L. A., & Mac Ian, P. S. (1995). Vicarious traumatization: an empirical study on the effects of trauma work on trauma therapists. *Professional Psychology: Research and Practice* 26: 558–65.

Petersen, A. H. (2021). *Can't Even: How Millennials Became the Burnout Generation.* New York: Mariner Books.

Compassion, Empathy, and Empathic Distress

Eisenberg, N. (2002). Empathy-related emotional responses, altruism, and their socialization. In: *Visions of Compassion: Western Scientists and Tibetan Buddhists Examine Human Nature.* New York: Oxford University Press, 131–64.

Eisenberg, N., Eggum, N. D., & Di Giunta, L. (2010). Empathy-related responding: associations with prosocial behavior, aggression, and intergroup relations. *Social Issues and Policy Review* 4(1): 143.

Goetz, J. L., & Simon-Thomas, E. (2017). The landscape of compassion: definitions and scientific approaches. In: Seppälä, E. M., Simon-Thomas, S., Brown, S. L., et al., eds. *The Oxford Handbook of Compassion Science.* Oxford: Oxford University Press, 3–15.

Goetz, J. L., Keltner, D., & Simon-Thomas, E. (2010). Compassion: an evolutionary analysis and empirical review. *Psychological Bulletin* 136(3): 351.

Jazaieri, H., Jinpa, G. T., McGonigal, K., Rosenberg, E. L., Finkelstein, J., Simon-Thomas, E., Cullen, M., Doty, J. R., Gross, J. J., & Goldin, P. R. (2013). Enhancing compassion: a randomized controlled trial of a compassion cultivation training program. *Journal of Happiness Studies* 14(4): 1113–26.

Mills, J., Wand, T., & Fraser, J. A. (2018). Examining self-care, self-compassion and compassion for others: a cross-sectional survey of palliative care nurses and doctors. *International Journal of Palliative Nursing* 24(1): 4–11. https://doi.org/10.12968/ijpn.2018.24.1.4

Rogers, C. R. (1975). Empathic: an unappreciated way of being. *Counseling Psychologist* 5(2): 2–10.

Shamay-Tsoory, S. G. (2009). Empathic processing: its cognitive and affective dimensions and neuroanatomical basis. In: Decety, J., & Ickes, W., eds. *The*

Social Neuroscience of Empathy. Cambridge: Massachusetts Institute of Technology Press, 215–32.

Titchener, E. B. (1909). *Lectures on the Experimental Psychology of the Thought-Processes*. New York: Macmillan.

Loss and Grief

Bartels, J. B. (2014). The pause. *Critical Care Nurse* 34(1): 74–75. https://doi.org/10.4037/ccn2014962

Critoph, D., & Smith, S. (2020). Care for people bereaved during the pandemic. *Cancer Nursing Practice* 19(6): 14–15. https://doi.org/10.7748/cnp.19.6.14.s10

Cunningham, T., Ducar, D. M., & Keim-Malpass, J. (2019). "The pause": a Delphi methodology examining an end-of-life practice. *Western Journal of Nursing Research* 41(10): 1481–98.

Endacott, R. (2019). "I cried too": allowing ICU nurses to grieve when patients die. *Intensive and Critical Care Nursing* 52: 1–2.

Feiler, B. (2016). The art of condolence. *New York Times*, October 2, 2016.

Hillis, S. D., Blenkinsop, A., Villaveces, A., Annor, F. B., Liburd, L., et al. (2021a). COVID-19-associated orphanhood and caregiver death in the United States. *Pediatrics* e2021053760.

Hillis, S. D., Unwin, H. J. T., Chen, Y., Cluver, L., Sherr, L., et al. (2021b). Global minimum estimates of children affected by COVID-19-associated orphanhood and deaths of caregivers: a modelling study. *The Lancet* 398(10298): 391–402.

Mannix, K. (2021). *Listen: How to Find the Words for Tender Conversations*. London: Harper Collins.

Miller, P., & Cutshall, S. (2001). *The Art of Being a Healing Presence: A Guide for Those in Caring Relationships*. Fort Wayne, IN: Willowgreen Press.

Neimeyer, R. A., ed. (2012). *Techniques of Grief Therapy: Creative Practices for Counseling the Bereaved*. New York: Routledge.

Sullender, R. S. (2010). Vicarious grieving and the media. *Pastoral Psychology* 59(2): 191–200.

Verdery, A. M., Smith-Greenaway, E., Margolis, R., & Daw, J. (2020). Tracking the reach of COVID-19 kin loss with a bereavement multiplier applied to the United States. *Proceedings of the National Academy of Sciences* 117(30): 17,695–701.

Moral Distress

American Association of Critical-Care Nurses (2006). *AACN Public Policy Position Statement: Moral Distress*. Aliso Viejo, CA: American Association of Critical-Care Nurses.

Antonsdottir, I., Rushton, C. H., Nelson, K. E., Heinze, K. E., Swoboda, S. M., & Hanson, G. C. (2021). Burnout and moral resilience in interdisciplinary healthcare professionals. *Journal of Clinical Nursing* 31(1–2): 1–13.

Carse, A., & Rushton, C. H. (2017). Harnessing the promise of moral distress: a call for re-orientation. *Journal of Clinical Ethics* 28(1): 15–29.

Carse, A., & Rushton, C. H. (2018). Moral distress. In: Rushton, C. H., ed. *Moral Resilience: Transforming Moral Suffering in Healthcare.* New York: Oxford University Press, 24–51.

Halifax, J. (2018). Contemplation by Design 2018 keynote: the strange and necessary case for hope. YouTube, November 1, 2018. https://www.youtube.com/watch?v=8xMNZVe2u-w

Hanna, D. R. (2004). Moral distress: the state of the science. *Research and Theory for Nursing Practice* 18(1): 73–93

Hilgers, L. (2022). Nurses have finally learned what they're worth. *New York Times Magazine,* February 15, 2022. https://www.nytimes.com/2022/02/15/magazine/traveling-nurses.html

Jameton, A. (1984). *Nursing Practice Issues.* Englewood Cliffs, NJ: Prentice Hall.

Litz, B. T., Stein, N., Delaney, E., Lebowitz, L., Nash, W. P., Silva, C., & Maguen, S. (2009). Moral injury and moral repair in war veterans: a preliminary model and intervention strategy. *Clinical Psychology Review* 29(8): 695–706.

Lorde, A. (2019). *The Black Unicorn.* London: Penguin.

Rushton, C. H. (2013). Principled moral outrage: an antidote to moral distress? *AACN Advanced Critical Care* 24(1): 82–89.

Rushton, C. H., Turner, K., Brock, R. N., & Braxton, J. M. (2021). Invisible moral wounds of the COVID-19 pandemic: are we experiencing moral injury? *AACN Advanced Critical Care* 32(1): 119–25.

Silverman, H. J., Kheirbek, R. E., Moscou-Jackson, G., & Day, J. (2021). Moral distress in nurses caring for patients with COVID-19. *Nursing Ethics* 28(7–8): 1137–64. https://doi.org/10.1177/09697330211003217

Thomas-Hawkins, C., Zha, P., Flynn, L., & Ando, S. (2022). Effects of race, workplace racism, and COVID worry on the emotional well-being of hospital-based nurses: a dual pandemic. *Behavioral Medicine* 48(2): 95–108.

Wiegand, D. L., & Funk, M. (2012). Consequences of clinical situations that cause critical care nurses to experience moral distress. *Nursing Ethics* 19: 479–87.

Williamson, V., Murphy, D., & Greenberg, N. (2020). COVID-19 and experiences of moral injury in front-line key workers. *Occupational Medicine* 70(5): 317–19.

CHAPTER 11

Continuing the Journey of Transformation and Healing

"It was bad, really bad. And traumatizing. I didn't recognize my emergency department. Beds and equipment were everywhere. The noise never stopped . . . code and monitor alarms, the beats and whooshes of ventilators. But there was also silence; patients' and families' voices were gone. I was in a war zone. When this is over, I'll deal with my trauma."

There is a sense of anxiety all new nurses have when starting their first job. Questions like, "Will I be able to handle it?" and "Will I be a good nurse?" fill my mind. The COVID-19 pandemic made it difficult for many new nurses; it also took a physical and mental toll on us.

I started my nursing career in September 2019, and by March 2020, my floor became a COVID unit and has been ever since. When I started taking care of patients with the virus, I was scared. Along with having a lot of anxiety, it did not help that this virus was so easily spread. We were all forced to social distance and stay away from our loved ones. At the end of March, my hospital offered hotel rooms for workers who took care of COVID patients. Since I was worried about bringing the virus back home to my family, I took that opportunity.

I spent four weeks in the hotel room, isolated from my friends, family, and society. It was a dark and depressing time. My hospital was at our peak with COVID patients.

Every day I was at work, we had rapid responses, patients getting intubated, or going to the ICU.

Every day, we were told to save our PPE supply, because we would never know when it would run out.

Every day, I was afraid that I might have the virus myself.

It hurt to see arguments on television about the severity of the virus and whether it was necessary to wear masks, to lock down, or to take other precautions. Imagine having to come to work with a continuous stream of patients taking their last breaths. I cannot fathom what the families of these patients had to go through; so many would say their goodbyes virtually. We nurses offered their last conversation and their last physical touch in this world...

Being a nurse in this pandemic has taught me a lot about the will of society but also the dark corners of this world. One day after work, I was at the grocery store and had my hospital badge on. A shopper saw my badge, and said, "You are the spreader; you shouldn't be here." As a nurse, I've learned that we need a hard outer shell. In this case, he penetrated right through. It hurt—a lot.

Rude comments have never bothered me, and I can quickly brush them off, but that comment stung. The situation intensified my feelings of anxiety and loneliness. I had no one to talk to, especially about what we health care professionals were going through. Who could understand death on a daily basis, and a society that was in turmoil? I was struggling mentally, and something as basic as a grocery store visit terrified me.

As nurses, we are constantly adapting to every situation. The one community that I could rely on, my nursing community, was there for me. We were blessed to have such support from the nursing staff, community, and patients.

A few months into the pandemic, we were approached by management to stop playing music when patients were discharged from the COVID ward. An employee from a different part of the hospital had complained. We saw the joy it brought to our patients at their worst times. My coworkers and I knew that we had to do something to continue this "tradition." We were selfish; the music was a motivator for us... it gave us hope that people can fight through this and that we could help them. So, we started playing our own music and brought pom-poms to cheer for our patients. Other times, we would go to the local park, let out some steam, and try to have some sort of sanity, at least for 30 minutes.

Our local community has also showed us lots of love. Every day we would get food donations from local restaurants. To me, this was such a compelling message of support. We knew these establishments were suffering, and yet they still made sure we were fed. Young students from neighboring schools wrote to us expressing their love and appreciation for our efforts. They called us heroes and were inspired by our efforts.

The biggest love we received was from the patients themselves. We were all going through the same feelings of isolation, and we became a pseudo-family. When I had to explain to my patients that we must cluster our care to decrease our exposure, they were understanding. Many of our patients would tell us how much of an angel we were to them, and to me, those words held the highest honor.

My floor still gets COVID patients, and we are exhausted and burnt out. We're anxious, angry, and being pushed to the limit. But I asked my colleagues, "If you could choose between working on a non-COVID unit or working on our unit with each other, what would you do?" All of my colleagues said the same thing: They would choose to work with their colleagues on our COVID unit.

In the beginning, I had trouble sleeping and brought my work home with me. I was having difficulty and not taking care of myself. I started therapy. I'm worried less about myself now, but I still need to practice not bringing my work home. It is a lot to handle. If I had the chance to go back to talk to my old self at the start of the pandemic, I would tell myself, "It's important to focus on my own mental health before I focus my energy on the patients." I tell all the new nurses on my ward the exact same thing: focus on you, so you can then focus on others!

Spring 2020: Kinara N. Patel, BSN, RN, Medical-Surgical/
COVID Unit, Somerset, New Jersey, United States

THE LANDSCAPE OF TRAUMA

•

As the story above so movingly captures, the fiercely precipitous arrival of COVID-19 disrupted life and nursing practice, in more ways than we could imagine. Stress and trauma became constant companions to nurses across the globe. The toxic consequences may be invisible at first, but each of these strange bedfellows causes us to respond in different ways.

In many cases, stress can be alleviated once a stressor is removed, but traumatic responses can linger after we are exposed to or witness actual or threatened death or serious injury, or work-related traumatic events (American Psychological Association, 2013). War, assault, death, and mass casualties are traumatic events. Throughout the pandemic, nurses have struggled with some if not all types of traumatic situations: alien landscapes, hazardous responsibilities, fear for their own lives and those of family members, as well as bearing witness to catastrophic illness and deaths in unprecedented numbers.

Before COVID, a stressful day might be a hectic 12 hours with lots of admissions, a few really sick patients, little chance to sit down, a small lunch of a refilled water bottle and two granola bars, and a cup of coffee right after huddle to catch up on charting before heading home. Then there's a quick stop at the grocery store or there's nothing for dinner. Slowly the stressors peel away when you leave work, and maybe you find a few peaceful moments with family, share a meal with warm-hearted conversation, and go to sleep.

What if that stressful day is repeated over and over again?

What if you see images that startle and terrify you?

What if you can't see or touch your family and friends?

Unlike stressors, traumatic events precipitate a cascade of physical and emotional responses, lasting well after the event ends. Traumatic events launch a neuroendocrine response that results in physiological and affective sequelae or peritraumatic symptoms, the emotional and physiological distress experienced during and/or immediately after a traumatic event.

For most of us, one, two, or even several of these reactions are common in the immediate aftermath of trauma. Symptoms can include intrusive memories or flashbacks; trying to avoid situations that remind you of the trauma; negative or distorted thoughts and mood; hyper-arousal that leaves you irritable, angry, and unable to sleep; and even the feeling that you are living through a surreal nightmare (American Psychological Association, 2013).

Each of us can have our own distinct reactions to trauma, depending on the situation, our life experiences, and coping skills. We can't ignore the past; previous traumas can add weight to new symptoms. But researchers have also found that past traumas can result in post-traumatic growth, which is the tendency to identify positive transformation after trauma exposure (Tedeschi et al., 2018).

As you may recall from your Psych 101 class, the hypothalamo-pituitary-adrenocortical (HPA) axis is our central stress response system. When the amygdala detects threat, it alerts the HPA axis, causing the release of glucocorticoids, which redirect the body's energy resources to meet real or anticipated threat. Glucocorticoids and the amygdala affect how we consolidate our memories, especially emotionally significant ones (McGaugh, 2004). Traumatic memories are intense, durable, and accurate, but they are also physiologically arousing, which can affect your sleep, concentration, and day-to-day activities. In contrast to their enhancing effects on memory consolidation, adrenal stress hormones may impair memory retrieval and working memory (Roozendaal and McGaugh, 2011). As the quote at the beginning of this chapter illustrates, the sights and sounds experienced by nurses working in the most challenging practice settings are likely to persist, at least for a short time. When traumatic memories cause long-term distress, posttraumatic stress disorder (PTSD) is a possibility.

Psychiatrist and pioneer in the trauma field Bessel van der Kolk reminds us that our bodies also carry trauma. In his global best-selling book The Body Keeps the Score, he reminds us that trauma reshapes both body and brain, compromising our capacities for joy and pleasure, engagement, self-control, and trust. Van der Kolk contends that we have to become familiar with and "befriend" the sensations in our bodies. We can expand our awareness of physical sensations and the way that our bodies interact with the world around us. Physical self-awareness is the first step as we let go of the traumas of the past. For nurses, awareness of bodily sensations is critical. Your ability to offer and receive physical touch has been significantly affected by this pandemic. Touching a patient's hand, hugging a colleague, and even embracing parents and children carried the threat of danger. As van der Kolk suggests, be mindful of your body, use breathwork to decrease hyperarousal, think about ways you can make up for lost time, and reclaim sensory experiences.

We know that nurses are no strangers to harrowing situations; many of you have experienced stressful practice settings long before the pandemic—forensic nurses caring for victims of sexual assault, the nurses of Liberia and Sierra Leone leading their communities through the Ebola epidemic, nurses from the Federal Emergency Management Agency (FEMA) deployed during natural disasters, Canadian nurses desperately trying to contain severe acute respiratory syndrome (SARS). Their lives were at risk, witnessing an overwhelming toll of human illness and injury, yet they moved forward. Much as so many of you are doing.

When nurses bear witness to critically ill patients, overwhelming clinical settings, depleted resources, and a health care environment that seems both ineffective and tone deaf, it takes a toll, no matter how well prepared you are. Nurses in many practice environments, not only the high-acuity settings or emergency departments, have been affected by this public health crisis. A study by the International Council of Nurses (2021a) found that almost 80% of their affiliate associations had nurses working during the COVID-19 response who experienced mental distress.

In Portugal, almost 8,000 nurses have been infected with the SARS-CoV-2 virus since the beginning of the COVID-19 pandemic, which represents about 10% of professionals registered in the Portuguese Nurses Order, from March 2020 until July 2021 (Ordem dos Enfermeiros, 2021). At the beginning of the pandemic, the Order of Nurses in France began "Nurses' Words," a forum on their website for nurses to give their testimony (Ordre National des Infirmiers, 2022). During that same period, French researchers (Azoulay et al., 2020) studied ICU clinicians. When compared to other providers, nurses had the highest rates of anxiety, depression, and peritraumatic dissociation. In Louhans, located in the central-eastern region of France, the Le Gouz clinic is the only mental health establishment in France to address the mental health needs of health care professionals (Ball, 2021). With an average stay of eight weeks, the 40-room center offers respite from the exhaustion in the lives of these professionals.

The International Council of Nurses has been calling for official statistics on infections and deaths among nurses for well over a year. In May 2021, the World Health Organization revealed that the COVID death toll of nurses and other health care workers between January 2020 and May 2021 officially reached 115,000; they also admitted that data collection was scant (International Council of Nurses, 2021b).

In early 2022, the US Senate and House of Representatives passed the Dr. Lorna Breen Health Care Provider Protection Act (H.R. 1667, 117th Cong. [2021–22]). The bill was named for an emergency department physician in New York City who died by suicide after working countless hours in the early days of the pandemic. This new law would authorize funding to create behavioral health programs to support health care professionals. The US Department of Health and Human Services will be required to evaluate and recommend strategies to reduce burnout and enhance resilience. To encourage health care professionals to seek professional support, the foundation will launch a nationwide information and awareness-building campaign.

COLLECTIVE TRAUMA, COLLECTIVE RESILIENCE
◆

It seems that the pandemic has caused collective trauma within the worldwide nursing community. When nurses bear witness to the trauma and pain of patients as well as the overwhelming changes in clinical settings, it can take a long-lasting toll, no matter how well prepared they are.

IN THEIR OWN WORDS

It was minutes before midnight. I walked into Ms. Johnson's room. I grabbed her hand and told her that I was there to give her midnight medicine. I secured the medication and stepped out of the room. I don't know what happened, but I cried, and cried some more. My goggles became moist and started to fog; I was worried that the moisture would break the seal on my PPE. When I doffed my PPE, I was drenched in sweat—a common occurrence in the "COVID cove." I went to the bathroom, washed my salty face, and freshened up. I asked myself why I was so emotional. What was it about Ms. Johnson, who by no means was the sickest or most severe case that I cared for? I asked myself why this had to be the outcome for poor Ms. Johnson. I began to think back on the hundreds of patients I cared for in New York, people from all walks, sick and dying and alone. I realized that I was hurting for Ms. Johnson and the many other patients who were sick and scared and alone. I realized that my heart hurt for the nurses at the bedside, fighting along with their patients for 12, 14, sometimes 16 hours, and it was still not enough for their patients to make it home to their loved ones.

I collected myself and returned to give her medication; I gave her a nice bath and braided her hair. Ms. Johnson remained stable during my entire shift. Before leaving for the day, I donned my PPE one last time to say goodbye to Ms. Johnson. I told her that she was beautiful and that she was loved, and I wished peace for her.

I met up with my best friend, and we walked out together. I shared with her that I had my "moment" that night. She knew exactly what I was talking about without me having to share a single detail. I told her that I felt defeated and that I wished there was more that I could do. She reminded me that sometimes things are out of our hands and that all we can do is our best, and to keep our compassion and love for this profession.

I made it home and sat in my driveway before going in the house. I called my mom and told her about my night. I cried again. Before hanging up, she said a prayer for me and all the health care personnel working during this pandemic. I stripped in the garage before going inside, where I was greeted by the well-rested faces of my children. We air hugged, and I went to shower. I washed all the ick off me and felt refreshed. Before going to sleep, I spent a little time with my family, listening to how my son cheated at Uno and how my daughter ate all the popcorn before their movie started. We ate breakfast together, and I told them all how much I loved and missed them when I went to work. My daughter tucked me in and wished me sweet dreams and peaceful rest. She told me that my patients still needed me and kissed my forehead.

The next night when I returned to work, I learned that Ms. Johnson coded and did not survive. Sadness momentarily came over me, then a sense of relief in knowing that her family was able to see her one last time and that she was finally resting in peace.

That night I reflected on my own family and my gratitude for their support and love throughout my nursing career and especially during this pandemic. I thought of the sacrifices made by my husband and children, and how just when I felt like I could not go any further, they were there to remind me that my patients need me. I thought about my colleagues on the front line and hoped that they too have a safe place to be vulnerable, to let it all out, and to have that moment.

Summer 2020: Felicia Permenter, BSN, RN, NBC-HWC, Intensive Care Unit, Brooklyn, New York, United States.

When psychological responses to a traumatic event permeate families, communities, society, and, in the case of the coronavirus pandemic, entire professions, we have to consider how we can recover from such sweeping devastation. We share the experience of shattered assumptions in our worldview and how we view our profession. The taken-for-granted beliefs and expectations about our lives and our connections to the world have evaporated. We've heard these shattered assumptions many times when nurses report, "I didn't sign up for this."

According to Hirschberger (2018), the process of healing is one that "begins with a collective trauma, transforms into a collective memory, and culminates in a system of meaning that allows groups to redefine who they are and where they are going" (1). In addition to redefining who we are and what we do, collective trauma brings opportunities for collective healing and building collective resilience.

Since early 2020, professional nurses have come together in ways we've not seen before, in countless settings, in diverse practices, from novices to seasoned veterans. As you read in the story above, it was the simple act of leaving work with a colleague, comforted by her support, and then being greeted by family at home that speaks volumes about our collective resilience. Nurses have joined together for a common purpose—support, perseverance, and, yes, survival. Some might argue that nurses haven't always been so welcoming to each other, as evidenced by the old cliché that nurses "eat their young." We beg to differ; nurses have always collaborated, but at this moment in history, something is different. You have raised your collective voices, and you have heard each other. And so has the rest of the world. We are witnessing a transformation, a sea change, in professional nursing and health care. In the words of one nurse, "I'm in awe of my coworkers. We have each other's backs. They are my family. I've never felt closer."

Resilience is the capacity to overcome adversity; not only to bounce back but to bounce forward, to grow (Walsh, 2020). It is not a personality trait or a static, unchanging part of us. Resilience evolves; it is a dynamic process that allows us to learn new coping strategies, reframe problems as challenges, seek social support, look for meaning, and connect to a larger whole. Humans are relational beings; we depend on each other, as we know that healing is forged over time and in community. Social connectedness is essential for health, well-being, and resilience (Haslam et al., 2018).

THE SCIENCE OF RESILIENCE AND POSTTRAUMATIC GROWTH

Resilience can be described as a stable trajectory of healthy functioning after an adverse event. It is a dynamic system that successfully adapts to disturbances that threaten the viability, function, or development of that system (Masten, 2014a, 2014b). Resilience harnesses resources to sustain well-being (Panter-Brick and Leckman, 2013). Resilience requires a conscious effort to move forward in an insightful, integrated, and positive manner as a result of lessons learned from an adverse experience (Southwick et al., 2014, 3).

Yehuda and Flory (2007) offer a provocative idea: trauma survivors who develop posttraumatic stress disorder (PTSD) may be just as resilient as trauma survivors who don't develop PTSD (Yehuda and Flory, 2007). In other words, resilience is not the opposite of PTSD. Think about your colleagues, nurses who have confronted the worst of the ever-changing pandemic. They may report trauma symptoms, but they move forward, creating new solutions to problems, supporting those around them, and delivering care. We do not leave our traumatic experiences and symptoms behind, yet anyone observing you and your colleagues would see a remarkably resilient group of people.

Our responses to stress and trauma take place in the context of our relationships with other human beings, the resources available to us, and the cultural, religious, organizational, community, and societal environments that surround us (Walsh, 2006; Sherrieb et al., 2010).

We all have a foundation of resilient behaviors, thoughts, and actions, many of them learned during our early years. As we move through life, there are opportunities to practice those behaviors, and perhaps even attend formal trainings. Resilience-building is a continuing, lifelong process (Cooper et al., 2020). It is likely that resilience exists on a continuum (Pietrzak and Southwick, 2011) and changes over time, a result of our development and interaction with the surrounding environment (Kim-Cohen and Turkewitz, 2012).

Researchers confirm that there is no single personality, genetic, epigenetic, developmental, demographic, cultural, economic, or social factor that has been shown to predict or enhance resilience by more than a small degree (Southwick et al., 2014). Without question, the capacity to be resilient can be enhanced and taught.

When human beings face adversity, they hold on to "meaning-making," but what really matters is the sense of hope that life does indeed make sense despite the messiness, violence, uncertainty, stress, worry, or despair (Panter-Brick and Eggerman, 2012). Instead of looking at the negative outcomes of trauma, clinicians and researchers are learning to simultaneously evaluate and teach ways to enhance resilience. The question now is: What goes right in people who negotiate potentially traumatic events with calm and self-control?

Finstad et al. (2021) point out that resilience, posttraumatic growth, and associated coping strategies are entwined in a complex relationship. Resilience allows stabilization in the face of adversity. The positive changes that occur during or after a traumatic event are posttraumatic growth. Fostering both resilience-building skills and growth-promoting skills can lead to enhanced self-efficacy, cognitive flexibility, and resilience. Greater resilience can lead to increased posttraumatic growth.

Earlier work by Calhoun and Tedeschi (2013) emphasizes how trauma does not always result in pathology; in the aftermath of trauma, there can be growth, newly supportive relationships, and greater self-awareness. How we respond to trauma depends for the most part on the situation or previous experiences. There might be factors that hinder posttraumatic growth (Henson et al., 2021). The flexibility of our responses is determined by the context, a repertoire of behaviors, and our ability to regroup using beneficial feedback (Bonanno and Burton, 2013).

(continued)

What does resilience look like in nurses and within the nursing profession? Cooper et al. (2020) systematically analyzed the concept of resilience as it relates to nurses, establishing a working definition of nurse resilience with the core attributes of social support, self-efficacy, work-life balance and self-care, humor, optimism, and a realistic outlook.

After trauma, resilience is enhanced by finding the places where there are strengths. Look around you. Your colleagues, family, and friends make the case for the power of collective resilience.

References

Bonanno, G. A., & Burton, C. L. (2013). Regulatory flexibility: an individual differences perspective on coping and emotion regulation. *Perspectives on Psychological Science* 8(6): 591–612.

Calhoun, L. G., Tedeschi, R. G. (2013). *Posttraumatic Growth in Clinical Practice*. New York: Routledge.

Cooper, A. L., Brown, J. A., Rees, C. S., & Leslie, G. D. (2020). Nurse resilience: a concept analysis. *International Journal of Mental Health Nursing* 29(4): 553–75.

Finstad, G. L., Giorgi, G., Lulli, L. G., Pandolfi, C., Foti, G., León-Perez, J. M., Cantero-Sánchez, F. J. & Mucci, N. (2021). Resilience, coping strategies and posttraumatic growth in the workplace following COVID-19: a narrative review on the positive aspects of trauma. *International Journal of Environmental Research and Public Health* 18(18): 9453.

Henson, C., Truchot, D., & Canevello, A. (2021). What promotes post traumatic growth? A systematic review. *European Journal of Trauma and Dissociation* 5(4): 100195.

Kim-Cohen, J., & Turkewitz, R. (2012). Resilience and measured gene-environment interactions. *Development and Psychopathology* 24: 1297–306.

Masten, A. S. (2014a). Global perspectives on resilience in children and youth. *Child Development* 85(1): 6–20. https://doi.org/10.1111/cdev.12205

Masten, A. S. (2014b). *Ordinary Magic: Resilience in Development*. New York: Guilford Press.

Panter-Brick, C., & Eggerman, M. (2012). Understanding culture, resilience, and mental health: the production of hope. In: Ungar, M., ed. *The Social Ecology of Resilience: A Handbook of Theory and Practice*. New York: Springer, 369–86.

Panter-Brick, C., & Leckman, J. F. (2013). Resilience in child development: interconnected pathways to wellbeing. *Journal of Child Psychology and Psychiatry* 54: 333–36. https://doi.org/10.1111/jcpp.12057

Pietrzak, R. H., & Southwick, S. M. (2011). Psychological resilience in OEF-OIF veterans: application of a novel classification approach and examination of demographic and psychosocial correlates. *Journal of Affective Disorders* 133(3): 560–68.

Sherrieb, K., Norris, F. H., & Galea, S. (2010). Measuring capacities for community resilience. *Social Indicators Research* 99(2): 227–47.

Southwick, S. M., Bonanno, G. A., Masten, A. S., Panter-Brick, C. A., & Yehuda, R. (2014). Resilience definitions, theory, and challenges: interdisciplinary perspec-

tives. *European Journal of Psychotraumatology* 5(1): 25338. https://doi.org/10.3402
/ejpt.v5.25338
Walsh, F. (2006). *Family Resilience.* New York: Guilford Press.
Yehuda, R., & Flory, J. D. (2007). Differentiating biological correlates of risk,
PTSD, and resilience following trauma exposure. *Journal of Traumatic Stress* 20(4):
435–47.

COLLECTIVE RESILIENCE

◆

The term "collective resilience" has its roots in several disciplines. In his book *Collective Trauma, Collective Healing* (2013), psychologist Jack Saul describes how communities and groups work together to heal and recover after traumatic events such as community disasters, mass casualties, and forced migration.

Psychologist and family therapist Froma Walsh (2016) rightly points out that resilience in response to traumatic life events doesn't suggest we take everything in stride and "just bounce back, quickly rallying and moving on unscathed" (904). Healing and resilience are forged gradually, over time and in community, "through struggles, suffering and setbacks" (Walsh, 2020). And we don't "get over" trauma or grief—we move through it. Collective resilience is fostered by shared beliefs, making meaning of our profession, the pandemic, and its challenges. Walsh emphasizes that it is possible to gain a positive, hopeful outlook, rising above distress and hardship by redefining values, transforming priorities and purpose, and creating deeper bonds.

Ryff and Singer (2008) point out the strong correlation between resilience and well-being. From the perspective of mental and physical health promotion, Ryff asks if well-being and resilience can be nurtured and facilitated. Furthermore, whether experiencing life disruptions or misfortunes, can a person learn through various strategies how to enhance well-being? Ryff and her collaborators have seen individuals thrive in the most difficult circumstances—those who encounter the greatest challenges maintain or even enhance their well-being (Ryff and Singer, 2008).

THE SCIENCE OF COLLECTIVE RESILIENCE

Our social environment is composed of families, communities, neighborhoods, work teams, organizations, and even entire professions, such as nursing. Social interactions with other members of our group, family members, or work colleagues have an especially important role in our health, well-being, and even the way we respond to stress. Our social identity is how we see ourselves within a specific group. Nurses have a shared social identity—internalizing a sense of shared group membership and the belief that one is part of an "us" that is bigger than "me" alone (Haslam et al., 2005).

Our social groups ground us and give us a sense of place, purpose, and belonging, leaving us with a positive sense of social identity and resulting in positive psychological consequences. There are strong relationships between social identity and health-related behavior, social support, and coping. The United Kingdom Community Life Survey was administered to more than 4,000 individuals by McNamara et al. (2021). They found that the relationship between community identity and well-being was mediated by social support and reduced loneliness.

Haslam et al. (2005) contend that our social identity, the group to which we belong, also plays a critical role in protecting us from negative and unhealthy reactions to stress. Their study found a strong positive relationship between social identity and both social support and life/job satisfaction. They also confirmed that there is a strong negative correlation between social identification and stress. Social support was the key, a significant mediator of the relationship between social identification and stress, and social identification and life/job satisfaction.

Such important effects can safeguard our well-being when it is threatened and can help us cope with the negative consequences of being a member of a devalued group. One study found that hospital staff who felt devalued were more cynical regarding the potential usefulness of a stress intervention program (O'Brien et al., 2004). Devalued groups were characterized by lower levels of organizational identification, and members of these groups felt their skills and expertise were underutilized or even ignored by their organization (Haslam et al., 2005).

Koen et al. (2011) contend that the resilience of an entire profession can be enhanced through promotion and adoption of psychosocial strategies, reducing stress and enhancing well-being at the individual and organizational levels.

Cleary et al. (2014) were among the first to apply the term "collective resilience" to the nursing profession. They argue that the responsibility for cultivating collective resilience in nursing falls not only on individual nurses, but also on their employers and professional groups. The significant changes in the profession and the ongoing public health crisis demand a new movement toward collective resilience. Another study specifically looked at nurses and vaccination practices, well before the pandemic of 2020 (Falomir-Pichastor et al., 2009). The researchers found that the more nurses identified with their nursing colleagues, the more they recognized vaccination as a professional duty, and as a result they were more likely to have been vaccinated in the past and intended to be vaccinated in the future. In *Critical Resilience for Nurses* (2017), Michael Traynor, professor of nursing policy at Middlesex University, London, focuses on the meaning of resilience in an atmosphere of staffing shortages, depleted resources, and financial and political demands. Resilience is viewed as a framework for not only facilitating and enhancing professional identity, but also for making significant change in the profession.

Using key lessons from the collective resilience literature, researchers from the United Kingdom and Switzerland developed a framework for how the constraints of pandemic social distancing could be reconciled with situations that preserve and enhance social cohesion and a sense of collective efficacy (Elcheroth and Drury, 2020). Social isolation has affected nurses in unforeseen and complicated ways. Nurses, unable to be with their own families, acted as "stand-ins" for their patients' families. And with personal protective equipment covering their faces and bodies, they reached out to colleagues for support and comfort. The very essence of social support was missing from their lives for days and months on end.

References

Cleary, M., Jackson, D., & Hungerford, C. L. (2014). Mental health nursing in Australia: resilience as a means of sustaining the specialty. *Issues in Mental Health Nursing* 35(1): 33–40.

Elcheroth, G., & Drury, J. (2020). Collective resilience in times of crisis: lessons from the literature for socially effective responses to the pandemic. *British Journal of Social Psychology* 59(3): 703–13.

(continued)

Falomir-Pichastor, J. M., Toscani, L., & Despointes, S. H. (2009). Determinants of flu vaccination among nurses: the effects of group identification and professional responsibility. *Applied Psychology* 58(1): 42–58. https://doi.org/10.1111/j.1464-0597.2008.00381.x

Haslam, S. A., O'Brien, A., Jetten, J., Vormedal, K., & Penna, S. (2005). Taking the strain: social identity, social support, and the experience of stress. *British Journal of Social Psychology* 44(3): 355–70.

Koen, M. P., van Eeden, C., & Wissing, M. P. (2011). The prevalence of resilience in a group of professional nurses. *Health SA Gesondheid* 16(1): https://doi.org/10.4102/hsag.v16i1.576

McNamara, N., Stevenson, C., Costa, S., Bowe, M., Wakefield, J., Kellezi, B., Wilson, I., Halder, M. & Mair, E. (2021). Community identification, social support, and loneliness: the benefits of social identification for personal well-being. *British Journal of Social Psychology* 60(4): 1379–402.

O'Brien, A. T., Haslam, S. A., Jetten, J., Humphrey, L., O'Sullivan, L., Postmes, T., Eggins, R., & Reynolds, K. J. (2004). Cynicism and disengagement among devalued employee groups: the need to ASPIRe. *Career Development International* 9(1): 28–44. https://doi.org/10.1108/13620430410518129

Traynor, M. (2017). *Critical Resilience for Nurses: An Evidence-Based Guide to Survival and Change in the Modern NHS.* New York: Routledge.

Communal coping occurs during times of shared stress or trauma, when collaborative problem-solving, emotional support, and group coping are used to navigate challenging circumstances (Bender et al., 2021). We've heard many nurses describe meaningful interactions with their peers characterized by expressions of gratitude and empathy, valuing colleagues, offering help and support, demonstrations of physical and emotional presence, and vulnerability. Bender et al. (2021) confirm the effectiveness of these collective rituals of healing: "rich, reciprocal, and attuned experiences of emotional connection were also presented alongside expressions of sorrow, frustration, and loss around these adapted modes of connecting." There is even a place for humor and lightheartedness in the emotional connection activities described by nurses, such as sharing memes, holding group competitions, composing music playlists, and a creating a family photo wall.

As you've read in this book, building resilience and enhancing one's well-being extends beyond the traditional approaches; in fact, resilience can be strengthened in unexpected ways. Nurses who are advocates and activists contribute to their profession and to the world around them. We need you now more than ever. But there is an even greater benefit—one that is personal. Taking action in one's profession or community is a potential antidote to vicarious trauma. We share our colleagues' stories of resilience and strategies for empowerment. We all have creative outlets, and creativity can enhance well-being and healing. Pennebaker and Smyth (2016) and DeSalvo (2020), who promote writing through trauma and discomfort, confirm these efforts.

But building resilience is not only a personal endeavor. Coping with trauma and stress means taking time to recognize what is happening in your life, and then practicing effective strategies that will protect and enhance your well-being—physical, emotional, and social. Your health is the number one priority; performing your job better in the face of more stress may be an added benefit, but it is not the primary reason for your recovery and healing.

It is time to share strategies with each other. You've already started. Some call this self-care. Instead, focus on well-being as your goal. Remember that well-being can be a shared goal and requires a collective approach, an approach that extends beyond individual efforts.

CANARIES IN THE COAL MINE
◆

Several authors have described nurses during the pandemic as canaries in a coal mine. In the late 1800s, miners in Canada, Great Britain, and the United States used canaries to detect carbon monoxide in the air of a coalmine. The birds, a sentinel species, could detect poisonous gas in the mine far sooner than humans could. If carbon monoxide filled the mine, the canary would fall to the bottom of the cage, allowing the miners to escape before the mine exploded. Soon the miners, who had grown fond of the birds and kept them as pets, built resuscitation cages. This small piece of history has great relevance for nurses.

Nurses have endured more than any other health care professional throughout the COVID-19 pandemic. They attempted to shore up a failing system that was not prepared to protect them. The answer is to not to build resuscitation cages, or to breed canaries that can handle increasing amounts of poisonous gas; the answer is to redesign the coal mine, the health care system.

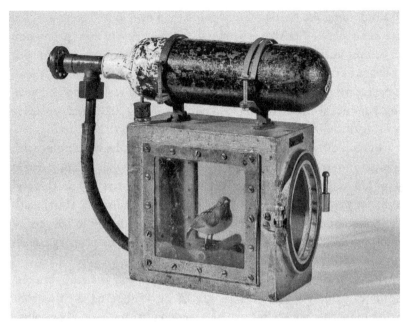

The World Health Organization's European policy framework identifies resilience as a key determinant for health and well-being (World Health Organization, 2013). Supportive people, activities, and environments are crucial for building resilience. Using the Ottawa Charter for Health Promotion (World Health Organization, 1986), Australian nurse researchers make the case for using this critical document to strengthen a resilient health care workforce (Wu and Oprescu, 2021). They develop planning strategies, key considerations, and outcomes for each of the five action areas of the charter: build healthy public policy, create supportive environments, strengthen community action, develop personal skills, and reorient health services. Clearly, this model embraces the importance of personal and collective resilience. It should involve multiple stakeholders, and it should incorporate resilience strategies into everyday activities, at work or at home.

Building collective resilience can be the way forward for nurses and the nursing profession. Personal resilience can flourish, meaning nurses will be more likely to recover when they are working in a supportive and validating community.

Becoming Your Best Self

Goal: To identify and practice resilience-enhancing strategies

Time and Place: Ongoing, at least once a week, wherever you are; carry your notebook, journal, or notes app with you.

What are the characteristics and qualities of resilience? A vast literature (Wu et al., 2013; Iacoviello and Charney, 2020) has identified key psychological factors held by resilient people or groups. The suggestions below are by no means exhaustive, but they do identify cognitive and behavioral components of the psychosocial factors associated with resilience, and it's a good place to start. These prompts have been developed over the years in our clinical practices and educational programming. Try a few of the strategies below.

▶ *Preserve and strengthen a positive view of yourself.* Keep a journal of your actions when dealing with challenging situations. Focus on your successes. You will develop confidence in your ability to meet challenging situations and trust your decision-making.

▶ *Seek out positive people, places, and events in the world around you.* Be mindful of how much you talk and read about sad cases at work, illness, and tragedy. Remember that the number of illnesses and accidents you see each day at work does not reflect what actually exists in the world. Tune in to the news once a day. Consider @Underthedesk news on Instagram or TikTok. This 60-second daily wrap-up breaks down politics, current events, and world news in a gentle way from a peaceful space (yes, it is actually from under a desk). Avoid doom-scrolling, and be aware when you have heard, seen, and read too much. This is good practice for everyone in your household, even children, who absorb far more than we realize.

  • For inspiration and feel-good stories, try following @tanks goodnews (tanksgoodnews.com) and @upworthy (upworthy.com).

▶ *Cultivate your ability to reexamine or reframe a situation,* and sidestep catastrophizing. Changing your focus can change the way you think about an event or situation. Allow for other interpretations, drop the negative thinking traps. You might not be able to erase or

(continued)

ignore a stressful experience, but you can reframe how you view the situation *and* how you respond. Look to the future after the immediate emotional landscape has shifted. Remember, problems are opportunities to create solutions.

▸ *Describe one problem* or difficult situation you've faced in the past six months:

_____

 Imagine yourself in 10 years looking back on this time. What would you say to your younger self?

_____

_____

▸ *Be curious and find opportunities for self-discovery. Learn something new.* Is there a new skill or talent you've always wanted to explore? What would it be?

_____

▸ *Look for meaning in both joyful and difficult times.* As Carol Ryff (2014) points out, embracing meaning in your life contributes to an overall sense of well-being. Ask yourself, "What I am supposed to learn from this?" How did you grow in that situation? Name the positives that emerged, whatever they might be. Recognize that while feeling vulnerable, you can experience personal growth, greater spirituality, and gratitude for your life and the people in it.

 List three things you discovered about yourself during a time of difficulty:

_____

_____

_____

▸ *Cultivate both cognitive and behavioral skills.* Actively seek support, guidance, and resources; recognize and name your needs. It takes courage to ask for help and support.

▸ *Recognize powerful emotions.* While it's important not to suppress emotions, realize when you may need to practice grounding, visualization, or breathwork in order to continue to function at work or even at home (switch on / switch off).

Describe how you might switch off an emotion: distraction, exercise, breath work:

_____

_____

▸ *Step by step, take action to deal with the challenges of daily living.* Recognize that even the smallest step is progress. These decisive actions will help keep worrying, or the urge to push the situation out of your mind and curl up in bed, at bay.

Name one or two actions you took during an unpleasant situation: _____

_____

▸ *Be aware of your needs.* Step back to rest, refuel, and reenergize yourself.

What will you do? Visualize it now: _____

_____

▸ *Don't hesitate to rely on yourself.* You have more strength than you realize!

Name your strengths. What do you do best? _____

_____

▸ *Nurture a positive view of yourself as a problem solver.* Keep a journal of your successes in dealing with difficult situations. You will develop confidence in your ability to solve problems and trust your instincts.

Name one problem you solved with or for another person:

_____

▸ *Develop realistic and measurable goals.* Keep moving toward these goals. There are no small accomplishments, only smaller steps that lead to your larger objective. Rather than identify a goal by

(continued)

the outcome, think of it in terms of a pledge of time, for example: "Today I will spend 45 minutes working on my paper for class." You may not have your paper finished, but you will have succeeded in achieving the goal of working on it for 45 minutes. Reflect on your accomplishments at the beginning and at the end of each day. Don't focus on what you failed to do; instead, ask yourself, "What one thing did I accomplish today that helps me move in the direction I want to go?"

Identify one long-term goal and two short-term objectives to reach that goal.

1. _____

   a. _____

   b. _____

▸ *Allow your goals to change.* Change might be uncomfortable, or you might think that some goals are unreachable. See a potential roadblock as a bridge to your next goal, not a barricade. Refocus on what you can change, and turn the roadblock into a temporary detour.

Name a goal that you felt you couldn't change or accomplish:

_____

How did you ultimately resolve that situation?

_____

▸ *Take GOOD care of yourself.* Be aware of your needs—physical, psychological, social, and spiritual. Spend time, on a regular basis, doing activities that soothe and calm or invigorate you. Taking care of yourself helps to keep your mind and body ready to deal with all kinds of situations.

Describe the last time you took a walk? Where did you go, and who was with you?

_____

▸ *Remember, you are not alone.* Discover and build your social support network—in your community, at work, at church, or in sports.

Reach out to others during their times of struggle; you will benefit as well. Don't be surprised if the person you thought would be the best listener isn't; new people may emerge as your supports. Be open to the possibilities. Connect with a resilient role model. Find your muse.

Name the people in your network of friends and at work:

_____

Now, name a few more:

_____

Who is the best listener?

_____

Who is the best problem-solver?

_____

Who makes the best coffee (or cookies)?

_____

▸ *Be hopeful.* Positivity and hope can be reinforced throughout our lives. Take cues from children and children's books such as Maya Angelou's remarkable poem and book *Life Doesn't Frighten Me* (2018). An optimistic outlook fosters the expectation that good things will happen in your life, and if bad things happen, you can handle it.

What or who gives you hope?

▸ *Express gratitude.* Who do you need to thank in your life? Practicing gratitude and expressing appreciation serve both the giver and the receiver.

Write a thank-you note to someone who gave you a meaningful gift, no matter how small, or how long ago.

Write to a colleague and express your gratitude for their help or presence during a challenging time.

Write a note of gratitude without using the word "thank."

(continued)

For more about resilience, see the following websites:

Personal Strategies for Engaging and Building Your Resilience from
the University of California, San Francisco: https://psychiatry
.ucsf.edu/copingresources/videos
Building Your Resilience from the American Psychological Association: https://www.apa.org/topics/resilience
Resilience Examples: What Key Skills Make You Resilient? from Positive Psychology: https://positivepsychology.com/resilience-skills

We've included some strategies to build your resilience, both personally and collectively. We are all relational beings; our interdependence
on each other is indispensable. Perhaps you are ready for something
more; maybe you've seen enough crisis, trauma, or overwhelming stress
to last a lifetime. Maybe you've seen it alone, or in your family, or with
your colleagues.

Crises are often followed by lessons learned. New knowledge and
skills are recruited into service when needed in the future. It is no acci-
dent that one of the first questions a therapist asks a new client is, "Have
you ever experienced anything like this before?" We do learn, even in
the most painful situations. Sometimes those previous lessons don't
work in new, more intense circumstances. Then it's time for reinforce-
ments. We will specifically focus on key questions that we've heard
many times in our practices: How do I know when I need professional
help? What does it look like, and where do I find it? Let's take a look at
this new terrain.

TAKING THE FIRST STEP

•

Many nurses have told us they've experienced traumatic stressors in
their practice; some even suspected they might have PTSD. They want
to get rid of those uncomfortable feelings, sleep better, and not be on
high alert all the time. We'd like to share a few thoughts on healing after
trauma.

The diagnosis of PTSD is based on the prerequisite of a traumatic event. Although most people in all walks of life are exposed to such events, the lifetime prevalence of PTSD in the United States is 6.7%, 7.2% in Australia, and 9.2% in Canada. For individuals who have been exposed to combat or traumatic events in humanitarian settings, rates of PTSD and anxiety may reach a prevalence of 30% to 40%. It is no surprise that nurses must endure many traumatic situations. Context is everything when it comes to trauma, and nurses are thrust into situations where they witness another person's most tragic moment—catastrophic illness, accidents, death, disaster, high-tech sensory overload, and desperate attempts at survival.

Since the fall of 2019, we have learned much more about trauma and PTSD symptoms among health care workers. In one study of nursing home workers in Italy, participants reported moderate to severe symptoms of anxiety (22%) and PTSD (43%) (Riello et al., 2020). The incidence of PTSD in nurses in China who were exposed to COVID-19 was 16.83% (Wang et al., 2020). In a recent analysis of PTSD symptoms in health care workers from three coronavirus outbreaks, the researchers reviewed 19 studies on the SARS 2003 outbreak, two on the MERS 2012 outbreak, and three on the COVID-19 outbreak (Carmassi et al., 2020). They found that risk and resilience factors included exposure level, position or role, years of experience, social and work support, organization, quarantine, age, gender, marital status, and coping styles. The authors suggested that these factors will provide critical information for planning timely and effective intervention strategies, focusing on enhancing resilience, and reducing adverse mental health outcomes among health care workers facing the current COVID-19 pandemic.

After years of research on prevention and treatment of PTSD, there is scientific certainty of effective treatment options. Bisson and Olff (2021) reviewed current evidence on prevention and treatment approaches, and found that nonpharmacological treatments were the most effective. These included cognitive behavioral therapy with a trauma focus (CBT-TF), cognitive processing therapy (CPT), cognitive therapy (CT), eye movement desensitization and reprocessing (EMDR), and prolonged exposure (PE). Pharmacological interventions may have their place for veterans of combat, but cognitive therapies are a first line of treatment for many. Approximately 50% to 60%

of individuals with PTSD recover within two years or less; a minority, specifically combat veterans, develop PTSD that becomes chronic (International Society for Traumatic Stress Studies Trauma and Public Health Task Force, 2015). It's important to note, however, that posttraumatic growth can be a viable and powerful outcome of trauma exposure (Hamam et al., 2021).

> *"Someone who has experienced trauma also has gifts to offer all of us—in their depth, their knowledge of our universal vulnerability, and their experience of the power of compassion."*
> *—Sharon Salzberg, Insight Meditation Society*

If you are concerned that you may be struggling with PTSD symptoms and it is interfering with your home or work life, or if others have expressed concern about you, it is time for an assessment. The Resources section of this book lists links to a number of global resources, hotlines, and organizations to answer your questions. We will also continue to add to these resources on our website.

Remember, you are not alone.

IN THEIR OWN WORDS
_____

> *"As a nurse, I have always been the caregiver and nurturer. Needing help for myself just did not fit with my self-image."*

It was a very bad year. I started January 2020 with a heightened anxiety level and continual state of distress related to the utter political turmoil percolating in our country over the previous year. What was happening to my country? What was happening within my own family and circle of friends? The deep divides disturbed me. The pandemic was taking hold of our lives. I was lucky enough to score a vaccine appointment for the end of that month. February rolled around and brought with it a serious and upsetting diagnosis for my husband, myelodysplastic syndrome. No wonder he was always so weak and falling down. In March, the class I was teaching in community nursing went completely online, and with it came unexpected challenges to design simulated "clinical experiences" for the students. But April was by far the worst. My father died alone in his nursing home after weeks of being without any family visits or communication with his children. Is it no wonder I slipped into a full depression for the first time in my life?

My depression took hold of me. My thoughts became cloudy, and I had a hard time concentrating. For the first time in my life, I could not read. I had no ability to focus. I was short-tempered. I made no attempt to keep in contact with my best friends, both of whom have been in my life for over 50 years. At the end of June, I retired from a 48-year career in nursing and nursing education—I no longer had the daily, engaging contact with students, faculty, and administration. I could not sleep. I woke up feeling hungover with exhaustion. I did not keep to a routine. I did very little beyond the absolute necessities of daily functions.

And then one sleepless night, it happened. Awake in my bed with my anxiety pulsing, I had my first thought of what it would be like to end my misery and cease to live. I immediately felt a bit of relief. I drifted off to sleep with my first "positive" thought in months.

Thoughts.

No one knows my feelings. And no one cares to know. No one ever asks.

Is life worth living?

I do not know.

The next day I tried to block out what I felt the night before. The pandemic was getting worse every day, so who was I to dwell on my own problems when so many other people were experiencing pain and loss? Former students of mine kept me abreast of their exhaustion of working in ICUs and EDs; one even became very ill with COVID-19 himself. Thoughts about my father's death persisted, and I began to believe that the pandemic did indeed play a part in his death. Even though we were told he died peacefully in his sleep, I felt that we had either been lied to or that his loneliness and lack of social contact with us, imposed by the guidelines set by the pandemic (confined to his room), contributed to his death.

Sometimes there is someone there.

But loneliness still grasps you in its cruel grip and squeezes out bitterness that flows over any promise of happiness.

Loneliness—the feeling of never really being understood.

Never really being valued by those that are right there with you.

Living in a solitary world where only you know your thoughts, your feelings, your worries, your dreams.

I slipped deeper and deeper into pain. One night I lay awake and fantasized about how I might actually end my life. I would want no mess for my husband to discover or my children to witness. I began to plan it out. Yes. I knew how I would "do it," an overdose of sleeping pills, but I did not have the resources. The thought of lying down and never having to get up again was very appealing to me. It gave me a false sense of control.

At some point I scared myself. I was having suicidal thoughts. Me. A nurse. A stable person. The strong one. The helper. The counselor. The advisor. Me. Suicidal thoughts. I was too ashamed and disturbed to confide this secret. It would be an admission of defeat and evidence of my weakness. Other people were truly suffering, and the pandemic was not getting any better, so my secret suffering should not matter by comparison. I felt unworthy of help.

I would not burden my husband by confiding in him because he was having his own challenges dealing with his new illness, and I think he felt that his mortality was slapping him in the face. So silent I would be. And lonely with my thoughts. So lonely. Until I could no longer be silent.

Lonely. Loneliness.

How misunderstood this feeling can be.

It is not being alone.

I started crying and could not stop. I had dark circles under my eyes and looked terrible. On a whim, I snapped a picture of myself and sent it to my adult children. Initially, they did not realize the gravity of my state of mind, but my daughter seemed so understanding that I began to tell her of my suicidal thoughts. She insisted that I tell my primary physician when I went in for my next regular visit that week. She was relentless.

A few days later, meekly and with no confidence, I told my primary care provider about my dark thoughts. She kicked into action. She was wonderful. She discussed a plan with me, and it was set up within an hour. I joined an online support group with my own personal coach. I had "work" to do, and I embraced it. I had an appointment to see a psychiatrist. Those steps alone brought me relief. It still took months to "get back" to my old self, but I did it. By December 2020, I felt nearly normal.

Why is it that I could not ask for help? As a nurse, I have always been the caregiver and nurturer. Needing help for myself just did not fit with my self-image. So, I rejected what I knew to be the most prudent course of action and instead chose a type of denial or delay. Nurses—we are people, too. With feelings and limits. Sometimes fragile, and always human. It was a very hard lesson to learn. It was a very hard year.

January 2020: Mary Jo Spicer Bugel, PhD, RN, NJ-CSN, Professor Emerita, Rutgers School of Nursing, Newark, New Jersey, United States

BEGINNING
•

Perhaps you've faced a crisis or overwhelming stress and, like the nurse storyteller above, you feel all alone. Or perhaps there is a family crisis, an illness, or death of a family member. You're doing okay. Just okay. Maybe you've been thinking that there might be something more you can do. Perhaps you want to shore up your resources if you're going through a personal or work crisis, or you hope to learn more about yourself when a nagging situation seems to require more attention. Perhaps you are still struggling with the challenging and sometimes terrifying work you've seen in your practice.

How do you know if your coping skills and strategies don't seem to be doing enough? When faced with a crisis, most of us use skills that we never knew we had, rising to the occasion and dealing with the situation as best we can. Trauma and loss are probably the most life-altering events you will face, often rendering you helpless or out of control. Relationships are stressed, sleep is impossible, and anxiety can leave you exhausted. While there are actions you can take to heal and promote your well-being, they may not be enough.

For most of us, it takes time to take the plunge and ask for assistance when it comes to our own mental health. Most health care providers have an easier time caring for others than asking for help. Often people begin to think about "talking to someone" well before they take the step of asking for a referral or making that first phone call. You may have already thought about trying counseling or psychotherapy, but for one reason or another, it just didn't happen. You're not questioning the value of counseling in general, but you're not sure it's right for you. You know that talking to an impartial person could be useful, especially if you feel you are burdening your friends with the dramas in your life. Perhaps an objective professional could help you see more clearly the issues preventing you from achieving your maximum well-being.

How do you know when it's time to take action and go to the next step? And once you determine that the time is right, how do you go about finding the right professional? You want someone who is a good fit for you, a good teammate, a competent trail guide. There are many resources that will make the choice easier for you. Let's take a look at a plan of action.

A PLAN OF ACTION

•

We've all read or heard media stories about nurses working on the front lines. Articles, news broadcasts, and documentaries show how these professionals work with the highest stress and greatest risk in the most frightening and fastest-paced environments. Couple those stories with images of nurses in full protective gear surrounded by life-saving equipment, and you may think that you haven't earned the title of frontline nurse because you are not working in those high-acuity settings. In fact, we've heard many nurses say that they feel guilty when anyone thanks them for their work, "After all, I only work in labor and delivery." There is much more to the title of frontline nurse than the media have us believe. Perhaps a new hashtag would say it best: #IAmTheFrontLine.

The Brookings Institute defines frontline workers as employees within essential industries (Tomer and Kane, 2020). These employees must physically show up for work while facing a variety of health risks in their workplaces, risks that include physical proximity to individuals and colleagues who may be exposed to viruses and other potentially hazardous conditions. We contend that the risks, physical and psychological, extend far beyond close physical proximity. Here are a few frontline nurses: the school nurse who has taken on hours of overtime, often unpaid, to follow up on symptomatic students and provide contact tracing; the newborn nursery staff who didn't know the COVID status of their patients and families, only to find out 24 hours later that the patient took antipyretics to hide COVID symptoms; and the hospice nurse who watched her patients die of loneliness, saw them not being touched, in the final stages of cancer or dementia, without their families.

You are all on the front line and have been exposed to any number of perilous situations. Not better or worse, but different. The underlying thread of uncertainty weaves through all practice settings. You are all entitled to seek and find care to preserve your mental health.

It's not too late.

You are not alone.

IN THEIR OWN WORDS

What brings you here today?

Everything—it hasn't stopped, there is no time to recoup. Regular patients are so much sicker and dying. It is nonstop—I can't do this ... my usual coping is not working. I don't see light at the end of the tunnel. Usually I can see the end of 12-hour shift, but tomorrow I have to get up and do the same thing. Terrible!

Spring 2020: Anonymous, Staff Nurse, Emergency Department, Western New York, United States

THE ACTION PLAN
•

Step 1: Psychoeducation

Learn as much as you can about how we human beings respond to stress, trauma, and loss. This book, while not all inclusive, is a good introduction. The Resources section contains many suggestions that may be helpful. We suggest two articles as a starting point: "Why Everyone Needs a Therapist," by Jeff Hayward (2020), and "The Five Myths of Self-Compassion," by Kristin Neff (2015). The international periodical *Psychology Today* and its website have a comprehensive glossary of terminology relevant to mental health practices.

Step 2: Awareness

*"I attended an online Zoom support group—for nurses.
I joined the call, but all I could do was cry. I related to all
that everyone said. Was I ready to share my feelings?
When are we ever really ready?"*

As we've mentioned previously, health care professionals, especially nurses, are hesitant to seek mental health resources and care. We often hear nurses ask, "What is wrong with me that I cannot cope with my work or my life?" They tell us that they are ashamed or embarrassed, often comparing themselves to their colleagues, quite certain that they are the only one struggling. We've often heard nurses acknowledge that they are going through a difficult time, but they will "wait until this is over."

The nursing profession and society in general have socialized nurses into thinking that they can do this important work without any consequences. For years, mental health professionals working with veterans and victims of sexual violence struggled with the trauma and stress of their clients. They didn't experience the trauma, but they heard their clients talk about their painful realities. As a result, mental health clinicians began to develop strategies to address secondary and vicarious trauma. Caring for another human being has consequences.

In the beginning of the pandemic, nurses just tried to survive and get through long shifts and overtime. Work, eat, sleep, and then repeat. There was no time to talk to someone about the stress of the moment. Six months later, when the first wave subsided, many nurses began to seek help.

Work-related stressors are not the only issues bombarding nurses. Dealing with families, children, parents, and siblings can take a toll. The work-life balance shifts and becomes unstable. It takes time and strategies to talk to family and right the ship. And you can't ignore your own personal history. Be aware of your own life experiences; they may need tending to again. Nurses may resist treatment, as they may be embarrassed or ashamed to seek help.

Remember, waiting is not usually a successful approach.

Step 3: Self-Assessment

"I've been experiencing low moods, mood swings, on-and-off decreased appetite since the first wave started. I don't have any prior history of mental health disorders. For a while, I didn't know what was wrong with me. My primary doc didn't screen for depression and minimized my concern about COVID-19 patients. She said to me, 'They don't all die.' Really, that's not what I'm seeing. One night another nurse had six patients. I was assigned eight. I couldn't do it. I had to ask for help. Am I being unfair? Am I being a baby?"

How do we recognize our own distress? Sometimes we cannot see what is so obvious to our partners, family, friends, and colleagues. There may be times that you are more concerned about your partner, coworker, or child. Nurses may not acknowledge the need for their own mental health care, but they certainly can recognize it in someone else. It's only human to talk ourselves out of getting help, perhaps assuming that the dark time will pass or get better. But maybe things will get worse.

Sometimes we have a friend or colleague who is such a great listener that we might think we don't need a professional resource. Friends and relatives are great supports, but if you find your friends becoming frustrated or too busy to listen, then it is time to talk to someone professionally. Friends try to help as much as they can, sometimes getting in over their heads. People who care about us usually find it difficult to admit they can no longer help us sort out our problems. Listen for cues. If you find yourself talking to the same person each morning for an hour, it could be time to find a professional resource.

And if you are one of those really good listeners and worried about a friend or colleague, take the advice Kathryn Mannix gives in her book *Listen*, and tell your friend, "I want to help you deal with this. Shall we look for someone who can give us expert advice?"

There are special considerations that merit talking with a professional, such as previous counseling or treatment, prior losses, a divorce, or earlier traumatic events. This is not to say your current distress is because of these past difficulties; rather, it is helpful to understand background experiences that might make you more vulnerable to new stressors. Approaches that were successful in the past may be useful going forward.

Talking with others in similar situations can be reassuring. This is especially valuable for nurses and other health care professionals. The pandemic has stretched many to the breaking point. As one nurse so clearly described, "My bucket is full; one more drop and it all spills over." We can learn from each other. You may even consider community support groups. Reach out to others, and let people reach out to you. You may have suggested professional help to those you care about in your own life, and their words may sound similar to the guidance you gave to them. Sometimes we need to be pushed to follow our own advice.

> *"In the past three years I've had a string of deaths—*
> *my grandpa, my grandmother, my cousin's wife. She was only*
> *35, my age, and died of metastatic cancer. I had a lot of trouble*
> *with grief, and I think I just put it away. My mother died from*
> *breast cancer when I was in high school, so many of my patients*
> *reminded me of that time. I had COVID over a year ago;*
> *I still don't have my complete sense of smell. I'm a big foodie.*
> *My friend thought she was making a joke and said, 'Wow,*
> *that's ironic, you of all people can't smell food!'*
> *It wasn't funny."*

Step 4: Evaluating and Accessing Services

Now it's time to dig in and do the research. You've made the decision to find a mental health provider, but how do you determine who will be the best fit for you? The Resources section and our companion website contain links to many international resources. Some are without charge or at minimal cost.

In the United States, numerous organizations and programs introduce nurses to mental health support through online groups and pro bono counseling services that prioritize health care providers. In New Jersey, The New Jersey Nursing Emotional Well-Being Institute and Schwartz Rounds offered a unique forum for convening and supporting professional nurses who are coping with the intense stress and increased demands of providing care during and after the pandemic. The twice-monthly virtual rounds provide support and opportunities to connect with one another. Virtual Schwartz Rounds sessions have become a welcomed source of support and respite for more than 1,700 nurses since December 2020.

The Emotional PPE Project began in the United States at the beginning of the pandemic. The online directory is for any health care provider affected by the COVID-19 crisis. Volunteer licensed mental health practitioners can be identified by state. Each of these experienced therapists pledges to provide free sessions. No insurance. No cost. Just a trained professional to talk to.

Mind.org in the United Kingdom provides advice and support to empower anyone experiencing a mental health problem. They also campaign to improve services, raise awareness, and promote understanding. Also in the United Kingdom is the Samaritans 24-hour / 7-days-a-week hotline for those who are struggling themselves, or for others worried about a friend or family member.

The Health Services of Ireland (HSE) provides all of Ireland's public health services in hospitals and communities across the country. Their employee assistance programs serve health care providers at no cost. Also available in Ireland is a listing of ecotherapy options through Nature Therapy Ireland.

As you begin the search for help, consider the questions below. Keep track of names, addresses, and key information.

Is mental health care free of charge in your state or country?
Do you have mental health insurance coverage?
Is there a limit on the number of sessions you can attend?
Is there a co-pay or fee that you must pay for the sessions?
Is there a directory of in-network and/or out-of-network
    providers?

If you do not have insurance, consider a professional who takes sliding scale payments, a community program, a faith-based program, or a university-based clinic. Perhaps one of the most comprehensive directories online is the *Psychology Today* website. The "Find a Therapist" tab lists an international directory with counselors, therapists, online services, and support groups in 14 countries. It can give you a good sense of the mental health programs and professionals available in your community. You can search for a therapist/counselor or online services by location, fees, insurance plans accepted, gender, and type of therapy. You can directly contact the professional by phone or by email through the website. In addition, the website provides articles that explore the process of finding a therapist, as well as a glossary of terms describing different types of therapy or counseling, and explanations of the credentials and licensures listed after the mental health professional's names. Areas of expertise and issues addressed include anxiety, depression, trauma, or grief; types of patients seen (adults, adolescents, families, LGBTQ, health professionals); and any additional preparation, certifications, and educational background. The therapist's personal statement allows you to learn more, and if they have a website, it is worth exploring as well.

Another directory in the United States is offered by the New Jersey Society of Psychiatric Advanced Practice Nurses. Founded in 1972, it is the first professional nursing body in the country to certify clinical nurse specialists in psychiatric nursing. Today, the society includes psychiatric advanced practice nurses: both psychiatric nurse practitioners and clinical nurse specialists in advanced practice nursing. The directory allows you to search for clinicians by location and areas of expertise, and you can contact them through the website.

Here are a few other questions you might want to consider:

Is this professional taking new clients?

What is their approach to counseling/therapy?

Do they prescribe medication? Most, if not all, therapists work with other mental health professionals who can prescribe medication and would refer you if there is a need.

To learn even more about potential counselors, check LinkedIn, your insurance directory, and professional organization websites. Consider contacting two or three professionals, develop a list of questions or points you want to ask, and identify your goals and what you are hoping to achieve.

Now, the hard part.

Step 5: Reaching Out

Gather contact information for the counselor or therapist. Most professionals can be reached by phone or email. Connect with them in the way you feel most comfortable. If you don't hear back from them in 48 hours, reach out again. If there is a waiting list, contact one or two additional professionals.

Give yourself time to decide who you would like to see; you don't have to make the decision right then and there on the phone. If you are in *urgent need* of mental health services, however, reach out to your primary care provider for a referral, or call 911 or an emergency hotline in your area. In the United States, if you or someone you know is suicidal or in emotional distress, you can call the new national 988 Suicide and Crisis Lifeline. It links to a suicide prevention network of over 200 crisis centers that provide 24-hour service, 7 days a week, through a toll-free hotline with the number 9-8-8. You can also chat with a trained crisis worker who is available 24 hours a day, 7 days a week. There are many international hotlines, such as the Heroes Aid website in Ireland, which also offers a 24-7 hotline in addition to other resources for health care providers. The Resources section lists additional hotlines, phone apps, and other resources for mental health needs, both immediate and long term.

Step 6: Telling a Friend or Colleague

Talk to your colleagues and friends. You are not alone.

Recognize that you can heal. You are not alone.

Find resources, share them with a colleague, and explore online groups and apps.

Practice self-compassion (nurturing and fierce), and read Kristin Neff's work.

A FEW FINAL THOUGHTS
◆

Recognize and acknowledge the stressor or crisis in your life and how it has affected you.

Accept the support of others; they would want your friendship and caring during their time of need. This is the first commandment of self-compassion.

Try to be flexible about demands on yourself; difficult times call for modifying your standards and commitments.

When approaching the problem at hand, break it down into small manageable parts, and take each step as it comes.

Don't expect too much of yourself at times of crisis. Nonessentials can be delayed.

Try to remain hopeful and patient; working one's way out of crisis and grieving takes time.

Think about these words from Sonya Jakubec, Canadian community mental health nurse and researcher: "We must reorient and relocate stress to address it in a more complete way. It is not only about the individual. Mental health does not exist simply in our brains ... but in our bodies, our communities and contexts."

◆

Your journey to well-being awaits you.

REFERENCES

American Psychiatric Association. (2013). *Diagnostic and Statistical Manual of Mental Disorders*, 5th ed. Arlington, VA: American Psychiatric Association.

Angelou, M., Basquiat, J. M., & Boyers, S. J. (2018). *Life Doesn't Frighten Me*. New York: Harry N. Abrams.

Azoulay, E., Cariou, A., Bruneel, F., Demoule, A., Kouatchet, A., et al. (2020). Symptoms of anxiety, depression, and peritraumatic dissociation in critical care clinicians managing patients with COVID-19: a cross-sectional study. *American Journal of Respiratory and Critical Care Medicine* 202(10): 1388–98.

Ball, S. (2021). France's "burnout" clinic: exhausted health workers seek respite from COVID front line. France 24 News, February 4, 2021. https://www .france24.com/en/video/20210402-france-s-burnout-clinic-exhausted -health-workers-seek-respite-from-covid-front-line

Bender, A., Berg, K. A., Miller, E. K., Evans, K. E., & Holmes, M. R. (2021). "Making sure we are all okay": healthcare workers' strategies for emotional connectedness during the COVID-19 pandemic. *Clinical Social Work Journal* 49(4): 445–55. https://doi.org/10.1007/s10615-020-00781-w

Bisson, J. I., & Olff, M. (2021). Prevention and treatment of PTSD: the current evidence base. *European Journal of Psychotraumatology* 12(1): 1824381. https:// doi.org/10.1080/20008198.2020.1824381

Carmassi, C., Foghi, C., Dell'Oste, V., Cordone, A., Bertelloni, A. A., Bui, E., & Dell'Osso, L. (2020). PTSD symptoms in healthcare workers facing the three coronavirus outbreaks: what can we expect after the COVID-19 pandemic. *Psychiatry Research* 292: 113312. https://doi.org/10.1016/j.psychres .2020.113312

DeSalvo, L. 2000. *Writing as a Way of Healing*. Boston: Beacon Press.

Hamam, A. A., Milo, S., Mor, I., Shaked, E., Eliav, A. S., & Lahav, Y. (2021). Peritraumatic reactions during the COVID-19 pandemic—the contribution of posttraumatic growth attributed to prior trauma. *Journal of Psychiatric Research* 132: 23–31.

Haslam, C., Jetten, J., Cruwys, T., Dingle, G. A., & Haslam, S. A. (2018). *The New Psychology of Health: Unlocking the Social Cure*. New York: Routledge.

Hayward, J. (2020). Why everyone needs a therapist. Medium, June 26, 2020. https://medium.com/@jeffhaywardwriting/why-everyone-needs-a -therapist-3704c7649f21

Hirschberger, G. (2018). Collective trauma and the social construction of meaning. *Frontiers in Psychology* 9: 1441.

Iacoviello, B. M., & Charney, D. S. (2020). Cognitive and behavioral components of resilience to stress. In: Chen, A., ed. *Stress Resilience*. San Diego, CA: Academic Press, 23–31.

International Council of Nurses. (2021a). *The COVID-19 Effect: World's Nurses Facing Mass Trauma, an Immediate Danger to the Profession and Future of Our Health Systems*. Geneva: International Council of Nurses.

International Council of Nurses. (2021b). ICN says 115,000 healthcare worker deaths from COVID-19 exposes collective failure of leaders to protect global workforce. October 21 2021, https://www.icn.ch/news/icn-says -115000-healthcare-worker-deaths-covid-19-exposes-collective-failure -leaders-protect

International Society for Traumatic Stress Studies Trauma and Public Health Task Force. (2015). *A Public Health Approach to Trauma: Implications for Science, Practice, Policy, and the Role of ISTSS*. Chicago: International Society of Traumatic Stress Studies. https://istss.org/getattachment/Education-Research /White-Papers/A-Public-Health-Approach-to-Trauma/Trauma-and-PH -Task-Force-Report.pdf.aspx

Mannix, K. (2021). *Listen: How to Find the Words for Tender Conversations*. London: William Collins.

McGaugh, J. L. (2004). The amygdala modulates the consolidation of memories of emotionally arousing experiences. *Annual Review of Neuroscience* 27: 1–28.

Neff, K. (2015). The five myths of self-compassion. *Psychotherapy Networker* 39(5): https://greatergood.berkeley.edu/article/item/the_five_myths_of _self_compassion

Ordem dos Enfermeiros. (2021). Cerca de 10% de Enfermeiros infetados com COVID-19. July 9, 2021, https://www.ordemenfermeiros.pt/noticias /conteudos/cerca-de-10-de-enfermeiros-infetados-com-covid-19/

Ordre National des Infirmiers. (2022). COVID-19: paroles d'infirmiers. Accessed September 12, 2022. https://www.ordre-infirmiers.fr/actualites-presse /actualite-covid-19/covid19-paroles-dinfirmiers.html

Pennebaker, J. W., & Smyth, J. M. (2016). *Opening Up by Writing It Down*. New York: Guilford Press.

Riello, M., Purgato, M., Bove, C., MacTaggart, D., & Rusconi, E. (2020) Prevalence of post-traumatic symptomatology and anxiety among residential nursing and care home workers following the first COVID-19 outbreak in northern Italy. *Royal Society Open Science* 7: 200880. http://dx.doi.org/10.1098/rsos.200880

Roozendaal, B., & McGaugh, J. L. (2011). Memory modulation. *Behavioral Neuroscience* 125(6): 797–824.

Ryff, C. D. (2014). Psychological well-being revisited: advances in the science and practice of eudaimonia. *Psychotherapy and Psychosomatics* 83(1): 10–28.

Ryff, C. D., & Singer, B. (2008). The integrative science of human resilience. In: *Interdisciplinary Research: Case Studies from Health and Social Science: Case Studies from Health and Social Science*. Oxford: Oxford University Press, 198–227.

Saul, J. (2013). *Collective Trauma, Collective Healing: Promoting Community Resilience in the Aftermath of Disaster*. New York: Routledge.

Tedeschi, R. G., Shakespeare-Finch, J., Taku, K., & Calhoun, L. G. (2018). *Posttraumatic Growth: Theory, Research, and Applications*. New York: Routledge.

Tomer, A., & Kane, J. W. (2020). *To Protect Frontline Workers during and after COVID-19, We Must Define Who They Are*. Washington, DC: Brookings Institution. https://www.brookings.edu/research/to-protect-frontline-workers-during-and-after-covid-19-we-must-define-who-they-are/

van der Kolk, B. A. (2015). *The Body Keeps the Score: Brain, Mind, and Body in the Healing of Trauma*. London: Penguin Books.

Walsh, F. (2016). *Strengthening Family Resilience*, 3rd ed. New York: Guilford Press.

Walsh, F. (2020). Loss and resilience in the time of COVID-19: meaning making, hope, and transcendence. *Family Process* 59(3): 898–911.

Wang, Y. X., Guo, H. T., Du, X. W., Song, W., Lu, C., & Hao, W. N. (2020). Factors associated with post-traumatic stress disorder of nurses exposed to corona virus disease 2019 in China. *Medicine* 99(26): e20965.

World Health Organization. (1986). *Ottawa Charter for Health Promotion, 1986*. No. WHO/EURO: 1986-4044-43803-61677. Geneva: World Health Organization Regional Office for Europe. https://apps.who.int/iris/bitstream/handle/10665/349652/WHO-EURO-1986–4044-43803–61677-eng.pdf?sequence=1

World Health Organization. (2013). *Health 2020: A European Policy Framework and Strategy for the 21st Century*. Geneva: World Health Organization Regional Office for Europe. https://apps.who.int/iris/handle/10665/326386

World Health Organization. (2021). Director-general's opening remarks at the World Health Assembly. May 24, 2021. https://www.who.int/director-general/speeches/detail/director-general-s-opening-remarks-at-the-world-health-assembly---24-may-2021

Wu, C. J., & Oprescu, F. I. (2021). Applying the Ottawa Charter to guide resilience-building programs for health care organizations. *Nursing and Health Sciences* 23(3): 665–69.

Wu, G., Feder, A., Cohen, H., Kim, J. J., Calderon, S., Charney, D. S., & Mathé, A. A. (2013). Understanding resilience. *Frontiers in Behavioral Neuroscience* 7(10). https://doi.org/10.3389/fnbeh.2013.00010

Afterword

We began writing this book more than two years ago. It has been a lab-
yrinthine journey through multiple seasons—winters of uncertainty,
springtimes of hope, restorative summers, and autumns of hesitant
beginnings.

In the natural world, each season of a tree has its purpose. Perhaps
we can view nursing in the same way—there are gifts we receive and
gifts we give with each season, much like the protective and resilient
Rowan tree.

Guardian, gate-keeper, path-protector,
you ward against the threat of evil
at the entrance to this house.

Stream-sentinel, rock-bound,
above a clefted torrent,
your tough roots purify the water.

In the glens, your red fruits
beckon blackbirds, thrushes,
to their astringent feast.

The barren seek your boughs
to bed beneath, assured conception
and a safe carriage.

Beltane sheep jump through rowan hoops,
and cattle rest, murrain-free,
with tail-tied twigs, in protected byres.

Your power, enchantress, is in your leafy shield;
a berried blessing, sanguine, steadfast.
Stand so for us, for all your green hands shade.

Colin Will, "Robin's Rowan," from *Recycled Cards*, 2011, Calder Wood Press, UK.
Reprinted with permission.

Acknowledgments

With Gratitude

The dark days of the COVID-19 pandemic were a relentless and jarring backdrop for this book. During the day, we worked with nurses and the general public; at night, we collected their stories, wrote, and dug into the research. Terrifying headlines and confusing public health warnings were our constant companions. If not for the nurses and colleagues who generously shared their experiences and support, it would have been an almost unthinkable task. We were led by nurses. They inspired, comforted, and created.

To Our Brilliant Team

There are so many people who have helped this book become a reality. We want to extend our deepest appreciation to all of you for your guidance and your friendship. Meghan Rabbitt took a first look and urged us to pilot an e-book for nurses. Our development editor and publishing guru, Allan Graubard, believed in our book from the very beginning and provided us with countless hours of support, suggestions, and guidance. Allan, we could not have done this without you. Many thanks go to our editor, Joe Rusko, for his guidance and critical recommendation to include nurses from across the globe—and of course for his good humor. Joe, we are so glad we've found a home at Johns Hopkins University Press. Our deepest gratitude to the team who brought our manuscript through the many stages of refinement: Mojie Crigler, Juliana McCarthy, Ashleigh McKown, and Jane Medrano. Not only did your questions and suggestions give us guidance, but they were also the signposts we needed to get to the finish line.

Thanks to Johnine Byrne, who helped us "see our words" with clarity and style, and to Susan Etu, who gave us important advice on capturing the eyes and ears of readers. In the midst of a new doctoral program, Kimberley Reda found time to help us discover and organize hundreds of resources.

We have only the highest praise for Carol Calkins, a dear friend and editing wizard who helped shape and reshape paragraphs, and made our sentences sing with inspiration and creativity. Not content with comments on paper or screen, Carol talked us through choices of words and phrases, listening to our voices for just the right message for our audience. To her we give our heartfelt gratitude.

To the many nurses, friends, and colleagues who talked with us and read our pilot e-book, thank you for giving us important feedback and suggestions for what became the pages in front of you: Susan Airey, Maureen Baker, Susan Barletta, Mary Jo Bugel, Cassandra Caggiano, Robin Cogan, Michelle Doyle, Suzanne Drake, Milagros Elia, Matt Farrell, Ed Lord, Sue Galina, Alison Glorioso, Saipriya Iyer, Tracy Jaworski-Lucas, Cathy McKeon, Nancy Chiocchi McMorrow, Michelle Neier, Jennifer Norton, Paige Panzer, Peg Pipchick, Danielle Rabbitt, Ellen Shave, Janice Smith, and Barbara Uihlein.

From the outset, our goal was to ensure that this book would meet the needs of nurses in the global community. We committed to being as inclusive as possible, and we asked these trailblazers to review our chapters and identify any blind spots or oversights. They did not disappoint.

We begin with profound thanks to Milagros Elia, who although based in the northeastern United States connected us to colleagues across oceans and miles. Spanning time zones, they talked with us, shared their stories, and reached out to their colleagues. Ed Lord and Suzi Tarrant from Wales opened our eyes to the value of nature as a healing instrument; Canadian Sonya Jakubec shared her glorious photos and a sense of how the interconnection of supportive environments influences well-being. In Great Britain, Hannah Grace Deller's incredible photographs served to raise the voices and images of UK nurses; Sarah Airriess connected us to Aileen Walsh, an expert on moral distress, who then introduced us to Debbie Critoph and her work on grief and loss during the pandemic. We met Lotta Carlson and Margaretha Jenholt Nobris from Sweden through longtime colleague Mary Jo Bugel. Vanessa Monteiro gave us her insightful observations about how Portuguese nurses survived the pandemic. Isabel Centeno wrote heartfelt and honest words about nurses in Mexico needing strategies to protect their well-being. Anna Fuhrmann, a pediatric nurse who was a leader of the Nurses Climate Challenge across Europe, introduced us to Neha Tawiri, a climate activist and passionate chest surgery nurse from India; also to Federica Pirro, a nurse climate champion who has worked in both Dublin, Ireland, and Turin, Italy, and shows us in her story that birthing a second baby can go hand in hand with delivering a groundbreaking climate change project.

Clodagh Connaughton launched Nurse A Tree (NAT) in Ireland with the goal of planting a tree for every nurse. She listened to our musings on the rowan tree, promptly researched more on this spiritual tower of strength in nature, and took beautiful photographs to further inspire us. Clodagh thought our book could be an amulet for nurses: to protect and ground us, to help avoid burnout.

To Lynette Goldtooth, our profound thanks for sharing your nursing journey as a Native American, the impact of COVID on the Navajo Nation in Arizona, and how you continue to persevere. You are an inspiration to all of us.

Like Karen Carroll, Katelyn McNair writes and speaks about #MeToo and the importance of speaking out for survivors of sexual violence—she understands the essence of activism. Kate, thank you for allowing us to share the words we wrote together several years ago.

We are so appreciative to Carole Geithner for her wonderful contributions. As a therapist and writer, she provided numerous writing resources for nurses. She understands completely how nursing, the humanities, and the arts are inextricably linked.

To Donna's colleagues at Nurses for America—the "Core"—Erin Hartnett, Eileen Gordon, Catherine Dodd, Carol Roe, Rosanne Farrell, and Sherry Pomeroy: Thank you for inspiring us with your passionate acts of courage and commitment. Congresswoman Lauren Underwood, we are in awe of your moving words. Your message will be heard loud and clear. We are honored to share your story in our book.

We are thankful for the wisdom of Robin Cogan, Jenny Gormley, and Kathy Hassey. They fiercely campaigned on behalf of school nurses, who were also on the front lines and needed to be heard.

We are so grateful to those who led the way in the field of psychological well-being and allowed us to share their groundbreaking work with the readers of our book: Tara Brach, Ethan Green, Carol Henderson, Dina Kaplan, Kirstin Neff, Carol Ryff, Dzung Vo, and Andrew Weil. To the artists, writers, poets, and singer-songwriters who showed us that creating may be the best therapy of all—Tara Beier, MK Czerwiec, DaLa, Cortney Davis, Hanna Grace Deller, Diane Carlson Evans, Kim Henry, Ruth Moody, and Megan Palmer—we are in awe of your gifts.

We offer our profound gratitude to two nursing leaders and scholars, Dr. Anne Hofmeyer and Dr. Sue Salmond, for their generous forewords that tell the story of nursing during a chaotic time from their personal and professional perspectives.

And, finally, to the many nurses who talked to us or wrote their stories, know that you were not only captivating storytellers, but also generous listeners. You graced us with your presence, inspired us, and gave us sustenance for bringing this book to life. We do not have adequate words to tell you how much we appreciate you: Alison Glorioso, whose image and powerful letter on Facebook triggered a sense of urgency unlike anything we've felt before; and Fredrick Apostadero, Kristen Bannister, Donna Barry, Mary Jo Bugel, Elyse Burch, Karen Carroll, Luis Carvajal, Christiam Fajardo, Amanda Grantham, Sue Hanly, Maryrose Huryk, Lisa Joseph, Kevin Moore, Claudia Nogueira, Suong Nguyen, Brittni Palmer, Kinara Patel, Felicia Permenter, Gail Pfeifer, Carol Roye, Neha Tiwari, and Lisa Wolf.

From Nicole

Writing a book is something I've always considered, but I certainly did not expect to accomplish it in my twenties and in the midst of a global pandemic. First, I would like to thank my coauthor, Donna Gaffney, for inviting me to join her in this project and take part in this journey of supporting courageous nurses. It is an honor and privilege to work alongside your brilliance. Your dedication to providing support and care to individuals in need is a true vocation.

I'm immensely grateful for my mom, Nancy Rabbitt Foster, who has always been my greatest champion. Through adversity and loss, she has taught me what true perseverance and strength looks like. Thank you for instilling the message that I am capable of anything I want to achieve in this one precious life.

Thanks go to my sister, Megan, who is fiercely loving and loyal in her own special way. Although she cannot read this book, her support is undeniable.

Although he is not physically present, I cannot continue without thanking my dad, Noel J. Foster, for being a constant source of presence and protection. I may not have inherited his red hair or blue eyes, but as the novice writer of the family, I hope to emulate him.

Thank you to the women who have supported and shaped me through the challenges and triumphs of my youth and adolescence, and have taught me what it means to show up fully in this world. This includes my former oncologist and friend Dr. Michelle Neier and the brilliant team at the Valerie Center in Morristown, New Jersey, who literally saved my life. My former tutor and current friend, Amanda Sherwin, taught me more than all the grade-level lesson books combined. To my cousin and editor extraordinaire, Meghan Rabbitt, thank you for your sage guidance and unwavering belief in my writing abilities.

Thank you to Project Write Now, the writing community that taught me to call myself a "writer" and believe it. I am forever grateful for the space you create and the wonderful instructors and students you bring together. Thank you to the wonderful writers—Jennifer Chauhan, Jennifer Gates, Lisa Hartsgrove, and Shanda McManus.

As I wrote this book, I thought of each and every nurse and health care professional in my life. I would like to acknowledge a few of the most courageous among them: Maureen Baker, Susan Barletta, Gina Flemming, Ed Ford, Shannon Holland, Cathy McKeon, Tricia Patterson, Bernadette Rabbitt, Danielle Rabbitt, and Barbara Uihlein.

Finally, to all those who have been a part of my getting there: my aunts and uncles and their significant others, Peggy Oblack, Bill Rabbitt, Mary Kay Wedel, and Patty Briskey; the kindest friends, Olivia Whitmer and Cassandra Caggiano; the most supportive cousins, Gillian Bonner and Shannon Wedel, and the countless other friends, family, and cousins whom I could fill up a chapter naming. Thank you.

From Donna

It has been years since my first book, *The Seasons of Grief: Helping Children Grow through Loss*, was published. After decades of writing chapters, articles, blog posts, and discussion guides, I wasn't sure if I had another book in me. The pandemic and my coauthor Nicole Foster changed all that. Once I looked at Nicole's new website, as suggested by my dear friend Peggy Oblack, I knew immediately that we had to work together. I asked Nicole if she would like to coauthor a book similar to the e-book posted on her website, but tailor it for nurses. I am so grateful that she said yes! As a health and wellness coach, Nicole brings content that blends so well with my own areas of expertise. Nicole, thank you for coming along on this journey.

I've been so fortunate to work with some of the most extraordinary professional nurses—clinicians, researchers, and educators. They were mentors, protégés, and, on many occasions, my soul mates. I understood early in my career that getting through the difficult times, including professional and personal challenges, was best met with a shared effort. Since March 2020, those words have never had more meaning. We all saw the need to reach out to each other during this catastrophic time.

I've known Anne Hofmeyer for more than a decade. We spent many hours on Zoom calls and writing long emails determining how we can best help nurses through the pandemic. Anne is not only an impressive writer but also a most compassionate nurse and friend. We collaborated on a number of projects, including the Rutgers webinar series. Anne brings a thoughtful and global perspective on these issues facing nurses today.

To my friend Ann Marie Mauro, who called me on a Saturday morning in March 2020 with an urgent request to offer a course at Rutgers University for their nursing students and alumni, thank you for thinking of me. My deepest admiration to Sue Salmond, who had the wisdom to assist nurses at Rutgers and throughout New Jersey offering virtual Schwartz Rounds and now the New Jersey Nursing Emotional Support Network. To Peg Pipchick, I am so grateful for your presence and guidance, and for being a part of our webinar series. Much appreciation to my colleagues Kathy Prendergast and Suzanne Drake at the Society of Advanced Practice Psychiatric Nurses in New Jersey.

It took me a while to figure out this "writing thing"; there were mentors along the way who taught me how to string together words in a manner that told a story with power and passion. LynNell Hancock at Columbia Journalism School taught me how to take my love of interviewing and craft a story that was clear and persuasive. Thank you, LynNell, for helping me through the intricacies of publishing nonfiction. As I struggled with the ethical dilemma of telling another nurse's story, I reached out to author and psychotherapist Milton Trachtenburg through the Authors' Guild. I haven't forgotten his powerful words: "Give these heroes a way to tell their stories through you, to you and with you. They will agree because they are stories that must be told."

Thank you, Milton. Dr. Shirley Smoyak, my graduate program director at Rutgers, was a firecracker of a nurse, never afraid to speak up or speak out. She wielded her red pencil on my papers with a vengeance. Shirley died in April 2022. I will never forget her.

I give my sincere thanks to my family and friends for all of their encouragement and support—phone calls, emails, texts, and much needed cheerleading that usually began with, "How's the book coming?" To Peggy Oblack, many thanks for connecting me with Nicole. Marsha Bagwell never let me forget the heart of the work I do, and how to capture its beauty in voice, words, and images. I am humbled by your spirit. To the brilliant writer-poet-screenwriter Joan Bauer, I give my sincere appreciation for our friendship and shared projects, past and future, and for always knowing what to say to get me "moving" when I feel stalled.

To my children, Ryan, Brendan, and Lauren and their partners, I give my love and appreciation for always being there to answer my questions and offer their thoughts and ideas despite being so busy with their own families and careers. To my grandchildren, Conner, Tyler, Sophia, Cavan, and Maddie, all budding writers and artists, thank you for allowing me to see nurses, helpers, and the pandemic through your eyes.

To my husband, Jack, my number one supporter, researcher, and reader, I give my deepest love and gratitude. You cleared the decks so I could write in the middle of a cross-country move during a pandemic— and brought me countless cups of coffee and tea. You added humor to the grueling process of peer review manuscript development with your keen quantitative sense by asking, "What percentage would you say you've completed?" I hope I can now say 100% done!

I am forever in debt to the courageous nurses who came forward to share their experiences with me over the years—in my practice, classes, letters and emails, workshops, and in our friendships. While not all of your stories are on these pages, they nevertheless form the heart of this book.

♦

To the many nurses whose stories we don't know, who have found the courage to continue in this profession: Thank you.

Resources

Introduction

Websites and Webinars

▸ Carol Ryff Publications, Institute on Aging, University of Wisconsin–Madison. https://aging.wisc.edu/ryff-publications/

▸ Hōkūle'a, the Polynesian Voyaging Society, seeks to perpetuate the art and science of traditional Polynesian voyaging and the spirit of exploration through experiential educational programs. https://www.hokulea.com/

▸ Midlife in the United States. http://www.midus.wisc.edu/

▸ MIDUS Newsletters. http://www.midus.wisc.edu/newsletter/index.php

▸ Photo Resource Hawaii has been providing authentic photos of Hawaii for publication since 1985. https://www.photoresourcehawaii.com/

Books and Articles

▸ Sze, D. (2017). Scientists define the 6 criteria of well-being. *Huffington Post,* December 6, 2017. https://www.huffpost.com/entry/scientists-determine-the_b_7457502

▸ Ryff, C. D., & Singer, B. (1996). Psychological well-being: meaning, measurement, and implications for psychotherapy research. *Psychotherapy and Psychosomatics* 65(1): 14–23.

▸ Ryff, C. D., & Singer, B. H. (2008). Know thyself and become what you are: a eudaimonic approach to psychological well-being. *Journal of Happiness Studies* 9(1): 13–39.

▸ Ryff, C. D., Heller, A. S., Schaefer, S. M., Van Reekum, C., & Davidson, R. J. (2016). Purposeful engagement, healthy aging, and the brain. *Current Behavioral Neuroscience Reports* 3(4): 318–27

Chapter 1. Becoming Self-Compassionate

Websites and Webinars

▸ Fierce (Motivating) Self Compassion. https://self-compassion.org/wp-content/uploads/2021/06/Motivating-Self-Compassion-Break.mp3

▸ How to Practice Self-Compassion: Eight Techniques and Tips. https://positivepsychology.com/how-to-practice-self-compassion/

▸ How Would You Treat a Friend Exercise. https://self-compassion.org/exercise-1-treat-friend/

▸ MonkeyMind's Easily Distracted. This website posts articles about the currents of the spiritual life, particularly where cultures meet. Patheos.com is an online destination to engage in the global dialogue about religion and spirituality, and to explore and experience the world's beliefs. https://www.patheos.com/blogs/monkeymind/

- ProQOL Helper Card. https://proqol.org/helper-pocket-card (Dr. Beth Hudnall Stamm developed this revised "pocket card" about caring for yourself in the face of difficult work for the current COVID-19 health crisis.)
- Self-Compassion and Mindfulness Resources. https://cultivatingself compassion.com/resources/
- Self-Compassion Training for Healthcare Communities (SCHC), Center for Mindful Self-Compassion. https://centerformsc.org/schc/
- Twelve-Point Self-Compassion Scale. https://self-compassion.org/wp-content/uploads/2020/01/ShortSCS.pdf

Videos

- Emotion Regulation and Grounding in the Midst of COVID-19. https://youtu.be/Mj9PcYbpF8U
- Mindful Healthcare Summit. https://www.mindfulhealthcaresummit.com/mhss-kristin-neff/
- Self-Compassion for Caregivers, by Kristin Neff. https://youtu.be/jJ9wGfwE-YE
- Self-Compassion Techniques from the American Nurses Association. https://youtu.be/ZIT6t1g7zIo

Books and Articles

- Goetz, J. L., & Simon-Thomas, E. (2017). The landscape of compassion: definitions and scientific approaches. In: Seppälä, E. M., Simon-Thomas, S., Brown, S. L., et al., eds. *The Oxford Handbook of Compassion Science.* New York: Oxford University Press, 3–16.
- Neff, K. (2015). *Self-Compassion: The Proven Power of Being Kind to Yourself.* New York: William Morrow.
- Neff, K. (2015). The 5 myths of self-compassion. *Psychotherapy Networker* 39(5).
- Neff, K., Knox, M., Long, P., & Gregory, K. (2020). Caring for others without losing yourself: an adaptation of the Mindful Self-Compassion Program for Healthcare Communities. *Journal of Clinical Psychology* 76: 1543–62. https://doi.org/10.1002/jclp.23007

Chapter 2. Managing Stress

Websites

- Lommasson, J. (2009). What We Carried, Fragments and Memories from Iraq and Syria. Presented by the Arab American National Museum for the Ellis Island National Museum of Immigration. https://whatwecarried.com/
- Stress Management Techniques from MindTools. https://www.mindtools.com/pages/main/newMN_TCS.htm

- The Bears: Helping People Talk about Emotions. https://innovativeresources
.org/resources/card-sets/bears-cards/
- The Stress Tip Sheet from the American Psychological Association. https://
www.apa.org/news/press/releases/2007/10/stress-tips
- What We Carried: Fragments and Memories from Iraq and Syria. https://
arabamericanmuseum.org/exhibition/what-we-carried/

Videos

- Managing Stress from Brainsmart. https://www.youtube.com/watch?v
=hnpQrMqDoqE
- Daily Habits to Reduce Stress and Anxiety with psychotherapist Emma
McAdam. https://youtu.be/7EX1Xnvvk5c
- The Awake Network's Mindful Healthcare Speaker Series: Kristin Neff.
YouTube video, June 2, 2020, https://www.mindfulhealthcaresummit.com
/mhss-kristin-neff/

Books and Articles

- Badeleh Shamooshaki, M. T. (2021). The effectiveness of mindfulness-based
stress reduction on nurses' job stress. *Iranian Journal of Psychiatric Nursing* 8(6):
53–61.
- Kabat-Zinn, J. (2003). Mindfulness-based interventions in context: past,
present and future. *Clinical Psychology: Science and Practice* 10(2): 144–56.
https://doi.org/10.1093/clipsy.bpg016
- Kabat-Zinn, J. (2013). *Full Catastrophe Living: Using the Wisdom of Your Body and
Mind to Face Stress, Pain and Illness.* New York: Random House.
- Kriakous, S. A., Elliott, K. A., Lamers, C., & Owen, R. (2021). The effectiveness
of mindfulness-based stress reduction on the psychological functioning of
healthcare professionals: a systematic review. *Mindfulness* 12(1): 1–28.
- Prelutsky, J. (2009). *What a Day It Was at School!* New York: Greenwillow Books.
- Suleiman-Martos, N., Gomez-Urquiza, J. L., Aguayo-Estremera, R., Cañadas-
De La Fuente, G. A., De La Fuente-Solana, E. I., & Albendín-García, L. (2020).
The effect of mindfulness training on burnout syndrome in nursing: a sys-
tematic review and meta-analysis. *Journal of Advanced Nursing* 76(5): 1124–40.

Apps

- Breathe + Simple Breath Trainer: offers guided breathing visualizations.
https://apps.apple.com/us/app/breathe-simple-breath-trainer
/id1106998959
- Happify: overcome negative thoughts, stress, and life's challenges. https://
www.happify.com/
- Insight Timer: app for sleep, anxiety, and stress. https://insighttimer.com/

- Lief: wearable stress relief using heart rate variability biofeedback and personalized wellness coaching. https://getlief.com/
- Moodfit: tracks moods and provides tools and exercises to help address negative emotions. https://www.getmoodfit.com/
- My Possible Self: tackle stress, anxiety, and loss. https://www.mypossible self.com/
- Personal Zen: reduce stress and anxiety, designed by a neuroscience researcher. https://personalzen.com/
- Sanvello: stress relief. https://www.sanvello.com/
- Shine: founded by a Black/Japanese woman who didn't see her experiences represented in mainstream wellness ("Our bodies, our skin color, our financial access, our past traumas—often felt otherized"). https://www.theshine app.com/

Podcasts

- Calmer You Podcast: features practical, expert interviews. https://www.calmer-you.com/podcast/
- Happier: hosted by Gretchen Rubin, author of the *Happiness Project* and *Better Than Before* https://gretchenrubin.com/podcasts/
- In Our Time: various academic topics to help calm and soothe listeners. https://podcasts.apple.com/us/podcast/in-our-time/id73330895

Chapter 3. Exploring Mindfulness and Meditation

Websites and Webinars

- Free Guided Meditations from UCLA Health. https://www.uclahealth.org /marc/mindful-meditations
- Meditation and Mindfulness—What You Need to Know, from the National Center for Complementary and Integrative Health. https://www.nccih.nih .gov/health/meditation-in-depth
- Mindful Healthcare Summit. https://www.mindfulhealthcaresummit.com /mhss-kristin-neff/
- Mindfulness Bristol: Living in the Here and Now. https://www.mindfulness bristol.co.uk/
- Mindspace Meditation. Enjoy mindful meditation through this UK website that offers programming and books for individuals, groups, and schools. https://www.mindspace.org.uk/
- Tara Brach's teachings blend Western psychology and Eastern spiritual practices, mindful attention to our inner life, and a full, compassionate engagement with our world. Her website contains practices, links to workshops, and more. https://www.tarabrach.com/

- The Path, founded by Dina Kaplan, teaches meditation for the modern mind. The Path has taught thousands of people to meditate around the world—in teacher trainings, retreats, private coaching, and courses. https://www.thepath.com/

Videos

- Loving-Kindness Meditation with Dr. Dzung Vo (at 13 minutes into the video; good for teens, too). https://www.youtube.com/watch?v=MM4ZkbaYvAI
- Loving-Kindness Meditation with Sharon Salzberg from Mindful.org. https://www.mindful.org/loving-kindness-takes-time-sharon-salzberg/
- Loving-Kindness Meditation from the University of New Hampshire. https://www.youtube.com/watch?v=sz7cpV7ERsM&t=1s
- Mindful Movement Loving-Kindness Meditation. https://www.youtube.com/watch?v=tY3NnodM3Ww
- Mindfulness of Breathing Exercise with Neuroscientist Amishi Jha from Mindful.org. https://www.mindful.org/the-mindfulness-of-breathing-exercise-with-neuroscientist-amishi-jha/
- Navy Seal Box Breathing Exercise. https://www.youtube.com/watch?v=FJJazKtH_9I

Books, Articles, and Handouts

- 4-7-8 Breath from Dr. Andrew Weil of the Arizona Center for Integrative Medicine. https://www.cordem.org/globalassets/files/academic-assembly/2017-aa/handouts/day-three/biofeedback-exercises-for-stress-2---fernances-j.pdf
- Hawken, J. (2015). *Mindfulness for a Broken Heart, Self-Compassion for Negative Mind-States.* Seattle: CreateSpace.
- The Top 5 Mindfulness Tips for Health Care Professionals. https://keltymentalhealth.ca/blog/2020/03/top-5-mindfulness-tips-health-care-professionals-during-covid-19-pandemic
- University of Wisconsin Integrative Health Program's guide to creating a gratitude practice, adapted from the original written by Shilagh A. Mirgain and Janice Singles. https://www.fammed.wisc.edu/files/webfm-uploads/documents/outreach/im/tool-creating-gratitude-practice.pdf

Apps

- Calm: tools, guided meditations, calming imagery, background noise, and a calendar to track meditations. https://www.calm.com/
- Exhale: the first emotional well-being app designed specifically for women who are Black, Indigenous, or of color. https://www.exhalesite.com/
- Headspace: provides support through a time of crisis, offering some meditations you can listen to any time. https://www.headspace.com/covid-19

▶ Insight Timer: the largest library of free guided meditations, including meditations for sleep and anxiety, and meditation timer. https://insighttimer.com/

▶ Meditation Studio by Muse: powered by more than 80 leading meditation experts, each of whom has created original, exclusive, and engaging guided meditations for you to experience right on your device, any time and anywhere. https://meditationstudioapp.com/

▶ UCLA Mindful: practice mindfulness meditation anywhere, any time with the guidance of the UCLA Mindful Awareness Research Center. https://apps.apple.com/us/app/ucla-mindful/id1459128935?ls=1

Podcasts

▶ *Yoga Girl Daily*: offers daily affirmations and practices. https://www.yogagirl.com/podcast/

Chapter 4. Sleeping Well

Websites and Webinars

▶ CBD for Sleep and Insomnia, from the American Sleep Association. https://www.sleepassociation.org/sleep-treatments/cbd/

▶ How Much Sleep Do I Need? Centers for Disease Control and Prevention. https://www.cdc.gov/sleep/about_sleep/how_much_sleep.html

▶ No Sleepless Nights. https://www.nosleeplessnights.com

Videos

▶ 30-Minute Body Scan Meditation for Beginners from Mindful.org. https://www.mindful.org/beginners-body-scan-meditation/

▶ 30-Minute Body Scan Meditation with Jon Kabat-Zinn. https://www.youtube.com/watch?v=_DTmGtznab4

Books and Articles

▶ Araç, S., & Dönmezdil, S. (2020). Investigation of mental health among hospital workers in the COVID-19 pandemic: a cross-sectional study. *Sao Paulo Medical Journal* 138(5): 433–40.

▶ Lee, S., Mu, C., Gonzalez, B. D., Vinci, C. E., & Small, B. J. (2021). Sleep health is associated with next-day mindful attention in healthcare workers. *Sleep Health* 7(1): 105–12. https://doi.org/10.1016/j.sleh.2020.07.005

▶ Walker, M. (2017). *Why We Sleep: Unlocking the Power of Sleep and Dreams.* New York: Simon and Schuster.

▶ Winter, W. C. (2017). *The Sleep Solution: Why Your Sleep Is Broken and How to Fix It.* New York: Penguin.

Apps

▶ Aura: breathwork for sleep is in their library of well-being resources. https://www.aurahealth.io/

▶ Calm: improve your sleep quality. https://www.calm.com/signup-flow?focus=sleep&goals=sleep_quality

▶ Headspace: exercises and resources to improve your sleep. https://www.headspace.com/sleep

▶ Insight Timer: a free app that provides meditation tracks for sleep. https://insighttimer.com/meditation-topics/sleep

▶ Noisli: a basic free plan offers different sounds to aid your sleep. https://www.noisli.com/

▶ Sleep Better: offers stories, tips, and strategies to help you sleep. https://www.bettersleep.com/sleep-better/

▶ Sleep Easy Insomnia Therapy: provides sleep programs, resources, sleep hygiene sessions developed by sleep expert Dr. Richard Shane. https://apps.apple.com/us/app/sleep-easy-insomnia-therapy/id1441338499

▶ Sleep Score: a free app that tracks and analyzes sleep patterns; also provides links to products that can help improve sleep. https://www.sleepscore.com/

▶ Slumber: an audio library of stories, meditations, soundscapes, and music designed to quiet the mind and transition to sleep. https://slumber.fm/

▶ WHOOP: monitor your sleep with personalized recommendations and coaching. https://www.whoop.com/experience/sleep/

Podcasts

▶ Nothing Much Happens: a seamless blending of storytelling with brain training methods that build better sleep habits over time. https://www.nothingmuchhappens.com/

Chapter 5. Nourishing Well

Websites and Webinars

▶ 100 Days of Real Food. Pledge 100 days without eating processed or refined food. https://www.100daysofrealfood.com/

▶ Aussie Food for Aussie families. https://delishdeliveries.com.au/

▶ Community Supported Agriculture (United Kingdom). https://communitysupportedagriculture.org.uk/

▶ Cookie + Kate. https://cookieandkate.com/

▶ Farm Direct (United Kingdom). https://farm-direct.com/

▶ Fine Fruits Direct (United Kingdom). https://www.finefruitsdirect.co.uk/

▶ Fruitezy (Australia). https://fruitezy.com.au/

▶ Gathering Dreams. https://gatheringdreams.com/

- I Love Fruits and Vegetables from Europe. https://ilovefruitandvegfrom europe.com/
- Minimalist Baker. https://minimalistbaker.com/
- Mindfulness and the Art of Chocolate Eating, Adam Dacey. https://www .mindspace.org.uk
- Olive Tomato. Elena Paravantes, award winning Registered Dietitian and Nutritionist provides a lifetime of experience being raised on the Mediterranean Diet. https://www.olivetomato.com/
- The Edgy Veg. https://www.theedgyveg.com/
- The Kitchen Girl. https://thekitchengirl.com/
- The Simple Veganista. https://simple-veganista.com/
- Urth Caffé. Loose leaf black, green, white, matcha green teas, and herbal infusions. https://www.urthcaffe.com/fine-teas

Books and Articles

- Bean, A. (2022). *The Complete Guide to Sports Nutrition*, 9th ed. London: Bloomsbury Sport.
- Buettner, D. (2017). *The Blue Zones Solution.* Washington, DC: National Geographic.
- Duyff, R. (2017). *Academy of Nutrition and Dietetics Complete Food and Nutrition Guide*, 5th ed. Eugene, OR: Harvest.
- Gehart, D. R. (2019). *Mindfulness for Chocolate Lovers: A Lighthearted Way to Stress Less and Savor More Each Day.* Lanham, MD: Rowman & Littlefield.
- Norwitz, N. G., & Naidoo, U. (2021). Nutrition as metabolic treatment for anxiety. *Frontiers in Psychiatry* 12:105.
- Pitchford, P. (2022). *Healing with Whole Foods*, 3rd ed. Berkeley, CA: North Atlantic Books.
- Pollan, M. (2009). *Food Rules: An Eater's Manual.* New York: Penguin.
- Selhub, E. (2020). Nutritional psychiatry: your brain on food. Harvard Health Blog, March 26, 2020. https://www.health.harvard.edu/blog/nutritional -psychiatry-your-brain-on-food-201511168626
- Trebole, E., & Resch, E. (2020). *Intuitive Eating: A Revolutionary Anti-Diet Approach.* New York: St Martin's Essentials.
- Willett, W. (2017). *Eat, Drink, and Be Healthy: The Harvard Medical School Guide to Healthy Eating.* Cambridge, MA: Free Press.

Apps

- Dr. Greger's Daily Dozen: details the healthiest foods and how many servings of each we should eat every day, without counting calories. https:// nutritionfacts.org/daily-dozen/

Chapter 6. Implementing Daily Movement and Exercise

Websites and Webinars

▸ Four Types of Exercise Can Improve Your Health and Physical Ability. National Institute on Aging. https://www.nia.nih.gov/health/four-types -exercise-can-improve-your-health-and-physical-ability

▸ UK Chief Medical Officers' Physical Activity Guidelines. https://assets .publishing.service.gov.uk/government/uploads/system/uploads /attachment_data/file/832868/uk-chief-medical-officers-physical-activity -guidelines.pdf

▸ What Is Dance/Movement? American Dance Therapy Association. https:// adta.memberclicks.net/what-is-dancemovement-therapy

Apps

▸ Couch to 5K. http://www.c25k.com/

▸ Daily Yoga. https://www.dailyyoga.com/#/

▸ Fitness Blender: hundreds of free, full-length workout videos; the most affordable and effective workout programs on the web; meal plans; and helpful health, nutrition, and fitness information. https://www.fitness blender.com/

▸ Fit On. https://app.fitonapp.com/

▸ Map My Run (United States). https://www.mapmyrun.com/us/

▸ Map My Run (worldwide). https://www.mapmyrun.com

▸ One Peloton: thousands of classes, expert-level instructors, and curated music, all in one place, with no equipment needed. https://www.onepeloton .com/app

▸ 7 Minute Workout. http://7minworkoutapp.net/#about

▸ Sworkit: at-home fitness and workouts. https://sworkit.com/

▸ Yoga Studio. https://yogastudioapp.com/

Chapter 7. Embracing Nature and the Outdoors

Websites and Webinars

▸ Actif Woods Wales: Woodland health and well-being activity groups. https://www.smallwoods.org.uk/en/coedlleol/what-we-do/projects /actif-woods-wales/

▸ Alberta Parks Inclusion Plan. https://albertaparks.ca/albertaparksca /visit-our-parks/inclusion-accessibility

▸ Alliance for Nurses for Healthy Environments: believes all humans have the right to healthy and safe environments. https://envirn.org/about/

- The Branching Out Programme (BOP)3 is run by Forestry Commission Scotland (FCS) with the goal of improving the health-related quality of life (HRQoL) of adults. https://issuu.com/gcvgreennetworkpartnership /docs/120815091752-a11e90dcad094577ab41d7394351e56e
- An Effective Approach for Personal Growth: Suzi Tarrant focuses on providing a warm and compassionate space where you can explore your life challenges and work toward healing and resolution, both online and outdoors. https://www.suzitarrant.com/
- Childhood by Nature: for parents, educators, and all caregivers of children, making it easier for all of us to raise kids the way nature intended— with an awareness of the natural world. https://childhoodbynature.com /aboutthissite/
- Children and Nature Network: a leading global movement to increase equitable access to nature so that children—and natural places—can thrive. https://www.childrenandnature.org/
- Dose of Nature around the World. https://www.doseofnature.org.uk /around-the-world
- Dose of Nature Prescription: a 10-week program that introduces individuals to the mental health benefits of spending time in nature. https://www .doseofnature.org.uk/doseofnatureprescriptions
- Dr. Frances E. Kuo, Natural Resources and Environmental Science Division, College of Agricultural, Consumer and Environmental Sciences, University of Illinois. https://nres.illinois.edu/directory/fekuo
- European Centre for the Environment and Human Health at Exeter University. https://www.ecehh.org/
- Global Consortium on Climate and Health Education: initiative whereby all health professionals throughout the world—doctors, nurses, public health practitioners, mental health practitioners, and allied health specialists— work together to prevent, reduce, and respond to the health impacts of climate change. https://www.publichealth.columbia.edu/research/global -consortium-climate-and-health-education/about
- Global Green and Healthy Hospitals: brings together hospitals, health systems, and health organizations from around the world under the shared goals of reducing the environmental footprint of the health sector and contributing to improved public and environmental health. https://www .greenhospitals.net/
- Green Exercise: research group at Essex University. https://www.essex.ac .uk/research-projects/green-exercise
- Healthcare Climate Council. https://climatecouncil.noharm.org/
- Healthcare without Harm. https://noharm-uscanada.org/
- Insight Timer: nature meditation. https://insighttimer.com/meditation -topics/naturalenvironment

- International Nature and Forest Therapy Alliance (INFTA). Implements and promotes forest therapy as an evidence-based public health practice. https://infta.net/
- Nacadia Therapy Garden, Copenhagen, Denmark. https://ign.ku.dk/terapihaven-nacadia
- Nature Connections Research Group at the University of Derby. https://www.derby.ac.uk/research/centres-groups/nature-connectedness-research-group/
- Nurses Climate Challenge. https://www.nursesclimatechallenge.org
- Nurses Drawdown. https://www.nursesdrawdown.org/
- Park Rx: what began as the home for the National ParkRx Initiative has grown into an information hub for Park Prescriptions, creating a space for knowledge-sharing in the practitioner community and providing a platform to share best practices, toolkits, and case studies. https://www.parkrx.org/
- Practice Green Health. https://practicegreenhealth.org/
- Project Drawdown. https://drawdown.org/
- Reconnect in Nature. http://reconnectinnature.org.uk
- Social and Economic Research Group, Institute of Forest Research, Forestray Commission, United Kingdom. https://www.researchgate.net/lab/Social-and-Economic-Research-Group-SERG-Liz-OBrien
- *The Lancet* Countdown on Health and Climate Change. https://www.thelancet.com/countdown-health-climate
- University of Glasgow's Institute of Health and Well-Being. https://www.gla.ac.uk/researchinstitutes/healthwellbeing/research/

Video and Audio Recordings

- A World of Calm video series. https://www.hbomax.com/series/urn:hbo:series:GX23urwuo4MNYwwEAAAPq
- Blue Planet documentary series. https://www.bbcearth.com/shows/blue-planet
- Calming Canadian Forest: a long-play (six-hour) nature soundscape for online listening. https://youtu.be/7MVQM5RoaL0
- Good Grief: a Canadian Television program created through a partnership between Mount Royal University and Alberta Parks that offers respite and support for those who are experiencing grieving and loss through an eight-week program that gives people the opportunity to take part in a series of gentle, guided walks along local nature trails. https://calgary.ctvnews.ca/guided-walks-help-grieving-families-cope-with-loss-1.3468967
- Peace in the Parks documentary. https://youtu.be/dkLSrzhwNzk
- Sounds of the Forest. https://timberfestival.org.uk/soundsoftheforest-soundmap/

▶ "Stillness": a soundtrack with nature sounds by a Montana cellist (three hours for relaxation or background for calm work). https://www.youtube.com/watch?v=4Xk-IXLcaSU

Books and Articles

For Children

▶ Cotton, K. (2017). *The Road Home*. New York: Abrams Books. Ages 5–7

▶ Covell, D. (2018). *Run Wild*. New York: Viking Books. Ages 5–7

▶ Dek, M. (2017). *A Walk in the Forest*. Princeton, NJ: Princeton Architectural Press. Ages 3–6

▶ Dyu, L., & Blackwell, A. (2019). *Earth Heroes*. London: Nosy Crow. Ages 8 and up

▶ Farrell, A. (2019). *The Hike*. San Francisco, CA: Chronicle Books. Ages 4–7

▶ Gray, R. (2015). *Flowers Are Calling*. Boston, MA: HMH Books. Ages 4–7

▶ Lloyd, M. W. (2016). *Finding Wild*. New York: Knopf. Ages 3–7

▶ Martin, M. (2017). *A River*. San Francisco, CA: Chronicle Books. Ages 5–8

▶ Schaefer, L. M. (2016). *Because of an Acorn*. San Francisco, CA: Chronicle Books. Ages 5–6

▶ Winter, J. (2019). *Our House Is on Fire: Greta Thunberg's Call to Save the Planet*. San Diego, CA: Beach Lane Books. Ages 3–6

▶ Wynne, P. J. (2016). *My First Book about Backyard Nature*. Mineola, NY: Dover. Ages 8–11

For Adults

▶ Allen, R. (2021). *Grounded: How Nature Can Improve Our Mental and Physical Well-Being*. London: Mortimer.

▶ Arvay, C. G. (2018). *The Healing Code of Nature: Discovering the New Science of Eco-Psychosomatics*. Louisville, CO: Sounds True.

▶ Demorest, S., Spengeman, S., Schenk, E., Cook, C., & Weston, H. L. (2019). The Nurses

▶ Climate Challenge: a national campaign to engage 5,000 health professionals around climate change. *Creative Nursing* 25(3): 208–15.

▶ Duncan, R. (2018). *Nature in Mind: SYSTEMIC THINKING and Imagination in Ecopsychology and Mental Health*. New York: Routledge.

▶ Glendinning, C. (1994). *My Name Is Chellis and I'm in Recovery from Western Civilization*. Boulder, CO: Shambhala.

▶ Hardman, I. (2020). *The Natural Health Service*. New York: Atlantic Press.

▶ Horowitz, A. (2015). *On Looking: A Walker's Guide to the Art of Observation*. New York: Scribner.

▶ Jakubec, S. L., Carruthers Den Hoed, D., & Ray, H. (2014). "I can reinvent myself out here": experiences of nature inclusion and mental well-being.

In: Altman, B. M. & Barnartt, S. N., eds. *Research in Social Science and Disability.* Environmental Contexts and Disability 8. Bingley, UK: Emerald Group, 213–29. https://doi.org/10.1108/S1479-354720140000008012

▸ Jakubec, S. L., Carruthers Den Hoed, D., Ray, H., & Krishnamurthy, A. (2016). Mental well-being and quality of life benefits of inclusion in nature for adults with disabilities and their caregivers. *Landscape Research* 41(6): 616–27. https://doi.org/10.1080/01426397.2016.1197190

▸ Jakubec, S. L., Carruthers Den Hoed, D., Ray, H., & Krishnamurthy, A. (2020). Grieving in nature: the place of parks and natural places in palliative and grief care. In: Quilley, S., and Zywert, K., eds. *Health in the Anthropocene: Living Well on a Finite Planet.* Toronto: University of Toronto Press.

▸ Jordan, M. (2014). *Nature and Therapy, Understanding Counselling and Psychotherapy in Outdoor Spaces.* New York: Routledge.

▸ McGeeney, A. (2016). *With Nature in Mind: The Ecotherapy Manual for Mental Health Professionals.* Menlyn, South Africa: Kingsley.

▸ Rust, M.-J. (2020). *Towards an Ecopsychotherapy.* London: Confer Books.

▸ Williams, F. (2017). *The Nature Fix: Why Nature Makes Us Happier, Healthier, and More Creative.* New York: W. W. Norton.

Apps

▸ Ecotherapy Wales on Instagram: @ecotherapy_wales

▸ Insight Timer: nature meditations and more. https://insighttimer.com/meditation-topics/naturalenvironment

Chapter 8. Finding Sanctuary in Words, Images, and Sounds

Websites, Webinars, and Virtual Presentations

▸ Arts and Caring for the Caregiver. https://heartsneedart.org/caring-for-the-caregiver/; https://heartsneedart.org/gratitudegrams/

▸ Artsy.net: lists the best places to take a ceramics class. https://www.artsy.net/article/artsy-editorial-best-places-ceramics-classes

▸ Ella Berthoud: bibliotherapist. http://www.ellaberthoud.com/

▸ Button Factory Arts in Canada: a free virtual art therapy program that offers nurses a chance to explore art mediums and connect outside the workplace. https://www.buttonfactoryarts.ca/

▸ Ceramic Arts Daily: free posts and videos to explore, as well as books and DVDs for sale, PDF files with tips and more (also free with registration), and subscriptions to ceramics magazines. https://ceramicartsnetwork.org/daily/

▸ Clay Times Magazine: offers a search tool to find classes in about 16 states. http://www.claytimes.com/index.html

▸ Community Building Art Works: connects veterans, health care providers, and civilians through workshops led by professional artists. https://cbaw.org/

- Mojie Crigler: writer. https://www.mojiecrigler.com/write-covid
- Health Humanities Consortium: promotes health humanities scholarship, education, and practices through interdisciplinary methods and theories that focus on the intersection of the arts and humanities, health, illness, and health care. https://healthhumanitiesconsortium.com/about/
- Carol Henderson: writer, teacher, editor, and coach who can help you learn to write with power and passion, in your own voice. http://carolhenderson .com/
- Institute of Poetic Medicine: awakening soulfulness in the human voice. https://poeticmedicine.org/
- Narrative Medicine Blog. https://narrativemedicine.blog/blog/virtual-live -sessions/
- "Nursing the Nation," by Molly Case: poem by spoken-word artist. http://www.mollycasespeaks.com/poetry-1
- James Pennebaker's COVID Project at the University of Texas at Austin. https://utpsyc.org/covid19/index.html
- Hunter Prosper: ICU Nurse tells Stories From a Stranger. https://www .tiktok.com/@hunterprosper
- *Poets and Writers* Magazine: find a group using their search tool. https://www .pw.org/groups
- *Pulse—Voices from the Heart of Medicine*: publishes and distributes first-person stories and poems, together with visual images or haikus, about health care. https://pulsevoices.org/
- *That Kindness: Nurses in Their Own Words*: a play by V (Eve Ensler) that draws on frank, impassioned interviews with nurses, "radical angels of the heart," in a soul-stirring portrait of kindness and activism amid crisis. https://www .facebook.com/watch/live/?ref=watch_permalink&v=416010976247724
- The Isolation Journals. https://www.theisolationjournals.com/
- *The Line*: crafted from firsthand interviews, this play by Jessica Blank and Erik Jensen features New York City medical first responders during the COVID-19 pandemic. https://www.dramatists.com/cgi-bin/db/single .asp?key=6305
- *The Nurse Antigone*: offered by Theater of War Productions, Sophocles's *Antigone* is an ancient play about a teenage girl who wishes to bury her brother, Polyneices, who recently died in a brutal civil war. https://theaterofwar.com /projects/the-nurse-antigone
- The Things They Carry Project: writing workshops to help health care workers and first responders process traumatic memories and make sense of their experiences. https://www.thingstheycarryproject.org/
- The Unprescription: reflective writing sessions for health care workers and their loved ones. https://beyondholistic.org/the-unprescription/

▸ Writing Medicine, by Laurel Braitman. https://www.laurelbraitman.com /writingmedicine

Videos and Audio Files

▸ Diane Carlson Evans: former army nurse and founder of the Vietnam Women's Memorial. https://www.youtube.com/watch?v=fPOA6-PM4cA

▸ "Hero and the Sage," by Tara Beier. https://www.youtube.com/watch?v =NQ8O1d7Kv7c

▸ "Kite," by Megan Palmer. https://www.youtube.com/watch?v=POmNdH ckkRg

▸ "One Voice," by Ruth Moody and sung by the Wailin' Jennys. https:// www.youtube.com/watch?v=y-24qGCvo7A

▸ "One Voice," sung by the US Navy Band. https://www.youtube.com/watch?v =6ZhvWki817o

▸ "Stop for a Minute," by Megan Palmer. https://www.meganpalmer.com /megan-palmer-transfer/2021/5/20/stop-for-a-minute

▸ The Ultimate Happy Playlist: curated by Jennifer Lee. https://open.spotify .com/playlist/1llkez7kiZtBeOw5UjFlJq

▸ "The Weight," by Robbie Robertson and sung by Dala. https://www.youtube .com/watch?v=2KfwglOMBHQ

▸ "The Weight," sung by Ringo Starr and Robbie Robertson (Playing for Change). https://www.youtube.com/watch?v=ph1GU1qQlzQ

Books and Articles

▸ Berthoud, E., & Elderkin, S. (2014). *The Novel Cure, from Abandonment to Zestlessness: 751 Books to Cure What Ails You*. London: Penguin.

▸ Carlson, D. (2020). *Healing Wounds: A Vietnam War Combat Nurse's 10-Year Fight to Win Women a Place of Honor in Washington, D.C.* Brentwood, TN: Permuted Press.

▸ Case, M. (2019). *How to Treat People: A Nurse's Notes*. New York: W. W. Norton.

▸ Crane, M. (2018). *Stories from the Tenth-Floor Clinic: A Nurse Practitioner Remembers*. Berkeley, CA: She Writes Press.

▸ Davis, C. (2004). *Leopold's Maneuvers*. Lincoln: University of Nebraska Press.

▸ Davis, C, & Schaefer, J. (1995). *Between the Heartbeats: Poetry and Prose by Nurses*. Iowa City: University of Iowa Press.

▸ Davis, J., & Schaefer, J. (2018). *Learning to Heal: Reflections on Nursing School in Poetry and Prose*. Kent, OH: Kent State University Press.

▸ Macduff, C. (2017). A brief historical review of poetry's place in nursing. *Journal of Research in Nursing* 22(6–7): 436–48.

▸ Pennebaker, J. W., & Smyth, J. M. (2016). *Opening Up by Writing It Down: How Expressive Writing Improves Health and Eases Emotional Pain*. New York: Guilford.

▸ Rosen, M. (2021). *Many Different Kinds of Love: A Story of Life, Death and the NHS.* London: Ebury Press.

▸ Schaefer, J. (2018). *Wild Onion Nurse: A Collection of 25 Years of the Poetry of Nursing in a College of Medicine Literary Journal.* Boca Raton, FL: CRC Press.

▸ Van Devanter, L., & Furey, J. A. (1991). *Visions of War, Dreams of Peace: Writings of Women in the Vietnam War.* New York: Grand Central Publishing.

▸ Zak, P. J. (2015). Why inspiring stories make us react: the neuroscience of narrative. Cerebrum, February 2, 2015. https://www.dana.org/article/why -inspiring-stories-make-us-react-the-neuroscience-of-narrative/

Apps

▸ Cove, Music for Mental Health: designed as a tool for young people who have experienced bereavement or loss to express how they feel by making music and storing it in a personal journal, adults may find Cove equally useful to express and capture a mood or emotion. http://www.cove-app.com

Chapter 9. Seeking Empowerment through Advocacy and Activism

Websites and Webinars

▸ Alliance of Nurses for Healthy Environments. https://envirn.org/about/

▸ American Nurses Association. (2017). Ethics and human rights statement. https://www.nursingworld.org/~4aef79/globalassets/docs/ana/ethics /anastatement-ethicshumanrights-january2017.pdf

▸ Barbara Glickstein Strategies: this public health nurse, health reporter, and media strategist trains national leaders in health care on how to be media makers in both traditional and digital media to advance the health of the public and public policy. https://www.barbaraglickstein.com/

▸ Canty, L., Nyirati, C., Taylor, V., & Chinn, P. L. (2022). An overdue reckoning on racism in nursing. *American Journal of Nursing* 122(2): 2022.

▸ Chinn, P. L. (2020). Nursing and racism: are we part of the problem or part of the solution? Nursology, June 16, 2020. https://nursology.net/2020/06/16 /nursing-and-racism-are-we-part-of-the-problem-or-part-of-the-solution -perhaps-both/

▸ Committee to Protect: a national mobilization of health care professionals and advocates who are building a pro-patient health care majority in Congress and in states so that we can live in an America where everyone has the health care they need to thrive. https://committeetoprotect.org/

▸ COVID Collaborative: a diverse and comprehensive team of leading experts in health, education, and the economy. https://www.covidcollaborative.us/

▸ Healthcare without Harm (Europe): connecting health care providers who are finding new ways to cut carbon emissions. https://noharm-europe.org/

▸ Healthcare without Harm (United States and Canada). https://noharm -uscanada.org/

- Health-e Voices: provide workshops and webinars to enhance the skills of health care providers. https://healthevoices.com/hcp.html
- Hidden Pain: information on child bereavement. https://www.covid collaborative.us/initiatives/hidden-pain
- National Nurses United. (2020). Thousands of nurses hold national day of action Aug. 5 to save lives during COVID-19 and beyond. August 3, 2020. https://www.nationalnursesunited.org/press/national-day-action-aug-5
- Nurse Manifest: a call to conscience and action. https://nursemanifest.com/
- Nurse Manifest: resources for nurses and activism. https://nursemanifest .com/resources/resources-for-activism/
- Nurses Climate Challenge: transforms health care worldwide by reducing its environmental footprint, becoming a community anchor for sustain-ability and a leader in the global movement for environmental health and justice. www.nursesclimatechallenge.org
- The Op-Ed Project: working to change who writes history, valuing radically inclusive society that moves toward freedom and justice. https://www .theopedproject.org/
- Rape, Abuse & Incest National Network. Hotline. https://www.rainn.org/
- The Relentless School Nurse: blog by Robin Cogan, MEd, RN, NCSN, FAAN. https://relentlessschoolnurse.com/therelentlessblog/
- The Truth about Nursing: seeks to increase public understanding of the cen-tral role nurses play in modern health care; to promote more accurate, bal-anced, and frequent media portrayals of nurses; and to increase the media's use of nurses as expert sources. https://www.truthaboutnursing.org/index .html#gsc.tab=0
- White Nurses, This Is on Us: Zoom series. https://nursemanifest.com/2022 /02/05/white-nurses-this-is-on-us-a-3-saturday-zoom-series-on-march-26 -april-2-and-april-9-2022-4-530-pm-eastern/

Books and Articles
- Buresh, B., & Gordon, S. (2013). *From Silence to Voice: What Nurses Know and Must Communicate to the Public*, 3rd ed. Ithaca, NY: IRL Press.

Chapter 10. Navigating the Challenges of the Health Care Landscape
Websites and Webinars
- Center to Advance Palliative Care (CAPC): a national organization dedicated to increasing the availability of quality health care for people living with a serious illness. CAPC provides health care professionals and organizations with the training, tools, and technical assistance necessary to effectively meet this need. https://www.capc.org/
- Healing Our Health System: the Schwartz Center for Compassionate Healthcare and the Dr. Lorna Breen Heroes' Foundation are working toward

an affiliation to create a comprehensive organization. Together, we will move the health care system forward in supporting its most valuable resource: its workforce. The health care system must better protect the well-being of the health workforce so that it can deliver high-quality, compassionate patient care. HealingOurHealthSystem.org

▸ James Clear: author of *Atomic Habits*, Clear issues his 3–2-1 *Newsletter* every Thursday, including three short ideas from Clear, two quotes from others, and one question for you to ponder. https://jamesclear.com/

▸ New Jersey Nursing and Emotional Well-Being Institute (NJ-NEW): supports nurses by providing statewide, research-based programming and direct support to address the emotional well-being of nurses, both on an individual and organizational level. NJ-NEW has positioned itself as the statewide lead and repository of programming and services: Stress First Aid Train the Trainer, Virtual Schwartz Rounds, and the NJ-NEW Well-Being Hub, a statewide learning collaborative and resource center serving individuals and health care organizations. NJ-NEW is also partnering with Nurse2Nurse, a confidential, peer-support helpline. https://njnew.org/

▸ Nurse Manifest: a call to action for nurses to make a difference in the world by having an overdue on racism in nursing; offers webinars and resources on the topics of activism and racism. https://nursemanifest.com/ongoing -overdue-reckoning-on-racism-in-nursing/launch-overdue-reckoning-on -racism-in-nursing/

▸ Project ECHO: this behavioral health provider resiliency program is free from the University of New Mexico, and it includes the Community Resiliency Model (CRM) and Zoom sessions every Monday (workgroups) and every other Monday (Rounds). These sessions offer continuing education credits without charge. The program is meant for behavioral health workers in any setting in the US and abroad. It is a response to the burnout of health care workers and is open to non-mental health workers as well. https://hsc .unm.edu/echo/partner-portal/programs/global/behavioral-health/

▸ Stress First Aid (SFA) offered by NJ-NEW: SFA is a framework of supportive and practical actions for nurses dealing with workplace stress. The program aims to assist nurses identify and address early signs of stress reactions in themselves and others. SFA seeks to enhance individual, unit, and system-wide resilience and to normalize the assessment and management of stress. https://njnew.org/programs/stress-first-aid/

▸ The ALL IN: Well-Being First for Healthcare: this campaign was developed by #FirstRespondersFirst and the Dr. Lorna Breen Heroes' Foundation. This website includes a Resilience Library, a curated list of resources to build resilient health care organizations. https://www.allinforhealthcare.org/

▸ The Compassion Institute: develops and delivers programs for institutions in the sectors of health, law enforcement, and public safety, and provides education for the general public; they also offer a free care package for health care professionals. https://www.compassioninstitute.com/healthcare /carepackage

▸ The Schwartz Center: provides education, training, and support to thousands of health care members in Australia, Canada, New Zealand, and the United States. In partnership with the Point of Care Foundation, more than 200 hospitals, hospices, and other health care organizations conduct the innovative Schwartz Rounds programs in Ireland, the United Kingdom, and the United States. The program unites caregivers from a range of disciplines to share experiences, learn from each other, and focus on the human dimension of health care. https://www.theschwartzcenter.org/

Videos

▸ "Reckoning with Racism in Nursing": this collection consists of 40 interviews with nurses of color and their allies. They were carried out in 2021 with nurses from around the United States. The collection spans decades of professional and personal experience of nurses of color, covering a large range of topics and concerns. https://www.rn-reckoning.org/the-collection

Books and Articles

▸ Duran, E. (2006). *Healing the Soul Wound: Counseling with American Indians and Other Native Peoples.* New York: Teachers College Press.

▸ Gaffney, D. (2020). Nurses are fighting for us. Their presence is a gift. The Hill, May 7, 2020. https://thehill.com/changing-america/opinion/496579 -nurses-have-always-been-there-through-pandemics-life-and-death

▸ Gaffney, D. (2021). Trauma, COVID-19 and collective resilience: a way forward for nursing. *New Jersey Nurse* 51(2): https://www.nursingald.com/publications /2213

▸ Gaffney, D., Primo, J., Sander, I., & Sandler, J. (2020). Kobe Bryant, children and grief. The Hill, January 27, 2020. https://thehill.com/changing-america /opinion/480076-kobe-bryant-children-and-grief

▸ Goleman, D. (2006). *Social Intelligence in the New Science of Social Relatedness.* London: Hutchinson.

▸ Halifax, J. (2018). *Standing at the Edge: Finding Freedom Where Fear and Courage Meet.* New York: Flatiron Books.

▸ Lewis, C. S. (2015). *A Grief Observed.* New York: HarperOne.

▸ Maslach, C. (2003). *Burnout: The Cost of Caring.* Cambridge, MA: Malor Books.

▸ National Academy of Medicine. (2019). *Taking Action against Clinician Burnout: A Systems Approach to Professional Well-Being.* Washington, DC: National Academies Press.

▸ Parks, T. (2020). What's different about the stress clinicians are facing, and what can help? Smart Brief, April 7, 2020. www.smartbrief.com/original/2020 /04/what's-different-about-stress-clinicians-are-facing-and-what-can-help

▸ Petersen, A. (2020). *Can't Even: How Millennials Became the Burnout Generation.* New York: Day Street Books.

▸ Solon, O. (2012). Compassion over empathy could help prevent emotional burnout—Tania Singer. *Wired Magazine*, July 12, 2012. https://www.wired.co .uk/article/tania-singer-compassion-burnout

▸ Threlkeld, C. (2021). Employee burnout report: COVID-19's impact and 3 strategies to curb it. Indeed, March 11, 2021. https://www.indeed.com/lead /preventing-employee-burnout-report

Chapter 11. Continuing the Journey of Transformation and Healing

Websites and Webinars

▸ American Psychological Association: building resilience. https://www.apa .org/topics/resilience

▸ Centre for Integrative Forest Therapy (Ireland). https://nadurforesttherapy .com/

▸ Dr. Lorna Breen Heroes Foundation: the foundation's mission is to reduce burnout of health care professionals and safeguard their well-being and job satisfaction. https://drlornabreen.org/

▸ Eco-therapy and nature therapy in Ireland. https://www.naturetherapy ireland.com/about-us

▸ Emotional PPE Project: a program that offers any provider in a health care–related field affected by the COVID-19 crisis mental health services from licensed mental health professionals, free of charge. https://emotionalppe .org/

▸ Greater Good Science Center: studies the psychology, sociology, and neuro-science of well-being and teaches skills that foster a thriving, resilient, and compassionate society. https://ggsc.berkeley.edu/

▸ International Association for Suicide Prevention: provides more than 1,600 services across the world that offer immediate emotional support and make them easily available; this association works directly with helplines to ensure that their data remains accurate and reliable. https://findahelpline .com/i/iasp

▸ Laya Healthcare: general practitioner / private health coverage. https://www .layahealthcare.ie

▸ Mind: mental health services in the United Kingdom, providing information and support, including skills to cope with coronavirus and to empower anyone experiencing a mental health problem. https://www.mind.org.uk/

▸ Pearlman, L. A., & McKay, L. (2008). *Understanding and Addressing Vicarious Trauma*. Pasadena, CA: Headington Institute. https://mutualaiddisaster relief.org/wp-content/uploads/2017/05/vtmoduletemplate2_ready_v2 _85791.pdf

▸ One Mind PsyberGuide: provides expert reviews on mental health apps (both credibility and user experience) and offers solid recommendations. https://onemindpsyberguide.org/

- *Psychology Today*: find a therapist in the United States. https://www.psychology today.com/us/therapists

- *Psychology Today*: find a therapist worldwide. https://www.psychologytoday .com/intl/counsellors?domain=content&cc=us&cl=en

- RAINN (Rape, Abuse & Incest National Network) is the US's largest anti-sexual violence organization. RAINN operates the National Sexual Assault Hotline (800.656.HOPE). https://www.rainn.org/

- Society of Psychiatric Advanced Practice Nurses: founded in 1972, this was the first professional nursing body in the United States to certify clinical nurse specialists in psychiatric nursing. https://psychapn.org/

- The School of Life: offers a wide range of products and services, including books, an app, online psychotherapy, and training. https://www.theschool oflife.com/

- University of California, San Francisco: personal strategies for engaging and building resilience. https://psychiatry.ucsf.edu/copingresources/videos

- University of California, San Francisco: useful wellness and mental health apps. https://psych.ucsf.edu/copingresources/apps

- US National Suicide Prevention Lifeline: 1-800-273-TALK (8255). https:// suicidepreventionlifeline.org/

- US substance abuse helpline and resources. https://www.samhsa.gov/

Books and Articles

- Duckworth, K. (2022). *You Are Not Alone: The NAMI Guide to Navigating Mental Health—With Advice from Experts and Wisdom from Real People and Families*. New York: Zando Books.

- Gottlieb, L. (2019). *Maybe You Should Talk to Someone: A Therapist, Her Therapist, and Our Lives Revealed*. Boston, MA: Houghton Mifflin.

- LeDoux, J. (2015). *Anxious: Using the Brain to Understand and Treat Fear and Anxiety*. London: Penguin.

- Schacter, D. (2008). *Searching for Memory: The Brain, the Mind, and the Past*. New York: Basic Books.

Apps and Online Therapy

An ever-increasing number of digital platforms and applications focus on mental health strategies and psychotherapy. These resources fall into two groups. First is therapy offered by licensed clinicians who practice in your geographic area and provide face-to-face and/or virtual sessions. A second type of therapy resource includes e-therapy-based apps, websites, or digital platforms that provide guidance and may even assign you a therapist. Virtual or remote therapies can be conducted by telephone, mail, text messaging, video conferencing, or online chat sessions.

Among the most popular are Talkspace and Better Help, both well-known apps that can help you find a licensed mental health professional or counselor.

Other mental health apps focus on a specific therapeutic strategy (cognitive behavioral therapy) or symptom management such as negative thinking, anxiety, and moods. The research on mental health apps continues to grow and is a consideration in how you might go about exploring these resources. A recent article on self-guided cognitive behavioral therapy apps in the *Journal of Medical Internet Research* assessed their features, functionality, and congruence with evidence (https://www.jmir.org/2021/7/e27619/). A downloadable chart comparing the apps is included in the article. A study conducted by a research team at Cornell Weill Medicine in the United States evaluated mobile apps used for depression self-management (https://www.ncbi.nlm.nih.gov/pmc /articles/PMC8075488/). They scored a number of commercially available apps, among them Sanvello, Talkspace, and Moodpath. A downloadable chart is also included in their paper.

Happify is an app designed to help with stress and worry. It contains games and activities that were created to help the user on a series of different "tracks" (or goals, such as self-confidence and coping with stress). The ultimate goal is to change patterns and develop healthier habits (https://www.happify.com/).

Moodnotes is a mood tracker and journaling app to capture your mood and help improve your thinking habits. Moodnotes empowers you to track your mood over time, avoid common thinking traps, and develop perspectives associated with increased happiness and well-being (https://www.thriveport .com/products/moodnotes/).

Psychological First Aid (PFA) was designed to assist responders who provide psychological first aid to adults, families, and children as part of an organized response effort. This app provides responders with summaries of PFA fundamentals, PFA interventions matched to specific concerns and needs of survivors, mentor tips for applying PFA in the field, a self-assessment tool for readiness to conduct PFA, and a survivors' needs form for simplified data collection and easy referral (https://apps.apple.com/us/app/pfa-mobile /id551079424).

Sanvello provides evidence-based solutions created by psychologists that use clinically validated techniques such as cognitive behavioral therapy (CBT). The app delivers CBT through a series of different activities, mediums, and tools for the user (https://www.sanvello.com/).

Stress First Aid is a community resource that provides guidance and resources for individuals dealing with stress, and for leaders, family members, friends, and coworkers who know someone who is currently dealing with emotional stress or is in a crisis situation (https://apps.apple.com/us/app /community-stress-first-aid/id466283645).

Note: We will continue to update our websites with the newest research findings and app recommendations for our readers.

Glossary

Activism. Taking informed, deliberate actions to bring caritative and universally beneficial values into the public sphere that challenge threats to human health and well-being.

Advocacy. Speaking on behalf of or in support of another person, place, or thing; advocacy is an essential element of the nursing mission to advance caritative values throughout the health professions.

Biophilia. From the ancient Greek word that refers to "love of life and the living world," this phrase now refers to our fundamental human need to affiliate with life and lifelike processes.

Blue spaces. Visible water areas, both natural and man-made, such as coastal waters, rivers, ponds, lakes, canals, and fountains.

Breathwork. A clinical identification of broad areas of breathwork: deep relaxation breathing, mindfulness breathwork, and yogic breathing.

Burnout. A gradual exhaustion, growing cynicism, and loss of commitment to work and relationships.

Caffeine. The natural chemical found in coffee, tea, cola, cocoa, and other products with stimulant effects on the central nervous system, heart, muscles, and blood control centers.

Chiropractor. A person who performs hands-on therapy concerned with the diagnosis and treatment of mechanical disorders of the musculoskeletal system, primarily the spine and its function.

Chronic stress. A prolonged feeling of stress that can negatively affect a person's health.

Circadian rhythm. The bodily clock that guides physical, mental, and behavioral changes (including sleep and wake cycles) within a 24-hour cycle.

Clinical practice. A set of techniques or methods that involve assessing, diagnosing, and treating the patient's psychological or physical conditions.

Collective resilience. Strength of purpose to overcome adversity expressed by a group, community, state, or nation(s).

Collective trauma. Trauma experienced collectively, within and across population types.

Compassion. The feeling that surfaces when witnessing another person's distress with a strong desire to help relieve attendant suffering.

Controlled-focus meditation. Focusing attention on an external or internal object, sound, or action, such as breathing during yoga movements.

COVID-19. An infectious disease caused by the SARS-CoV-2 virus.

Deep relaxation breathing. Diaphragmatic breathing; an effective way to decrease anxiety and train the mind to relax by staying attentive to the breath.

Ecopsychology. The blending of ecology and psychology into a unified perspective on how humans relate to nature; the integration of ecological theories within the practice of psychotherapy.

Emotional intelligence (EI). Skill in perceiving, understanding, and managing emotions and feelings.

Empathic distress fatigue. A strong aversion and self-oriented response to the suffering of others, accompanied by the desire to withdraw from a situation to protect oneself from negative feelings.

Empathy. The ability to understand and share the feelings of others without prejudice or predisposition.

Employee assistance program (EAP). A voluntary, work-based program that offers free confidential assessments, short-term counseling, referrals, and follow-up services to employees who have personal and/or work-related problems affecting mental and emotional well-being.

Empowerment. The process of becoming stronger and more confident, especially in controlling one's life and claiming one's rights.

Endurance (aerobic) activities. Activities that increase breathing and heart rate if done for more than two minutes at a time; improves heart health, lungs, and circulatory system; builds strength, balance, and flexibility.

Essential oils. Natural aromatic oils used for their immediate effect on the olfactory system.

Eudaimonia. An ancient Greek term that refers to living well and actualizing one's potential.

Evidence-based practice. The integration of empirical research evidence with clinical expertise and patient value.

Family APGAR. A scale that measures appearance, pulse, grimace, activity, and resolve to assess adult satisfaction with social support received from the family.

Fierce self-compassion. Activating compassion to achieve goals in a dynamic fashion.

Gratitude practice. A technique that helps to validate the benefits of gratitude; in other words, counting one's blessings.

Green spaces. Rural and urban areas that incorporate forests, landscapes, wilderness areas, farms, and gardens into parks and backyards.

Grounding. A mental technique to focus awareness during crisis situations, starting from the soles of the feet up.

Herbal tea. Natural tea that helps to calm the body and mind.

Loving-kindness meditation. A way to cultivate a propensity for kindness by mentally sending goodwill, kindness, and warmth toward others by silently repeating a series of mantras.

Mantra. A sacred utterance or invocation consisting of a numinous sound, syllable, word, or group of words in Sanskrit, although mantras can be created in any language.

Meditation. An ancient practice that focuses on training awareness and concentration to achieve a clear, calm, and relaxed mind.

Mental health. Refers to a person's psychological well-being.

Mindfulness. The nonjudgmental observation of the present moment or present internal or external stimuli.

Mindfulness-based cognitive therapy. A technique used to help treat depression.

Mindfulness-based stress reduction (MBSR). Programs that reduce stress using meditation, yoga, breathing exercises, and social support modalities.

Mindfulness breathing. A technique that involves a strong focus on mindfulness and an awareness of one's breathing and associated sensations.

Model of psychological well-being. This model from Carol Ryff identifies six essential elements: self-acceptance, growth, positive relationships, autonomy, purpose, and environmental mastery.

Moral apathy. A denial, lack of caring, or willful ignorance that makes it possible to ignore situations that cause harm to others.

Moral distress. An element of burnout, moral distress occurs when you are not able to fulfill your caritative obligations because of value conflicts, ineffective communication, lack of teamwork or organizational oversight, or poor staffing policies.

Moral injury. Initially identified in military personnel, moral injury refers to unprecedented traumatic events that affect a person when failing to protect or bear witness to those events.

Moral outrage. A principled response to conflictive or compromising situations; grounded in reflection, knowledge, and compassion.

Open monitoring meditation. Focusing awareness on the present moment rather than on distractions; accepting stray thoughts, bodily sensations, and emotions without judgment.

Personal protective equipment (PPE). Protective gear worn to minimize exposure to hazards in the workplace.

Posttraumatic growth. The tendency to identify positive transformation after exposure to trauma.

Practice. Being present with purpose, skills, and readiness to act as required or desired.

Resilience. The capacity to overcome adverse situations and to sustain or attain well-being.

Secondary traumatic stress. The emotional duress that occurs when a person hears about or encounters a traumatic event experienced by another person.

Self-care. Activities that provide for and support an individual's needs biologically, psychologically, and socially.

Self-compassion. The expression of compassion for others turned to self, especially during times of perceived inadequacy, failure, or suffering.

Social justice. In nursing, this concept embraces equal access for all people to health, well-being, rights, economic standing, and opportunities.

Strength training. Also known as "resistance activities"; builds muscles and can be done with weights, resistance bands, or body weight at a gym, at home, or other location of choice.

Stress. A feeling of emotional or physical tension in response to an event or thought that makes the person feel frustrated, angry, or nervous.

Stressor. The agent, structure, or event that causes stress.

Subjective well-being. A person's sense of living a meaningful and fulfilling life with happiness, satisfaction, and contentment.

Systemic injustice. The continuance of unjust, divisive activities that sustain inequalities systemically between races, genders, age groups, and other identifiers.

Tender self-compassion. Being tender to oneself.

Traumatic event. Major life events that cause physical and psychological trauma, precipitating a cascade of physical and emotional responses that sustain long after the causative event ends.

Vicarious trauma. The distressing change in worldview held by nurses who are repeatedly exposed to the trauma of others.

Visualization. An act of mental imagery that can reduce stress by exploring an experience with closed eyes in a calm, safe space.

Wayfinding. Ancient Polynesian manner of navigating across the oceans with non-instrumental tools, such as mental mapping, star gazing, and sensitivity to the environment.

Yoga. An ancient tradition that combines breathing exercises, meditation, and physical postures to achieve a state of relaxation and balance of mind, body, and spirit. Regular practice of yoga promotes strength, endurance, and flexibility, and facilitates characteristics of friendliness, compassion, and greater self-control.

Yogic breathing. Known as "pranayama," yogic breathing aims to increase vital energy in the body and mind. It involves controlling the breath with specific patterns and variations in rates of respiration.

Index